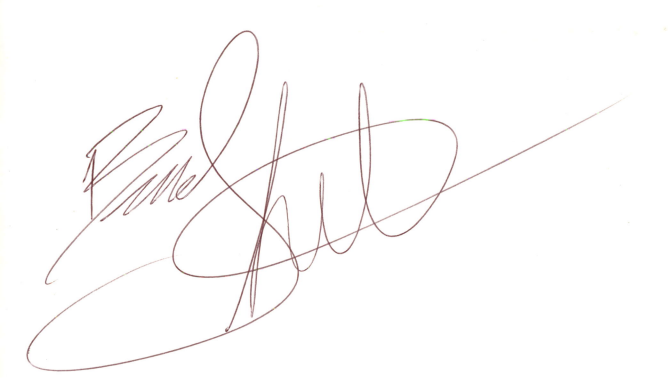

BRADY

PARAMEDIC CARE: Principles & Practice

PATIENT ASSESSMENT

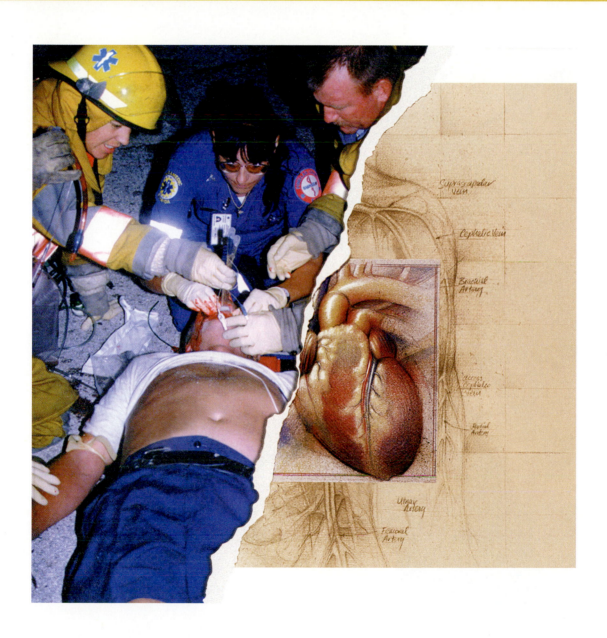

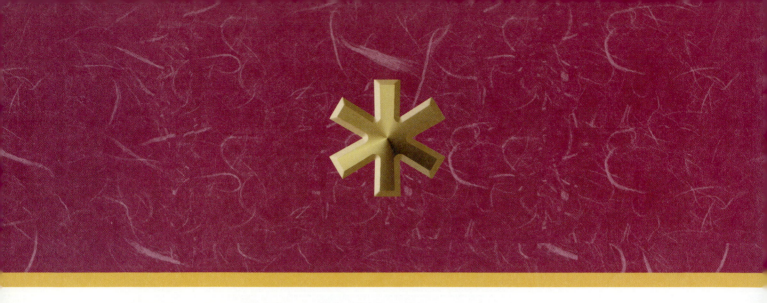

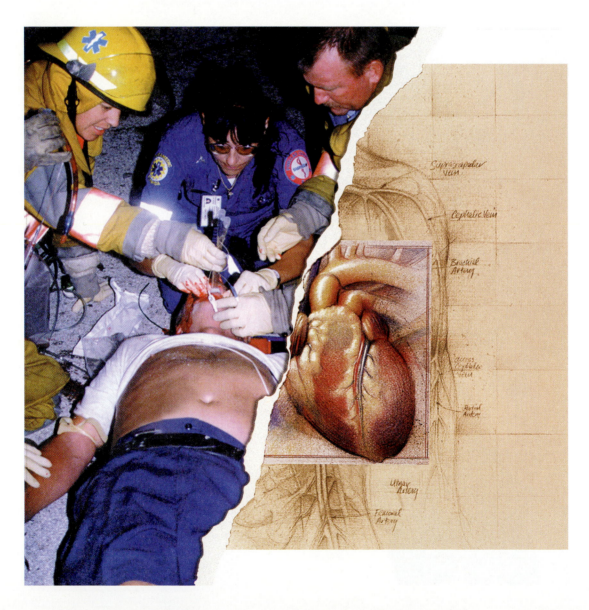

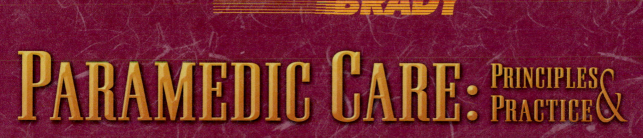

PARAMEDIC CARE: PRINCIPLES & PRACTICE

PATIENT ASSESSMENT

BRYAN E. BLEDSOE, D.O., F.A.C.E.P., F.A.A.E.M., F.A.E.P., EMT-P

Emergency Department Staff Physician
Baylor Medical Center—Ellis County
Waxahachie, Texas
and
Clinical Associate Professor of Emergency Medicine
University of North Texas Health Sciences Center
Fort Worth, Texas

ROBERT S. PORTER, M.A., NREMT-P

Senior Advanced Life Support Educator
Madison County Emergency Medical Services
Canastota, New York
and
Flight Paramedic
AirOne, Onondaga County Sheriff's Department
Syracuse, New York

RICHARD A. CHERRY, M.S., NREMT-P

Clinical Assistant Professor of Emergency Medicine
Director of Paramedic Training
SUNY Upstate Medical University
Syracuse, New York

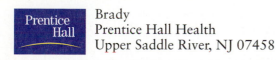

Brady
Prentice Hall Health
Upper Saddle River, NJ 07458

Library of Congress Cataloging-in-Publication Data

Bledsoe, Bryan E., 1955-
    Paramedic care: principles & practice / Bryan E. Bledsoe, Robert S. Porter,
Richard A. Cherry
        p. ; cm.
    Includes index.
    ISBN 0-13-021597-X (alk. paper)
    1. Emergency medicine. 2. Emergency medical technicians. I. Porter,
Robert S., 1950-   II. Cherry, Richard A.   III. Title
    [DNLM: 1. Emergency Medical Services—methods. 2. Emergency Medical
Technicians, WX 215 B6465p 1999]
    RC86.7B5964 2000
    616.02'5—dc21   99-055264

Publisher: Julie Alexander
Acquisitions editor: Laura Edwards
Managing development editor: Lois Berlowitz
Development editors: Sandra Breuer, John Joerschke
Managing production editor: Patrick Walsh
Editorial/production supervision: Larry Hayden IV
Senior production manager: Ilene Sanford
Marketing manager: Tiffany Price
Marketing coordinator: Cindy Frederick
Interior design: Jill Yutkowitz
Cover design: Rob Richman
Cover photography: Eddie Sperling
Cover illustration: Malcolm Farley
Managing photography editor: Michal Heron
Assistant photography editor: Mary Jo Robertiello
Interior photographers: Michael Gallitelli, Michal Heron,
    Richard Logan
Page makeup: Carlisle Communications, Inc.

©2000 by Prentice-Hall, Inc.
Upper Saddle River, New Jersey 07458

Printed in the United States of America
10 9 8 7 6 5 4 3 2

ISBN 0-13-021597-X

Prentice-Hall International (UK) Limited, London
Prentice-Hall of Australia Pty. Limited, Sydney
Prentice-Hall Canada Inc., Toronto
Prentice-Hall Hispanoamericana, S.A., Mexico
Prentice-Hall of India Private Limited, New Delhi
Prentice-Hall of Japan, Inc., Tokyo
Prentice-Hall (Singapore) Pte Ltd
Editora Prentice-Hall do Brasil, Ltda., Rio de Janeiro

Art Acknowledgments

Rolin Graphics, Plymouth, Minnesota

Photo Acknowledgments

All photographs not credited adjacent to the
photograph were photographed on assignment
for Brady/Prentice Hall Pearson Education.

Organizations: We wish to thank the following
organizations for their valuable assistance in
creating the photo program for this edition:

Rural-Metro Medical Services, Syracuse, NY
North Area Volunteer Ambulance Corps
    (NAVAC), North Syracuse, NY

Models
For their assistance as models, our gratitude to
the following EMS professionals:

Darlene Button, Susan Cherry, Brian Locastro,
Jay Scott, John Woods, Paul Voutsinas

Technical Advisor: Acknowledgment for
providing extraordinary technical support during
the photo shoots to:

Richard A. Cherry, M.S., NREMT-P
Clinical Assistant Professor
Upstate Medical University
Syracuse, NY

SPECIAL NOTES

This book is respectfully dedicated to the EMTs and paramedics who toil each day in an environment that is unpredictable, often dangerous, and constantly changing. They risk their lives to aid the sick and the injured, driven only by their love of humanity and their devotion to this profession we call emergency medical services.

B.E.B.

To those who answer the call to care on cold, dark, and rainy nights.

R.S.P.

"At one time or another in everyone's lives the inner fire goes out. Then it is burst into flame by an encounter with another human being." Rudyard Kipling just described what my wife Sue has meant to me.

R.A.C.

Content Overview

Below is a brief content description of each chapter in *Patient Assesssment*.

CHAPTER 1   THE HISTORY   2

* Provides the basic components of a complete health history
* Discusses how to effectively conduct an interview
* Provides suggestions for communicating with difficult patients, hostile patients, and patients with language barriers

CHAPTER 2   PHYSICAL EXAM TECHNIQUES   26

* Presents the techniques of conducting a comprehensive physical exam
* Includes in each section a review of anatomy and physiology

CHAPTER 3   PATIENT ASSESSMENT IN THE FIELD   170

* Offers a practical approach to conducting problem-oriented history and physical exams

CHAPTER 4   CLINICAL DECISION MAKING   234

* Provides the basic steps for making clinical decisions
* Discusses how to think critically in emergency situations

CHAPTER 5   COMMUNICATIONS   250

* Discusses communication, the key component that links every phase of an EMS run
* Includes several examples of typical radio medical reports

CHAPTER 6   DOCUMENTATION   270

* Describes how to write a Prehospital Care Report (PCR)
* Offers examples of the various narrative writing styles

Detailed Contents

SERIES PREFACE   xiii
PREFACE TO VOLUME 2   xv
ACKNOWLEDGMENTS   xvii
ABOUT THE AUTHORS   xix

NOTICES   xxi
PRECAUTIONS ON BLOODBORNE
PATHOGENS AND INFECTIOUS
DISEASES   xxiii

CHAPTER 1

THE HISTORY   2

Introduction   5
Establishing Patient Rapport   5
  Setting the Stage   5
  The First Impression   6
  Introductions   7
  Asking Questions   8
  Language and Communication   9
    Facilitation   9
    Reflection   9
    Clarification   9
    Empathy   10
    Confrontation   10
    Interpretation   10
    Asking about Feelings   10
  Taking a History on Sensitive Topics   10
The Comprehensive Patient History   11
  Preliminary Data   11
  The Chief Complaint   11
  The Present Illness   12
    Onset   12
    Provocation/Palliation   12
    Quality   13
    Region/Radiation   13
    Severity   13
    Time   13
    Associated Symptoms   13
    Pertinent Negatives   13
  The Past History   13
    General State of Health   14
    Childhood Diseases   14
    Adult Diseases   14
    Psychiatric Illnesses   14
    Accidents or Injuries   14
    Surgeries or Hospitalizations   14
  Current Health Status   14
    Current Medications   15
    Allergies   15
    Tobacco   15
    Alcohol, Drugs, and Related Substances   15
    Diet   16
    Screening Tests   16
    Immunizations   16

    Sleep Patterns   16
    Exercise and Leisure Activities   16
    Environmental Hazards   16
    Use of Safety Measures   16
    Family History   16
    Home Situation and Significant
      Others   16
    Daily Life   17
    Important Experiences   17
    Religious Beliefs   17
    The Patient's Outlook   17
  Review of Systems   17
    General   17
    Skin   17
    Head, Eyes, Ears, Nose, and
      Throat (HEENT)   17
    Respiratory   18
    Cardiac   18
    Gastrointestinal   18
    Urinary   18
    Male Genital   18
    Female Genital   18
    Peripheral Vascular   18
    Musculoskeletal   18
    Neurologic   19
    Hematologic   19
    Endocrine   19
    Psychiatric   19
  Special Challenges   19
    Silence   19
    Overly Talkative Patients   19
    Patients with Multiple Symptoms   20
    Anxious Patients   20
    Patients Needing Reassurance   20
    Anger and Hostility   20
    Intoxication   21
    Crying   21
    Depression   21
    Sexually Attractive or Seductive Patients   21
    Confusing Behaviors or Histories   21
    Limited Intelligence   22
    Language Barriers   22
    Hearing Problems   22
    Blindness   23
    Talking with Families or Friends   23

CHAPTER 2

PHYSICAL EXAM TECHNIQUES   26

Physical Examination Approach and Overview   28
   Examination Techniques   29
     Inspection   29
     Palpation   30
     Percussion   31
     Auscultation   32
     Measurement of Vitals   33
       Pulse   33
       Respiration   34
       Blood Pressure   35
       Body Temperature   37
   Equipment   37
     Stethoscope   37
     Sphygmomanometer   38
     Ophthalmoscope   39
     Otoscope   39
     Scale   39
     Additional Equipment   40
   The General Approach   40
Overview of a Comprehensive Examination   41
   The General Survey   41
     Appearance   41
       Level of Consciousness   41
       Signs of Distress   41
       Apparent State of Health   42
       Vital Statistics   42
       Sexual Development   42
       Skin Color and Obvious Lesions   42
       Posture, Gait, and Motor Activity   42
       Dress, Grooming, and Personal
         Hygiene   42
       Odors of Breath or Body   42
       Facial Expression   42
     Vital Signs   43
       Pulse   43
       Respiration   43
       Blood Pressure   43
       Temperature   46
     Additional Assessment Techniques   46
       Pulse Oximetry   46
       Cardiac Monitoring   47
       Blood Glucose Determination   48
Anatomical Regions   49
   The Skin   49
     Color   50
     Moisture   50
     Temperature   51
     Texture   51
     Mobility and Turgor   51
     Lesions   51
   The Hair   53
   The Nails   55
   The Head   57
   The Eyes   59

The Ears   65
The Nose   67
The Mouth   70
The Neck   74
The Chest and Lungs   77
   Posterior Chest Examination   79
   Anterior Chest Examination   82
The Cardiovascular System   83
The Abdomen   89
   Abdominal Organs   90
     Digestive   90
     Urinary   90
     Female Reproductive   91
     Male Reproductive   91
     Cardiovascular   92
     Lymphatic   93
   Abdominal Examination   93
The Female Genitalia   95
The Male Genitalia   98
The Anus   99
The Musculoskeletal System   100
   The Extremities   104
     Hands and Wrists   104
     Elbows   106
     Shoulders   110
     Ankles and Feet   115
     Knee   118
     Hips   119
   The Spine   124
The Peripheral Vascular System   128
The Nervous System   133
   Mental Status and Speech   134
     Appearance and Behavior   134
     Speech and Language   136
     Mood   136
     Thought and Perceptions   136
     Insight and Judgment   137
     Memory and Attention   137
   The Cranial Nerves   137
     CN-I   140
     CN-II   141
     CN-III   141
     CN-III, IV, VI   141
     CN-V   144
     CN-VII   145
     CN-VIII   145
     CN-IX, X   145
     CN-XI   145
     CN-XII   147
   The Motor System   147
   The Sensory System   151
   Reflexes   153
     Biceps   153
     Triceps   154
     Brachioradialis   154
     Quadriceps   154
     Achilles   155
     Plantar   155

Physical Examination of Infants and Children 158
    Building Patient and Family Rapport 158
    General Appearance and Behavior 158
        Infants (Newborn to One Year) 159
        Toddlers (One–Three years) 159
        Preschoolers (Three–Six Years) 159
        School-age (Six–Twelve Years) 160
        Adolescents (Thirteen–Eighteen Years) 160
    Anatomy and the Physical Exam 160
        General Appearance 160
        Head and Neck 160
        Chest and Lungs 162
        Cardiovascular 163
        Abdomen 163
        Musculoskeletal 164
        Nervous System 164
Recording Examination Findings 164

CHAPTER 3

PATIENT ASSESSMENT IN THE FIELD 170

Scene Size-Up 174
    Body Substance Isolation 175
    Scene Safety 176
    Location of All Patients 182
    Mechanism of Injury 184
    Nature of the Illness 185
The Initial Assessment 185
    Forming a General Impression 186
    Mental Status 187
        Alert 188
        Verbal 188
        Pain 188
        Decorticate 188
        Unresponsive 188
    Airway Assessment 189
    Breathing Assessment 194
    Circulation Assessment 195
    Priority Determination 198
The Focused History and Physical Exam 200
    The Major Trauma Patient 200
        Mechanism of Injury 200
        Rapid Trauma Assessment 202
        Head 203
        Neck 203
        Chest 204
        Abdomen 205
        Pelvis 208
        Extremities 208
        Posterior Body 211
        Vital Signs 211
        The History 211
    The Isolated Injury Trauma Patient 212
    The Responsive Medical Patient 213
        The History 213
        Chief Complaint 213
        History of the Present Illness 214

Past Medical History 214
    Current Health Status 214
Focused Physical Exam 214
    Chest Pain/Respiratory Distress 215
        HEENT 215
        Neck 215
        Chest 215
        Cardiovascular 215
        Abdomen 216
        Extremities 216
    Altered Mental Status 216
        HEENT 216
        Chest 217
        Abdomen 217
        Pelvis 217
        Extremities 217
        Posterior Body 217
        Neuro 217
    Acute Abdomen 218
        HEENT 218
        Chest 218
        Abdomen 218
        Posterior Body 218
    Baseline Vital Signs 218
    Additional Assessment Techniques 219
        Pulse Oximetry 219
        Cardiac Monitoring 219
        Blood Glucose Determination 219
    Emergency Medical Care 219
The Unresponsive Medical Patient 220
The Detailed Physical Exam 222
        Head 222
        Eyes 222
        Ears 223
        Nose and Sinuses 223
        Mouth and Pharynx 223
        Neck 223
        Chest and Lungs 223
        Cardiovascular System 226
        Abdomen 226
        Pelvis 226
        Genitalia 226
        Anus and Rectum 226
        Peripheral Vascular System 226
        Musculoskeletal System 228
        Nervous System 228
            Mental Status and Speech 228
            Cranial Nerves 228
            Motor System 228
            Reflexes 228
            Sensory System 228
    Vital Signs 228
    Recording Exam Findings 228
Ongoing Assessment 229
    Mental Status 229
    Airway Patency 229
    Breathing Rate and Quality 229
    Pulse Rate and Quality 231

Skin Condition 231
Transport Priorities 231
Vital Signs 231
Focused Assessment 231
Effects of Interventions 231
Management Plans 232

CHAPTER 4

CLINICAL DECISION MAKING 234

Introduction 236
Paramedic Practice 237
Patient Acuity 237
Protocols and Algorithms 238
Critical Thinking Skills 240
Fundamental Knowledge and Abilities 240
Useful Thinking Styles 242
Reflective vs. Impulsive 242
Divergent vs. Impulsive 242
Anticipatory vs. Reactive 243
Thinking Under Pressure 243
Mental Check List 243
Stop and Think 244
Scan the Situation 244
Decide and Act 244
Maintain Control 244
Reevaluate 244
The Critical Decision Process 244
Form a Concept 245
Interpret the Data 245
Apply the Principles 246
Evaluate 246
Reflect 246
Putting It All Together 247

CHAPTER 5

COMMUNICATIONS 250

Introduction to Communication 252
Basic Communication Model 253
Verbal Communication 254
Written Communication 255
Terminology 256
The EMS Response 257
Detection and Citizen Access 257
Call Taking and Emergency Response 258
Prearrival Instruction 259
Call Coordination and Incident
Recording 259
Discussion with Medical
Direction Physician 259
Transfer Communications 260
Communication Technology 260
Radio Communication 261
Simplex 261
Duplex 261

Multiplex 262
Trunking 262
Digital Communication 262
Alternative Technologies 263
Cellular Telephone 263
Facsimile 263
Computer 263
New Technology 264
Reporting Procedures 265
Standard Format 265
General Radio Procedures 266
Model Verbal Reports 267
Regulation 268

CHAPTER 6

DOCUMENTATION 270

Introduction 272
Uses for Documentation 273
Medical 273
Administrative 274
Research 274
Legal 274
General Considerations 274
Medical Terminology 275
Abbreviations and Acronyms 275
Times 285
Communications 285
Pertinent Negatives 286
Oral Statements 286
Additional Resources 286
Elements of Good Documentation 287
Completeness and Accuracy 287
Legibility 287
Timeliness 289
Absence of Alterations 289
Professionalism 290
Narrative Writing 290
Narrative Sections 290
Subjective Narrative 290
Objective Narrative 291
Head-to-Toe 291
Body Systems 292
Assessment/Management 292
General Formats 293
SOAP 293
CHART 294
Other Formats 294
Patient Management 294
Call Incident 295
Special Considerations 296
Patient Refusals 296
Services Not Needed 297
Mass Casualty Incidents 298
Consequences of Inappropriate Documentation 299
Closing 300

Series Preface

Congratulations on your decision to further your EMS career by undertaking the course of education required for certification as an Emergency Medical Technician-Paramedic! The world of paramedic emergency care is one that you will find both challenging and rewarding. Whether you will be working as a volunteer or paid paramedic, you will find the field of advanced prehospital care very interesting.

This textbook will serve as your guide and reference to advanced out-of-hospital care. It is based upon the 1998 United States Department of Transportation EMT-Paramedic National Standard Curriculum and is divided into five volumes. The first volume is entitled *Introduction to Advanced Prehospital Care* and addresses the fundamentals of paramedic practice, including pathophysiology, pharmacology, medication administration and advanced airway management. The second volume, *Patient Assessment,* builds on the assessment skills of the basic EMT with special emphasis on advanced patient assessment at the scene. The third volume of the series, *Medical Emergencies,* is the most extensive and addresses paramedic level care of medical emergencies. Particular emphasis is placed upon the most common medical problems; respiratory and cardiovascular emergencies. *Trauma Emergencies,* the fourth volume of the text, discusses advanced prehospital care from the mechanism of injury analysis to shock/trauma resuscitation. The last volume in the series addresses *Special Considerations/Operations* including neonatal, pediatric, geriatric, home health care, and specially challenged patients, and incident command, ambulance service, rescue, hazardous material, and crime scene operations. These five volumes will help prepare you for the challenges of prehospital care.

SKILLS

The psychomotor skills of fluid and medication administration, advanced airway care, ECG monitoring and defibrillation, and advanced medical and trauma patient care are best learned in the classroom, skills laboratory, and then the clinical and field setting. Common advanced prehospital skills are discussed in the text as well as outlined in the accompanying procedure sheets. Review these before and while practicing the skill. It is important to point out that this or any other text cannot teach skills. Care skills are only learned under the watchful eye of a paramedic instructor and perfected during your clinical and field internship.

HOW TO USE THIS TEXTBOOK

Paramedic Care: Principles & Practice is designed to accompany a paramedic education program that follows the 1998 United States Department of Transportation *Emergency Medical Technician-Paramedic: National Standard Curriculum.* The education program should include ample classroom, practical laboratory, in-hospital clinical, and prehospital field experience. These educational experiences must be guided by instructors and preceptors with special training and experience in their areas of participation in your program.

It is intended that your program coordinator will assign reading from *Paramedic Care: Principles & Practice* in preparation for each classroom lecture and discussion section. The knowledge gained from reading this text will form the foundation of the information you will need in order to function effectively as a paramedic in your EMS system. Your instructors will build upon this information to strengthen your knowledge and understanding of advanced prehospital care so that you may apply it in your practice. The in-hospital clinical and prehospital field experiences will further refine your knowledge and skills under the watchful eyes of your preceptors.

In preparing for each classroom session, read the assigned chapter carefully. First, review the chapter objectives. They will identify important concepts to be learned from the reading. Read the Case Study to get a feeling of why a chapter is important and how the knowledge it contains can be applied in the field. Read the chapter content carefully, while keeping the chapter objectives in mind. Read the You Make the Call feature and answer the questions to assure you understand the application of the knowledge presented in the chapter. Last, re-read the chapter objectives and be sure that you are able to answer each one completely. If you cannot, reread the section of the chapter to which the objective relates. If you still do not understand the objective or any portion of what you have read, ask your instructor to explain it at your next class session.

Ideally, you should read this entire text series at least three times. The volume chapter should be read in preparation for the class session, the entire volume should be read before the division or course test, and the entire text series should be reread before the program final exam and/or certification testing. While this might seem like a lot of reading, it will improve your classroom performance, your knowledge of emergency care, and ultimately, the care you provide to emergency patients.

The workbook that accompanies this text can also assist in improving classroom performance. It contains information, sample test questions, and exercises designed to assist learning. Its use can be very helpful in identifying the important elements of paramedic education, in exercising the knowledge of prehospital care, and in helping you self-test your knowledge.

Paramedic Care: Principles & Practice presents the knowledge of emergency care in as accurate, standardized, and clear a manner as is possible. However, each EMS system is uniquely different, and it is beyond the scope of this text to address all differences. You must count heavily on your instructors, the program coordinator, and ultimately the program medical director to identify how specific emergency care procedures are applied in your system.

The authors of the 1998 U.S. DOT *EMT-Paramedic National Standard Curriculum* have made one thing perfectly clear. They are no longer interested in training programs that prepare technicians, or skilled tradesmen, at the paramedic level. Twenty-first century paramedics are practitioners of emergency field medicine and professional health care clinicians. The expanded curriculum provides both a broad-based medical education and a specific, intensive training program. They designed it to prepare paramedics to perform their traditional role as providers of emergency field medicine. They also have provided a much broader foundation in anatomy and physiology, patient assessment, pathophysiology of disease, and pharmacology. This dual-purpose curriculum will allow paramedics to expand their roles in the health care industry. This change in philosophy marks a new beginning for the paramedic field. *Patient Assessment* reflects that philosophy.

This book provides paramedic students with the principles of patient assessment. The first two chapters present the techniques of conducting a comprehensive history and physical exam. The remaining chapters discuss ways to integrate the techniques learned in the first two chapters to real patient situations. Like the entire curriculum, this book is both broad-based and specific.

Chapter 1 "The History" provides the basic components of a complete health history. The components include the chief complaint, the present history, the past history, the current health status, and the review of systems. It is comprehensive and not meant to be used in its entirety in emergency field situations. It also discusses how to effectively conduct an interview and use nonverbal communication skills to elicit vital information from your patients. In addition, it provides suggestions for communicating with difficult patients, hostile patients, and patients with language barriers.

Chapter 2 "Physical Exam Techniques" presents the techniques of conducting a comprehensive physical exam. Like the history, it is complete and not intended for all situations. With time and clinical experience you will learn which components of the history and physical exam are appropriate to assess and manage your particular situation. If you are hired to conduct pre-employment physical exams, you may use the history and physical exam in its entirety. If you are assessing and managing a critical patient in the field, you will select those components most appropriate for your situation. Topics in this chapter include assessing the skin; the head; the neck; the chest along with the respiratory and cardiovascular systems; the abdomen and digestive system; the extremities and musculoskeletal system; the peripheral vascular system; and how to conduct a comprehensive neurological exam. With each section is a review of the anatomy and physiology of the areas you are examining.

Chapter 3 "Patient Assessment in the Field" offers a practical approach to conducting problem-oriented history and physical exams. It deals with ways to use your new skills to assess patients in the field. With time and clinical experience, you will learn which components are appropriate for different situations. Topics include scene safety; the initial assessment; the focused history and physical exam for the following types of patients: responsive medical patient, unresponsive medical patient, trauma patient with significant mechanism of injury, and the trauma patient with an isolated injury; the detailed physical exam, and the ongoing assessment.

Chapter 4 "Clinical Decision Making" provides the basic steps for making clinical decisions. It describes each step in detail and discusses how to think critically in emergency situations. Topics include forming a concept, interpreting the data, applying principles of emergency medicine, evaluating your treatment plan, and reflecting on your care after the emergency response. This chapter is unique to emergency medical services textbooks.

Chapter 5 "Communications" deals with verbal communication. Communication is the key component that links every phase of an EMS response and helps ensure a continuity of care. Topics include the principles of communication, communication during the different phases of an EMS response, communication technology, and giving a medical report. We have provided several examples of typical radio medical reports.

Chapter 6 "Documentation" deals with writing a Prehospital Care Report, or PCR. Topics include the use of medical terminology and abbreviations, the elements of a good report, writing the narrative, and dealing with patient refusals. Again, we have provided examples of the various narrative writing styles.

This volume, *Patient Assessment,* describes how to conduct a comprehensive history and physical exam and document your findings appropriately. It also describes how to perform a problem-oriented patient assessment on a real patient in the field, report your findings to your medical direction physician, and document the response on your PCR. It represents the philosophy of the new paramedic curriculum and helps the student prepare to meet the challenge of being a twenty-first century paramedic. Good luck!

Brady's *Paramedic Care: Principles & Practice* is a five-volume series designed to provide educational enrichment as prescribed by the 1998 U.S. DOT *EMT–Paramedic National Standard Curriculum.* Volume 1, *Introduction to Advanced Prehospital Care* presents the foundations of paramedic practice as well as an introduction to pathophysiology, pharmacology, medication administration, and airway management and ventilation. Volume 2, *Patient Assessment* adds the cognitive and psychomotor skills of patient assessment, communications, and documentation. This knowledge base expands as the series applies it to the medical patient in Volume 3, *Medical Emergencies* and to the trauma patient in Volume 4, *Trauma Emergencies.* Volume 5, *Special Considerations/Operations* enriches these general patient care concepts and principles with applications to special patients and circumstances we commonly see as paramedics. The product of this complete and integrated series is a set of principles of paramedic care you will be required to practice in the 21st century.

Acknowledgments

We wish to thank the following groups of people for their assistance on developing this volume of *Paramedic Care: Principles & Practice*.

DEVELOPMENT AND PRODUCTION

The task of writing, editing, reviewing, and producing a textbook the size of *Paramedic Care: Principles & Practice* is complex. Many talented people have been involved in developing and producing this new program.

First, the authors would like to acknowledge the support of Julie Alexander and Laura Edwards. Their belief in us and support of EMS has allowed us to assure that *Paramedic Care: Principles & Practice* will be in the forefront of paramedic education. Special thanks go to Sandra Breuer, who served as Project Coordinator for this new paramedic series, and John Joerschke, Development Editor for this volume. The extraordinary efforts of these exceptionally dedicated editors are deeply appreciated.

The challenges of production were in the very capable hands of Patrick Walsh and Larry Hayden, who skillfully supervised all production stages to create the final product you now hold. In developing our art and photo program we were fortunate to work with yet additional talent, leaders within their professions. Most of the staged photographs are by Michal Heron of New York City, whose commitment to excellence never falters. The new art was drafted by Rolin Graphics of Plymouth, Minnesota.

REVIEW BOARDS

Our special thanks to Joseph J. Mistovich, chairperson and Associate Professor, Department of Health Professions, Youngtown State University, Youngstown, Ohio, for his review of *Patient Assessment*. His knowledge of the new paramedic curriculum, experience, and high standards proved to be significant contributions to text development.

Our special thanks also to Dr. Howard A. Werman, Associate Professor, Department of Emergency Medicine, The Ohio State University College of Medicine and Public Health, Columbus, Ohio. Dr. Werman's reviews were carefully prepared, and we appreciate the thoughtful advice and keen insight he offered.

INSTRUCTOR REVIEWERS

The reviewers of *Paramedic Care: Principles & Practice* have provided many excellent suggestions and ideas for improving the text. The quality of the reviews has been outstanding, and the reviews have been a major aid in the preparation and revision of the manuscript. The assistance provided by these EMS experts is deeply appreciated.

Linda M. Abrahamson, RN, EMT-P
EMS Education Coordinator
Will Grundy EMS
Silver Cross Hospital
Joliet, IL

Brenda Beasley, RN, BS, EMT-P
EMS Program Director
Calhoun College
Decatur, AL

Ed Carlson, Med, REMT-P
Department of EMS Education
University of South Alabama
Mobile, AL

Chuck Carter, RN, NREMT-P, CEN
Mississippi State Department of Health
Division of EMS
Jackson, MS

Claudette Dirzanowski, EMT-P
Certified Instructor/Examiner for the
    State of Texas, AHA, ARC, PHTLS
Sweeney Community Hospital and
    Brazosport College
Sweeney, TX

Bob Elling, MPA, REMT-P
Director, Institute of Prehospital
    Emergency Medicine
Hudson Valley Community College
Troy, NY

Catherine Pattison, RN, MSN, EMT-B
EMS Program Administrator
Bishop State Community College
Mobile, AL

Steven A. Weinman, RN, BSN, CEN
Instructor, Emergency Department
New York Presbyterian Hospital
New York Cornell Campus
New York, NY

About the Authors

BRYAN E. BLEDSOE, D.O., F.A.C.E.P., F.A.A.E.M., F.A.E.P., EMT-P

Dr. Bryan Bledsoe is an emergency physician with special interest in prehospital care. He received his B.S. degree from the University of Texas at Arlington and received his medical degree from the University of North Texas Health Sciences Center / Texas College of Osteopathic Medicine. He completed his internship at Texas Tech University and residency training at Scott and White Memorial Hospital / Texas A&M College of Medicine. Dr. Bledsoe is board-certified in emergency medicine and family practice. He is presently a Ph.D. candidate at Charles Sturt University at Wagga Wagga, New South Wales, Australia.

Prior to attending medical school, Dr. Bledsoe worked as an EMT, paramedic, and paramedic instructor. He completed EMT training in 1974 and paramedic training in 1976, and worked for 6 years as a field paramedic in Fort Worth, Texas. In 1979, he joined the faculty of the University of North Texas Health Sciences Center and served as coordinator of EMT and paramedic education programs at the university. Dr. Bledsoe is active in emergency medicine and serves as medical director for several EMS agencies and educational programs.

Dr. Bledsoe has authored several EMS books published by Brady including *Paramedic Emergency Care, Intermediate Emergency Care, Atlas of Paramedic Skills, Prehospital Emergency Pharmacology,* and *Pocket Reference for EMTs and Paramedics.* He is married to Emma Bledsoe. They have two children, Bryan and Andrea, and live in Midlothian, Texas, a suburb of Dallas. He enjoys saltwater fishing and listening to Jimmy Buffett.

ROBERT S. PORTER, M.A., NREMT-P

Robert Porter has been teaching in Emergency Medical Services for 25 years and currently serves as the Senior Advanced Life Support Educator for Madison County, New York, and as a Flight Paramedic with the Onondaga County Sheriff's Department helicopter service, AirOne. Mr. Porter is a Wisconsin native and received his Bachelor's degree in education from the University of Wisconsin. He completed his Paramedic training at Northeast Wisconsin Technical Institute in 1978 and earned a Master's Degree in Health Education at Central Michigan University in 1990.

Mr. Porter has been an EMT and EMS educator and administrator since 1973 and obtained his National Registration as an EMT-Paramedic in 1978. He has taught both basic and advanced level EMS courses in the states of Wisconsin, Michigan, Louisiana, Pennsylvania, and New York. Mr. Porter served for more than ten years as a paramedic program accreditation-site evaluator for the American Medical Association and is a past chair of the National Society of EMT Instructor/Coordinators. He has published numerous articles in EMS periodicals and has authored Brady's *Paramedic Emergency Care, Intermediate Emergency Care, Tactical Emergency Care,* and *Weapons of Mass Destruction: Emergency Care* as well as the workbooks accompanying this text, *Paramedic Emergency Care,* and *Intermediate Emergency Care.* When not writing or teaching, Mr. Porter enjoys offshore sailboat racing, historic home restoration, and listening to Dr. Bryan Bledsoe complain about the Texas heat.

Richard A. Cherry, M.S., NREMT-P

Richard Cherry is Clinical Assistant Professor of Emergency Medicine and Director of Paramedic Training at SUNY Upstate Medical University in Syracuse, NY. His experience includes years of classroom teaching and emergency field work. A native of Buffalo, Mr. Cherry earned his Bachelor's degree and teaching certificate at nearby St. Bonaventure University in 1972. He taught high school for the next 10 years while he earned his Master's degree in Education from Oswego State University in 1977. He holds a permanent teaching license in New York State.

Mr. Cherry entered the emergency medical services field in 1974 with the De-Witt Volunteer Fire Department where he served his community as a firefighter and EMS provider for over 15 years. He took his first EMT course in 1977 and became an ALS provider two years later. He earned his paramedic certificate in 1985 as a member of the area's first paramedic class. He still answers emergency calls for Brewerton Ambulance.

Mr. Cherry has authored several books for Brady. Most notable is *EMT Teaching: A Common Sense Approach*. He has made presentations at many state, national, and international EMS conferences on a variety of teaching topics. In addition to his paramedic teaching, he is course director, instructor, and instructor trainer for ACLS, PALS, and PHTLS courses conducted for physicians, residents, nurses, medical students, and other house staff. He lives in Parish, New York with his wife Sue, a paramedic with Rural-Metro Medical Services, their children, and many pets.

Notices

It is the intent of the authors and publishers that this textbook be used as part of a formal paramedic education program taught by a qualified instructor and supervised by a licensed physician. The care procedures presented here represent accepted practices in the United States. They are not offered as a standard of care. Paramedic-level emergency care is to be performed only under the authority and guidance of a licensed physician. It is the reader's responsibility to know and follow local care protocols as provided by medical advisors directing the system to which he or she belongs. Also, it is the reader's responsibility to stay informed of emergency care procedure changes.

NOTICE ON DRUGS AND DRUG DOSAGES

Every effort has been made to ensure that the drug dosages presented in this textbook are in accordance with nationally accepted standards. When applicable, the dosages and routes are taken from the American Heart Association's Advanced Cardiac Life Support Guidelines. The American Medical Association's publication *Drug Evaluations,* the *Physician's Desk Reference,* and the Appleton & Lange *Health Professionals Drug Guide 2000* are followed with regard to drug dosages not covered by the American Heart Association's guidelines. It is the responsibility of the reader to be familiar with the drugs used in his or her system, as well as the dosages specified by the medical director. The drugs presented in this book should only be administered by direct order, whether verbally or through accepted standing orders, of a licensed physician.

NOTICE ON GENDER USAGE

The English language has historically given preference to the male gender. Among many words, the pronouns "he" and "his" are commonly used to describe both genders. Society evolves faster than language and the male pronouns still predominate in our speech. The authors have made great effort to treat the two genders equally, recognizing that a significant percentage of paramedics and patients are female. However, in some instances, male pronouns may be used to describe both male and female paramedics and patients solely for the purpose of brevity. This is not intended to offend any readers of the female gender.

NOTICE ON PHOTOGRAPHS

Please note that many of the photographs contained in this book are taken of actual emergency situations. As such, it is possible that they may not accurately depict current, appropriate, or advisable practices of emergency medical care. They have been included for the sole purpose of giving general insight into real-life emergency settings.

NOTICE ON CASE STUDIES

The names used and situations depicted in the case studies throughout this program are fictitious.

Precautions on Bloodborne Pathogens and Infectious Diseases

Prehospital emergency personnel, like all health care workers, are at risk for exposure to bloodborne pathogens and infectious diseases. In emergency situations it is often difficult to take or enforce proper infection control measures. However, as a paramedic, you must recognize your high-risk status. Study the following information on infection control before turning to the main portion of this book.

Infection control is designed to protect emergency personnel, their families, and their patients from unnecessary exposure to communicable diseases.

Laws, regulations, and standards regarding infection control include:

* *Centers for Disease Control (CDC) Guidelines.* The CDC has published extensive guidelines regarding infection control. Proper equipment and techniques that should be used by emergency response personnel to prevent or minimize risk of exposure are defined.

* *The Ryan White Act.* The Ryan White Act of 1990 allows emergency personnel to find out if they were exposed to an infectious disease while rendering patient care. Employers are required to name a "designated officer" to coordinate communications with the treating hospital.

* *Americans with Disabilities Act.* This act prohibits discrimination against individuals with disabilities including those with contagious diseases. It guarantees equal employment opportunities and job protection if the infected individual can perform essential job functions and does not pose a threat to the safety and health of patients and coworkers.

* *Occupational Safety and Health Administration (OSHA) Regulations.* OSHA recently enacted a regulation entitled Occupational Exposure to Bloodborne Pathogens that classifies emergency response personnel as being at the greatest risk of occupational exposure to communicable diseases. This regulation requires employers to provide hepatitis B (HBV) vaccinations free of charge, maintain a written exposure control plan, and provide personal protective equipment (PPE). These requirements primarily apply to private employers. Applicability to local and state governmental employees varies by locality. Many states have developed their own OSHA plans.

* *National Fire Protection Association (NFPA) Guidelines.* This is a national organization that has established specific guidelines and requirements regarding infection control for emergency response agencies, particularly fire departments and EMS services.

BODY SUBSTANCE ISOLATION PRECAUTIONS AND PERSONAL PROTECTIVE EQUIPMENT

Emergency response personnel should practice *Body Substance Isolation (BSI),* a strategy that considers ALL body substances potentially infectious. To achieve this, all emergency personnel should utilize *Personal Protective Equipment (PPE).*

Appropriate PPE should be available on every emergency vehicle. The minimum recommended PPE includes the following:

* *Gloves.* Disposable gloves should be donned by all emergency response personnel BEFORE initiating any emergency care. When an emergency incident involves more than one patient, you should attempt to change gloves between patients. When gloves have been contaminated, they should be removed as soon as possible. To properly remove contaminated gloves, grasp one glove approximately one inch from the wrist. Without touching the inside of the glove, pull the glove half-way off and stop. With that half gloved hand, pull the glove on the opposite hand completely off. Place the removed glove in the palm of the other glove, with the inside of the removed glove exposed. Pull the second glove completely off with the ungloved hand, only touching the inside of the glove. Always wash hands after gloves are removed, even when the gloves appear intact.

* *Masks and Protective Eyewear.* Masks and protective equipment should be present on all emergency vehicles and used in accordance with the level of exposure encountered. Masks and protective eyewear should be worn together whenever blood spatter is likely to occur, such as arterial bleeding, childbirth, endotracheal intubation, invasive procedures, oral suctioning, and clean-up of equipment that requires heavy scrubbing or brushing. Both you and the patient should wear masks whenever the potential for airborne transmission of disease exists.

* *HEPA Respirators.* Due to the resurgence of tuberculosis (TB), prehospital personnel should protect themselves from TB infection through use of a high-efficiency particulate air (HEPA) respirator, a design approved by the National Institute of Occupational Safety and Health (NIOSH). It should fit snugly and be capable of filtering out the tuberculosis bacillus. The HEPA respirator should be worn when caring for patients with confirmed or suspected TB. This is especially true when performing "high hazard" procedures such as administration of nebulized medications, endotracheal intubation, or suctioning on such a patient.

* *Gowns.* Gowns protect clothing from blood splashes. If large splashes of blood are expected, such as with childbirth, wear impervious gowns.

* *Resuscitation Equipment.* Disposable resuscitation equipment should be the primary means of artificial ventilation in emergency care. Such items should be used once, then disposed of.

Remember, the proper use of personal protective equipment ensures effective infection control and minimizes risk. Use ALL protective equipment recommended for any particular situation to ensure maximum protection.

Consider ALL body substances potentially infectious and ALWAYS practice body substance isolation.

Welcome to Paramedic Care

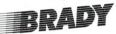

ONE LAKE STREET
UPPER SADDLE RIVER, NJ 07458

Dear Paramedic Instructor,

Brady, Your Partner in Education, is pleased to present *Paramedic Care: Principles & Practice*—a comprehensive series developed specifically to meet the new U.S. DOT National Standard Curriculum for EMT-Paramedics.

We recognize that for many of you the new curriculum represents a dramatic change in the way your paramedic course will be taught. *Paramedic Care: Principles & Practice* was developed specifically to help both you and your students succeed. Written in a student-friendly, easy-to-understand style, our new series consists of five volumes:

- Volume 1: *Introduction to Advanced Prehospital Care*
- Volume 2: *Patient Assessment*
- Volume 3: *Medical Emergencies*
- Volume 4: *Trauma Emergencies*
- Volume 5: *Special Considerations/Operations.*

The texts in this series are designed to work in tandem to cover all the objectives in the eight modules of the new U.S. DOT curriculum. However, each volume may also be used individually to help you tailor your course to state and local protocols.

Our high-quality instructor materials provide everything you need to help get your new curriculum course up and running. The Instructor's Resource Manual will contain lecture outlines and lesson plans that cover the new curriculum, along with student handouts and suggestions for class activities.

The *Paramedic Care* series also offers the latest multimedia technology to enhance and enrich your students' classroom experiences and to help you manage your classes more efficiently. The series' accompanying Companion Website contains chapter-by-chapter interactive student quizzes and links to related EMS sites for students. The Companion Website also offers downloadable instructor resources, teaching tips, links to curriculum-related websites, and an online syllabus builder. Our partnership with Victory Technology brings you *MedMedic*, an interactive CD-ROM tied chapter by chapter to each of the books. These new CDs include video, interactive student quizzes, and animations.

We wish you the best of luck as you transition to the new paramedic curriculum.

Sincerely,

Julie Levin Alexander
Vice President and Publisher

BRADY
Your Partner in Education

EMPHASIZING PRINCIPLES

Chapter Objectives with Page References

Each chapter begins with clearly stated **Objectives** that follow the new DOT Paramedic curriculum. Students can refer to these objectives while studying to make sure they understand the material fully. Page references after each objective indicate where relevant content is covered in the chapter.

Content Review

Content Review summarizes important content and gives students a format for quick review.

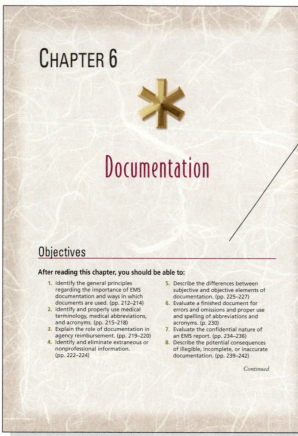

CHAPTER 6

Documentation

Objectives

After reading this chapter, you should be able to:

1. Identify the general principles regarding the importance of EMS documentation and ways in which documents are used. (pp. 212–214)
2. Identify and properly use medical terminology, medical abbreviations, and acronyms. (pp. 215–218)
3. Explain the role of documentation in agency reimbursement. (pp. 219–220)
4. Identify and eliminate extraneous or nonprofessional information. (pp. 222–224)
5. Describe the differences between subjective and objective elements of documentation. (pp. 225–227)
6. Evaluate a finished document for errors and omissions and proper use and spelling of abbreviations and acronyms. (p. 230)
7. Evaluate the confidential nature of an EMS report. (pp. 234–236)
8. Describe the potential consequences of illegible, incomplete, or inaccurate documentation. (pp. 239–242)

Continued

Key Points

Key Points in the margins help students identify and learn the fundamental principles of paramedic practice.

Key Terms

Reinforcement of **Key Terms** helps students master new terminology.

Content Review

FACILITATING BEHAVIORS
- Stay calm
- Plan for the worst
- Work systematically
- Remain adaptable

Be like the duck—cool and calm on the water's surface, while paddling feverishly underneath.

Except for safety concerns, never allow anything to distract you from your most important job—assessing and caring for your patient.

* **reflective** acting thoughtfully, deliberately, and analytically.

* **impulsive** acting instinctively without stopping to think.

* **divergent** taking into account all aspects of a complex situation.

USEFUL THINKING STYLES

As a paramedic, you will face confusing emergencies that would challenge even the most knowledgeable, analytical care provider. You must be able to stay calm and not panic. Your self-control in the face of extreme chaos will set the example for other team members to follow. Even when you are struggling to maintain your composure—especially then—never let others know. The key is focusing on the task and blocking out the distractions. Be like the duck—cool and calm on the water's surface, while paddling feverishly underneath.

Assume and plan for the worst, and always err on the side of benefitting your patient. For example, if you are deliberating whether to immobilize your patient, initiate advanced life support procedures, or administer oxygen, just do it! It is better to err by providing care than by withholding it. Be pessimistic! Anticipate all potential bad side effects of your treatments and prepare "plan B." For example, as you deliver a bronchodilating drug to your severe asthmatic patient, anticipate that it will not work and mentally prepare to intubate him and perform positive pressure ventilation. Or while you are administering atropine to your patient with symptomatic bradycardia, plan ahead for external cardiac pacing and dopamine, if atropine therapy fails to restore adequate circulation.

Establish and maintain a systematic assessment pattern. Practice your assessments until they become second nature, and you will avoid skipping and missing steps. Be disciplined and stay focused, especially when you are confronted with a complex emergency scene. For example, your patient lies moaning on the ground in a pool of blood. Bystanders are screaming at you to help him; others are trying to tell you what happened. The police are gathering the story and trying unsuccessfully to talk with your patient. You must gain control of this scene. You do so by focusing on your patient and performing a systematic assessment. Use common acronyms (MS-ABC, OPQRST, SAMPLE) or make up your own to help you remember the key elements of your assessment. Except for safety concerns, never allow anything to distract you from your most important job—assessing and caring for your patient.

The different situations you encounter will require a variety of management styles. Adapting your styles of situation analysis (reflective vs. impulsive), data processing (convergent vs. divergent), and decision making (anticipatory vs. reactive) to each situation will enable you to provide the best possible care in every case.

Reflective vs. Impulsive Some situations call for you to be **reflective**, take your time, and figure out what is wrong with your patient. You have a patient who complains of "not feeling well." She has a long history of cardiac, renal, respiratory, and diabetic problems. Since she is in no real distress and is hemodynamically stable, you can take your time to determine her primary problem. Other situations call for immediate action. They require you to make an instinctive, **impulsive** decision and manage your patient's life-threatening condition. For example, if your patient presents apneic and pulseless, you will immediately begin CPR and prepare for rapid defibrillation. If he presents with a spurting artery, you will at once take measures to control the hemorrhage. If he is choking and has a weak, ineffective cough, you will quickly perform the Heimlich maneuver. You have to think fast in these situations.

Divergent vs. Convergent To process the data you receive from your patient and the scene, you can use either a divergent approach or a convergent approach. The **divergent** approach considers all aspects of a situation before arriving at a solution. It is insightful and works well when you are confronted with complex

4 CHAPTER 1 *The History*

...try ha... ...own ...dio ...t 5-1). These wo... ...orten air time and transmit thoughts and ideas quickly. For exam... ...opy, 10-4, and *roger* mean "I heard you and I understand what you said." Using industry terminology appropriately is an important part of effective communication. It provides a common *means* of communicating with other *emergency* care professionals.

communicating with other emergency care professionals.

Table 5-1	COMMON RADIO TERMINOLOGY
Term	**Meaning**
Copy, 10-4, roger	I understand
Affirmative	Yes
Negative	No
Stand by	Please wait
Repeat	Please repeat what you said
Land-line	Telephone communications
Rendezvous	Meet with
LZ	Landing zone (helicopter)
ETA	Estimated time of arrival
Over	I am finished with my transmission
Mobile status	On the air, driving around
Stage	Wait before entering a scene
Clear	End of transmission
Unfounded	We cannot find the incident/patient
Be advised	Listen carefully to this

Tables and Illustrations

Tables and **illustrations** offer visual support to enhance students' understanding of paramedic principles and practice.

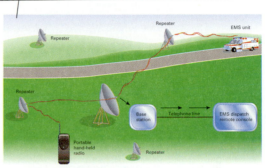

FIGURE 5-2 Example of an EMS system using repeaters.

a large geographical expanse can place repeaters strategically throughout its service area. These devices receive transmissions from a low-powered source and rebroadcast them at a higher power (Figure 5-2).

Your regional EMS system may consist of ma... ...y agencies that have conducted business for decades on different r... ...frequencies. Cit... ...radio band... ... ...

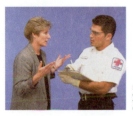

FIGURE 1-3 If the patient cannot provide useful information, gather it from family members or bystanders.

BLINDNESS

Blind patients present special problems. They need you to identify yourself immediately, since they cannot see your uniform. Always announce yourself and explain who you are and why you are there. If possible, take your patient's hand to establish a personal contact and to show him where you are. Remember that nonverbal communication such as hand gestures, facial expressions, and body language, are useless in these cases. Your voice is your only tool for effective communication.

TALKING WITH FAMILIES OR FRIENDS

You will often encounter patients who cannot give you any useful information. In these cases, find a third party who can augment the patient history and offer a useful adjunct to the patient's answers (Figure 1-3). The typical case is the postictal patient who cannot describe his seizure activity to you. Another example is learning from his friend that your patient's wife died in an automobile accident just three weeks ago. Now you better understand why your patient appears depressed and suicidal. Make sure that patient confidentiality is a priority when you accept personal information from a family member, friend, or bystander.

SUMMARY

This chapter dealt with taking a good history. While it presented the patient history in its entirety, common sense will determine which parts are appropriate for a given situation. Most of a paramedic's work is patient contact. It is making a connection with people in crisis. Patients most often comment on the attitudes of their paramedics. How well did they relate to them? Did they make them feel at ease? Did they care for them? Patients rarely comment on a paramedic's technical skills. Top-notch paramedics are technically skillful and treat all their patients with dignity and compassion. This begins with the history.

Good patient interaction can lead to good patient outcomes, improved patient satisfaction, and better adherence to treatment. As a paramedic you have

Summar...

End-of-Chapter Summary

Each end-of-chapter **Summary** reviews the main topics covered.

...) Past Hi...
c) Current He...
d) Review of Systems

FURTHER READING

Bates, Barbara, Lynn S. Bickley, and Robert A. Hoekelman. *A Guide to Physical Examination and History Taking.* 6th ed. Philadelphia: J.B. Lippincott, 1995.

Coulehan, John L. and Marian R. Block. *The Medical Interview: Mastering Skills for Clinical Practice.* 3rd ed. Philadelphia: F.A. Davis, 1997.

Epstein, Owen, et al. *Clinical Examination.* St. Louis: Mosby, 1997.

Lipkin, Mack Jr., Samuel M. Putnam, and Aaron Lazare. *The Medical Interview: Clinical Care, Education, and Research.* New York: Springer, 1994.

Seidel Henry M. *Mosby's Guide to Physical Examination.* 3rd ed. St. Louis: Mosby, 1994.

Willms, Janice L., Henry Schniederman, and Paula S. Algranati. *Physical Diagnosis: Bedside Evaluation of Diagnosis and Function.* Baltimore: Williams & Wilkins, 1994.

ON THE WEB

Visit Brady's Paramedic Website through www.brady books.com/paramedic.

Further Reading and On the Web

Each chapter ends with recommendations for books and journal articles. Links to relevant websites plus a link to the text's Companion Website can be found at **www.bradybooks.com/paramedic.**

EMPHASIZING PRACTICE

Case Study

Case Studies draw students into the reading and create a link between text content and real-life situations and experiences.

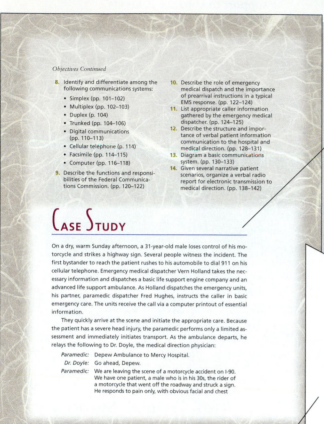

Objectives Continued

8. Identify and differentiate among the following communications systems:
   - Simplex (pp. 101–102)
   - Multiplex (pp. 102–103)
   - Duplex (p. 104)
   - Trunked (pp. 104–106)
   - Digital communications (pp. 110–113)
   - Cellular telephone (p. 114)
   - Facsimile (pp. 114–115)
   - Computer (pp. 116–118)
9. Describe the functions and responsibilities of the Federal Communications Commission. (pp. 120–122)
10. Describe the role of emergency medical dispatch and the importance of prearrival instructions in a typical EMS response. (pp. 122–124)
11. List appropriate caller information gathered by the emergency medical dispatcher. (pp. 124–125)
12. Describe the structure and importance of verbal patient information communication to the hospital and medical direction. (pp. 128–131)
13. Diagram a basic communications system. (pp. 130–133)
14. Given several narrative patient scenarios, organize a verbal radio report for electronic transmission to medical direction. (pp. 138–142)

CASE STUDY

On a dry, warm Sunday afternoon, a 31-year-old male loses control of his motorcycle and strikes a highway sign. Several people witness the incident. The first bystander to reach the patient rushes to his automobile to dial 911 on his cellular telephone. Emergency medical dispatcher Vern Holland takes the necessary information and dispatches a basic life support engine company and an advanced life support ambulance. As Holland dispatches the emergency units, his partner, paramedic dispatcher Fred Hughes, instructs the caller in basic emergency care. The units receive the call via a computer printout of essential information.

They quickly arrive at the scene and initiate the appropriate care. Because the patient has a severe head injury, the paramedic performs only a limited assessment and immediately initiates transport. As the ambulance departs, he relays the following to Dr. Doyle, the medical direction physician:

Paramedic: Depew Ambulance to Mercy Hospital.
Dr. Doyle: Go ahead, Depew.
Paramedic: We are leaving the scene of a motorcycle accident on I-90. We have one patient, a male who is in his 30s, the rider of a motorcycle that went off the roadway and struck a sign. He responds to pain only, with obvious facial and chest

...wing ...cumstan... ...t of... ...of injury may als... ...p rehabilitation ...provide better therapy. Your PCR becomes an important document tha... ...elps ensure your patient's continuous effective care.

Prehospital Care Report

			MILEAGE		USE MILITARY TIMES
Agency Name	ARLINGTON RESCUE		END	2 4 4 9 6	CALL REC'D 0 7 0 5
Dispatch Information	CARDIAC		BEGIN	2 4 4 7 6	ENROUTE 0 7 0 7
Call Location	124 CYPRUS ST 2nd FLOOR		TOTAL	0 0 0 2 0	ARRIVED AT SCENE 0 7 1 9

CHECK ONE: ☑ Residence ☐ Health Facility ☐ Farm ☐ Indust. Facility ☐ Other Work Loc. ☐ Roadway ☐ Recreational ☐ Other — LOCATION CODE 0 1 2 4   FROM SCENE 0 7 3 8

CALL TYPE AS REC'D — MECHANISM OF INJURY
☑ Emergency ☑ MVA (✓ seat belt used) N/A ☐ Knife — AT DESTIN 0 7 5 4
☐ Non-Emergency ☐ Fall of ___ feet ☐ Machinery — IN SERVICE 0 8 1 0
☐ Stand-by ☐ Unarmed assault — IN QUARTERS 0 8 3 2
☐ GSW

FIGURE 6-1 The run data in a prehospital care report is vital to your agency's efforts to improve patient care.

Uses for Documentation 12

Documentation

Covered thoroughly throughout the text, **proper documentation techniques** are critical to ensuring provider protection on the job as well as patient safety during the transition of care.

You Make the Call

Promoting critical thinking skills, each **You Make the Call** presents a hypothetical situation that requires students to apply principles to actual practice. Suggested responses are found at the back of the text.

YOU MAKE THE CALL

A call comes into your unit for a "possible heart attack" on State Route 11. You and your partner climb into Palermo Rescue, a nontransport first-response vehicle. Your response time is about ten minutes. Upon arrival, a family member meets you. He leads you into the den of a small farm house. Here you see your patient sitting in an overstuffed chair. You note that your patient is a 69-year-old male in obvious distress.

You begin questioning your patient to develop a history. As he speaks, you immediately notice that he has difficulty breathing. He complains of severe chest pain, which began about 30 minutes ago. With his hand, he indicates that the pain is pressure-like and substernal. He also indicates that it radiates to his left arm and jaw. He describes a history of heart disease, including two prior heart attacks. Three years ago, he had cardiac bypass surgery. He currently takes Lanoxin, Lasix, Capoten, and an aspirin a day. He is allergic to Mellaril.

You and your partner complete your assessment. Your patient says he weighs about 250 pounds. He is alert, but anxious. He exhibits jugular venous distention and bibasilar crackles. His abdomen is nontender. His distal pulses are good. Vital signs include: blood pressure 210/110 mmHg, pulse of 70 per minute and regular, and respirations of 20 breaths per minute and mildly labored. Pulse oximetry is 93% on supplemental oxygen. During your assessment, your patient becomes progressively more dyspneic. The transporting ambulance arrives and the paramedic asks you to give a radio report to the receiving hospital based on your assessment while she prepares her patient for transport.

- Based on the information above, organize and prepare your radio report to inform the receiving hospital of your patient's condition.

See Suggested Responses at the back of this book.

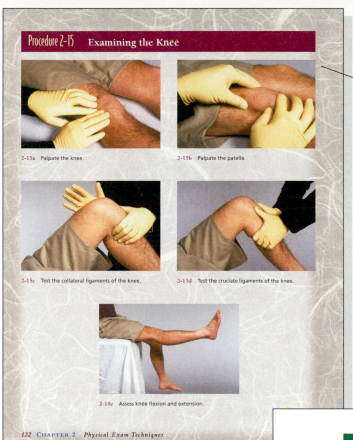

Procedure 2-15   Examining the Knee

2-15a   Palpate the knee.

2-15b   Palpate the patella.

2-15c   Test the collateral ligaments of the knee.

2-15d   Test the cruciate ligaments of the knee.

2-15e   Assess knee flexion and extension.

122   CHAPTER 2   Physical Exam Techniques

Procedure Scans

Newly photographed **Procedure Scans** provide step-by-step visual support on how to perform skills included in the DOT curriculum.

Patient Care Algorithms

Clearly presented **algorithms** provide graphic "pathways" that integrate assessment and care for medical or trauma emergencies. These visual summaries give students a step-by-step flow of assessment and emergency care procedures.

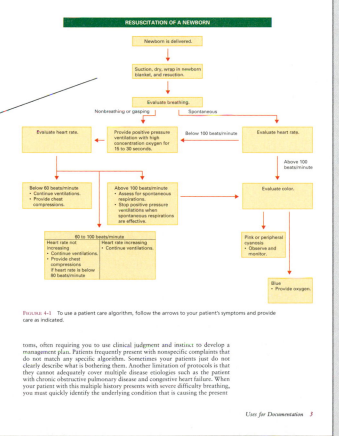

FIGURE 4-1   To use a patient care algorithm, follow the arrows to your patient's symptoms and provide care as indicated.

toms, often requiring you to use clinical judgment and instinct to develop a management plan. Patients frequently present with nonspecific complaints that do not match any specific algorithm. Sometimes your patients just do not clearly describe what is bothering them. Another limitation of protocols is that they cannot adequately cover multiple disease etiologies such as the patient with chronic obstructive pulmonary disease and congestive heart failure. When your patient with this multiple history presents with severe difficulty breathing, you must quickly identify the underlying condition that is causing the present

Uses for Documentation   3

TEACHING & LEARNING PACKAGE

FOR THE INSTRUCTOR

Instructor's Resource Manual

The Instructor's Resource Manual for each volume contains everything needed to teach the 1998 U.S. DOT National Standard Curriculum for Paramedics. It fully covers the DOT curriculum with:

• time estimates for various topics
• listing of additional resources
• lecture outlines
• student activities handouts
• answers to student review questions
• case study discussion questions.

The manual is also available on disk so instructors can customize resources to their individual needs.

PowerPoint® Presentations on CD-ROM

This CD-ROM offers PowerPoint® presentations that contain word slides and images organized by chapter. The entire presentation is fully customizable.

Computerized Test Bank

The Computerized Test Bank contains textbook-based questions in a format that enables instructors to select questions based on topic area and degree of difficulty.

FOR THE STUDENT

Student Workbook

A student workbook with review and practice activities accompanies each volume of the *Paramedic Care* series. The workbooks include multiple-choice questions, fill-in-the-blank questions, labeling exercises, case studies, and special projects, along with an answer key with text page references.

MedMedic CD-ROM

Tied chapter by chapter to each of the volumes in the *Paramedic Care* series, this interactive CD-ROM set contains videos, student quizzes, and animations.

ONLINE RESOURCES

Paramedic Care Companion Website: www.bradybooks.com/paramedic

This free site, tied chapter-by-chapter to the five texts, reinforces student learning through interactive online study guides, quizzes based on the new curriculum, and case studies, as well as links to important EMS-related Internet resources. The *Paramedic Care* Companion Website also includes instructor resources, such as a bridge guide to help instructors transition to the new curriculum, links to EMS-related sites (including a site to download the new curriculum), and teaching tips. Instructors can also use the site to create a customized syllabus.

EMS Supersite: www.bradybooks.com/ems

Brady's EMS Supersite is a free, one-stop Web resource for both students and instructors offering:

• Online Brady catalog
• Links to all Brady Companion Websites
• Interactive case studies
• Case Study of the Month
• Useful EMS-related links
• Games, puzzles, and activities
• Test-taking tips
• Test writing and teaching tips
• Sample chapters and multimedia demos.

For information on additional media to support the series, please contact your Brady representative:
1-800-638-0220

OTHER TITLES OF INTEREST

ANATOMY & PHYSIOLOGY

GUY, Learning Human Anatomy, Second Edition (0-8385-5657-4)

Organized by body regions, this popular text helps students learn human anatomy. Its outline format and easy-to-remember illustrations make it ideal for review and a perfect introductory gross anatomy text.

MARTINI et al., Essentials of Anatomy and Physiology, Second Edition (0-13-082192-6)

A one-semester/one-quarter anatomy and physiology text for students in allied health, physical education, and other programs requiring an overview of the human body's systems. An extensive instructor support package is available.

CARDIAC/EKG

BEASLEY, Understanding EKGs (0-8359-8571-7)

This text is a direct, basic approach to EKG interpretation that presents all the essential concepts for mastering the basics of this challenging field, while assuming no prior knowledge of EKGs.

BEASLEY, Understanding 12-Lead EKGs (0-13-027281-7)

This comprehensive, reader-friendly text teaches beginning students basic 12-lead EKG interpretation.

MISTOVICH et al., Advanced Cardiac Life Support (0-8359-5050-6)

Straightforward and easy to follow, this text offers clear explanations, a colorful design, and covers all of the core concepts covered in an advanced cardiac life support course.

PAGE, 12-Lead ECG for the Acute Care Provider (0-13-022460-X)

This full-color text presents EKG interpretation in a practical, easy-to-understand and user-friendly manner. Practice cases are included throughout the text.

For a complete listing of additional Brady titles, visit us on the Web: www.bradybooks.com

WALRAVEN, Basic Arrhythmias, Fifth Edition (0-8359-5305-X)

This classic bestseller covers all the basics of EKG and includes appendices on Clinical Implications of Arrhythmias, Cardiac Anatomy & Physiology, 12-Lead EKG, Basic 12-Lead Interpretation and Pacemakers.

MATHEMATICS

BENJAMIN-CHUNG, Math Principles and Practice: Preparing for Health Career Success (0-8359-5272-X)

This easy-to-follow text provides basic math skills for students or practicing health care professionals. It employs a common sense approach that builds on basic math skills to facilitate the understanding of more complex math calculations.

TIGER, Mathematical Concepts for Clinical Sciences (0-13-011549-5)

This book is geared for all entry-level clinical science curricula and presents material in a step-by-step approach that emphasizes the understanding of concepts, not the memorization of numbers and formulas.

MEDICAL

DALTON et al., Advanced Medical Life Support (0-8359-5179-0)

This groundbreaking text offers a practical approach to adult medical emergencies. Each chapter discusses realistic methods that a seasoned EMS practitioner would use.

MEDICAL TERMINOLOGY

FREMGEN, Medical Terminology: An Anatomy & Physiology Systems Approach (0-8359-4991-5)

In this full-color text-workbook, Bonnie F. Fremgen uses an integrated body systems approach and reader-friendly writing style to teach medical terminology.

LILLIS, A Concise Introduction to Medical Terminology (0-8385-4321-9)

A basic introduction to over 700 commonly used medical terms and word elements to help students learn the terminology they need to succeed.

(continued on next page)

OTHER TITLES OF INTEREST

MEDICAL TERMINOLOGY *(continued)*

RICE, Medical Terminology with Human Anatomy, Fourth Edition (0-8385-6274-4)

Providing comprehensive coverage of all aspects of medical terminology, the Fourth Edition of this popular text is arranged by body systems and specialty areas. Rice makes learning easy and interesting by presenting important prefixes, roots, and suffixes as they relate to each specialty or system.

RICE, The Terminology of Health and Medicine (0-8385-6260-4)

This self-study text presents learning concepts in numbered frames—with a series of statements on the right side of the page and the answers provided in a column on the outside. Terms are arranged by body system.

PATHOPHYSIOLOGY

BURNS, Pathophysiology (0-8385-8084-X)

Students will master the basics of general disease processes—as well as major diseases of the body system—by using the only pathophysiology text that offers a programmed approach with questions within each frame that test comprehension, and self-tests at the end of each section.

KENT/HART, Introduction to Human Disease, Fourth Edition (0-8385-4070-8)

This is the perfect text for any student seeking a reliable and concise overview of human disease. Each chapter contains most frequently encountered and serious problems, symptoms, signs and tests, specific diseases, and review questions.

MULVIHILL, Human Disease, Fourth Edition (0-8385-3928-9)

This popular book comprehensively covers mechanisms of disease and health problems, as well as commonly occurring diseases. Normal anatomy and physiology is reviewed at the beginning of each chapter.

For a complete listing of additional Brady titles, visit us on the Web: www.bradybooks.com

PEDIATRICS

EICHELBERGER, Pediatric Emergencies, Second Edition (0-8359-5123-5)

This text was developed to provide a standard of prehospital pediatric emergency care for both basic and advanced providers.

MARKENSON et al., Pediatric Prehospital Care (0-13-022618-1)

Written for all levels of EMS providers, this text presents a physiological approach to rapid and accurate pediatric assessment, identification of potential problems, establishing treatment priorities with effective on-going assessment, and rapid and safe transport.

PHARMACOLOGY

GRAJEDA-HIGLEY, Pharmacology (0-8385-8136-6)

This pharmacology handbook combines a systems approach with cartoon-type illustrations for a unique and user-friendly physiological presentation of pharmacological concepts.

MIKOLAJ, Drug Dosage Calculations (0-8359-4994-X)

This practical volume gives readers all the tools needed to solve virtually every type of dosage and calculation problem they will encounter in the workplace.

SHANNON, The Health Professional's Drug Guide 2000 (0-8385-0424-8)

This drug guide provides health care professionals with accurate, easily accessible information about their patients' medications. Comprehensive yet user-friendly, this handy resource includes important clinical implications for hundreds of drugs, including adverse reactions, interactions and side effects.

TRAUMA

CAMPBELL, Basic Trauma Life Support for Paramedics and Advanced Providers, Fourth Edition (0-13-084584-1)

Brady's best selling BTLS text provides a complete course that covers all the skills necessary for rapid assessment, resuscitation, stabilization and transportation of the trauma patient.

PARAMEDIC CARE: Principles & Practice

PATIENT ASSESSMENT

BRADY

CHAPTER 1

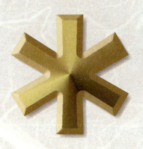

The History

Objectives

After reading this chapter, you should be able to:

1. Describe the techniques of history taking. (pp. 5–11)
2. Discuss the importance of using open- and closed-ended questions. (p. 8)
3. Describe the use of, and differentiate between, facilitation, reflection, clarification, empathetic responses, confrontation, and interpretation. (pp. 9–10)
4. Describe the structure, purpose, and how to obtain a comprehensive health history. (pp. 5–24)
5. List the components of a comprehensive history of an adult patient. (pp. 11–19)

CASE STUDY

En route to a call, paramedic supervisor John Bigelow reviews the key elements of a medical interview in his head. John is precepting paramedic student Maryann Conrad and wants to be a positive role model. As they approach the scene John quickly sizes it up. Nothing seems unusual. To the best of his knowledge, the scene is safe.

According to the dispatch information, John and Maryann are responding to evaluate an elderly man with abdominal pain. Upon first meeting his patient, John notices that he is in no real distress and appears stable. John does an initial assessment and then demonstrates taking a comprehensive patient history for Maryann. He introduces himself and Maryann and asks for his patient's name, which he will use throughout the interview.

John begins with a general question. "What seems to be the problem today, Mr. O'Donnell?"

"My stomach hurts," Mr. O'Donnell replies.

John begins exploring the history of the present illness with questions like "What were you doing when it started? Did it come on suddenly? Does anything make it worse or better? Can you describe how it feels? Can you point to the area that hurts? Does the pain travel anywhere else? How bad is it? On a scale of one to ten, with ten being the worst pain you have ever felt, how

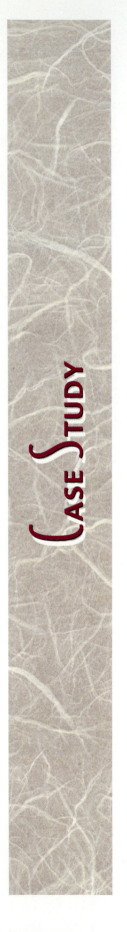

would you rate this pain? When did it start? Is it constant or does it come and go? Are you nauseous and have you vomited? Have you experienced a change in your bowel habits? Do you have any difficulty breathing?"

It seems that Mr. O'Donnell's pain came on suddenly after he ate this afternoon. He describes it as a sharp pain in the upper right quadrant that radiates to the right shoulder area. As Mr. O'Donnell answers John's questions, John leans forward, listening intently and often repeating Mr. O'Donnell's words. Maryann watches and learns.

John begins forming his differential field diagnosis, which includes hepatitis, acute myocardial infarction, pneumonia, aneurysm, cholecystitis, gastritis, pancreatitis, and peptic ulcer disease. He continues with the history. "Mr. O'Donnell, have you ever been treated for this problem in the past? Are you being treated for any other problems right now? Do you have diabetes, heart disease, breathing problems, kidney problems, stomach problems? Have you been injured recently? Have you had any surgeries? Does this problem usually happen right after eating? Are you taking any medications for it right now? Are you allergic to any medications? Do you smoke? Do you drink? How often do you drink? Did you drink any alcohol today? Does this problem get worse when you drink? What did you eat today?"

John learns that Mr. O'Donnell commonly has experienced pain after eating fatty foods. When John learns that his patient also drinks moderately every other day, he begins thinking about gall bladder disease. He decides to proceed to the review of body systems, beginning with the gastrointestinal system. He learns that Mr. O'Donnell often has indigestion and protracted episodes of pain and that his stools are clay colored. He also has noticed a yellowish tint to his eyes and that he feels feverish. Mr. O'Donnell denies vomiting blood or having blood in his stools. Hearing this, John suspects that his patient has cholecystitis. He conducts a focused physical exam and directs Maryann to take vital signs.

En route to St. Joseph's Hospital, John has Maryann conduct a detailed physical exam while he watches. At the hospital John reports to the ED attending, Dr. Zehner, who agrees with his preliminary diagnosis of gall bladder disease. Following an assessment that includes labs and an ultrasound, Dr. Zehner calls for the surgical service. After the call, John reviews the key points of taking a comprehensive patient history with Maryann. He explains how it helped him obtain important pieces of information that allowed him to focus the physical exam and led to his correct field diagnosis.

INTRODUCTION

In the majority of medical cases, you will base your field diagnosis on the patient history. Clearly, how you conduct the patient interview and the questions you ask will determine how much relevant medical information your patient reveals. In medical cases, obtaining an adequate history of your patient's **chief complaint**, recent illnesses, and significant past medical history is as important as, if not more important than, the physical exam. The information you gather will direct the physical exam and reveal clues to your patient's problem. Although we present the history by itself in this chapter, you will most likely conduct it simultaneously with parts of the physical exam.

The ability to elicit a good history is the foundation for providing good care to patients you have never met before. To conduct a good interview you must gain your patient's trust in just a very short time. Then you must ask the right questions, listen intently to your patient's answers, and respond accordingly. In this chapter we will discuss both the verbal and nonverbal components of taking a comprehensive medical history.

We present the medical history in its entirety, as a well-structured, yet flexible, tool having several component procedures that are conducted in order. In reality, your patient's answers will alter the sequence of your questioning, and some of the information in this chapter will not readily adapt itself to prehospital emergency medicine. As you gain clinical experience, you will learn which components of the history are appropriate to the particular situations you encounter. Whether your patient is critical or stable, the situation determines the length and completeness of the interview. For example, complicated medical cases require a close investigation of your patient's chief complaint and past history. Trauma cases, on the other hand, are generally sudden events not precipitated by medical conditions and require only a modified approach to history taking.

The interview is the focal point of your relationship with your patients. It establishes the bonding necessary for effective and efficient patient care. By asking a series of well-designed questions you begin to build a profile of your patients. You also should have a good understanding of their problems and a list of causes (**differential field diagnosis**) to explain their signs and symptoms. Often, learning about your patient's history, medications, and even their lifestyle will reveal clues to your final field diagnosis.

* **chief complaint** the reason the ambulance was called.

The ability to elicit a good history lays the foundation for good patient care.

* **differential field diagnosis** the list of possible causes for your patient's symptoms.

ESTABLISHING PATIENT RAPPORT

Your patients will form an opinion about you within the first few minutes, so you must establish a positive rapport quickly. This is not always easy. The situation, the patient, and the conditions will determine your ability to establish rapport. You can do several things, however, to facilitate this task. By asking them the right questions you will discover their chief complaint and their symptoms. By responding to them with empathy, you will win their trust and encourage them to discuss freely their problems with you. Their answers will also help you decide which areas require in-depth investigation and on which body systems to focus.

SETTING THE STAGE

Sometimes you will assess a patient from a long-term care facility. If your patient's chart is available, as in a nursing home or extended care facility, review it before conducting the interview. Quickly note his age, sex, race, marital status, address, and occupation. The insight into your patient's life experiences that you begin developing with this information may provide subtle clues to help steer your questioning. Determine any past medical problems or previous referrals for the same condition. Note any treatments rendered and their effects. On emergency scenes, review the first responder's run sheet. Look for the chief complaint, a brief history including a current medication list, and vital signs. Be careful not to let your patient's chart, his past medical history, or someone else's first impression bias your possible field diagnoses. Always accept such information gratefully, but briefly reconfirm it with the patient and conduct your interview with an open mind.

If possible, conduct the interview in a quiet room, alone, with no distractions. Since you are asking your patient to divulge very intimate information, privacy encourages open communication. It should be a place where you and your patient can sit down and comfortably talk about his current problem and past experiences. Unfortunately, on emergency runs, you conduct the patient interview in a variety of settings beyond your control from the kitchen floor to a busy street corner or a crowded bus. Often the back of your ambulance is where your patient will disclose important personal information to you. Some patients, however, will still be reluctant to reveal intimate information to a nonphysician in the emergency setting. Paramedics are often surprised at the hospital when their patients tell a different story to the physician in the emergency department, but this is common. To maximize your chances of obtaining a good history, practice the following techniques for developing better patient rapport.

THE FIRST IMPRESSION

Present yourself as a caring, compassionate, competent, and confident health care professional.

When you arrive on the scene, your patient, his family, and bystanders will form an impression of you. You have only a few precious minutes to make that impression a positive one. If you expect your patient to trust you with very private information, you must establish a positive, trusting relationship. Present yourself as a caring, compassionate, competent, and confident health care professional. Because this first impression will be based largely on your appearance, your dress and grooming will play an important role in the paramedic-patient relationship. Your appearance should suggest neatness, cleanliness, pride, and professionalism. Your uniform should be clean and pressed, your shoes or boots polished, your hands and nails clean, and your hair well groomed.

Your voice, body language, gestures, and especially eye contact should communicate that you care about your patient's problems. Your questioning process should make the patient comfortable, confident in your care, and supportive of your control of the situation. Position yourself at his eye level and focus your attention on him. Give his requests and concerns high priority, even if they are not medically significant. For example, if your patient complains of being cold, cover him with a blanket. Beyond making him feel warmer, it may also increase his confidence in your desire and ability to help. If you cannot care for a complaint immediately, express your concern and assure him you will either take care of it shortly or get him to a setting where it can be cared for.

A calm, reassuring voice and demeanor can put even the most apprehensive patient at ease.

A calm, reassuring voice and demeanor can put even the most apprehensive patient at ease. Remember that while his problems may not seem extraordinary to you, they may be extremely disturbing to him. You are accustomed to handling emergency situations; he is not. You are not horrified by a gory scene; he probably is. You deal with life-threatening emergencies everyday; he probably never does. Understanding these differences helps you to display an appropriate demeanor and begin your interview.

INTRODUCTIONS

As you enter, immediately make eye contact with your patient and maintain it as you conduct the interview. Eye contact is the most important form of nonverbal communication. It tells your patient, "I am sincerely interested in you and your problems." Always keeping in mind that your personal safety takes the highest priority in any emergency, quickly determine whether you should enter your patient's personal space (18 inches to 3 feet). Then kneel, crouch, or sit beside him and address him from eye level or lower to reassure him that he still has some control. Avoid standing over him, which appears threatening or indifferent.

Wear an identification badge. Introduce yourself by name, title, and agency. For example, "Hi, my name is Jay. I'm a paramedic with Brewerton Ambulance. What's your name?" Use your patient's name frequently during the interview. Ask him how he wishes to be called—for instance, "Mr. MacCormack," "Nicholas", or "Nick"—and respect his wishes. Avoid using slang terms such as, *honey, toots, dude, chief, pops,* or *babe* that your patient might construe as disrespectful and demeaning. This short verbal exchange reveals a wealth of information on your patient's respiratory status, level of consciousness, hearing, and speech abilities, and on any language barriers.

Be aware of other forms of nonverbal communication. Your job is to gain your patient's trust and cooperation in order to assess and care for him effectively. You do so by demonstrating sincerity through both verbal and nonverbal communication. Patients will detect inconsistencies in what you say and how you say it. Your tone of voice, facial expressions, and body language convey your true attitudes. Your actions must match your words. Touch is a powerful communication tool. Used properly, it conveys compassion, caring, and reassurance to your already apprehensive patient. Make contact by shaking hands or offering a comforting touch (Figure 1-1). This yields the additional benefit of enabling you to begin your assessment. For example, touching your patient's wrist allows you to make personal contact while quietly assessing his pulse and skin condition. Of course, you should try to get a sense of how your patient reacts to touch. It may make some patients feel threatened or uncomfortable. Avoid touching hostile, paranoid, or combative patients.

Eye contact is the most important form of nonverbal communication.

Make contact by shaking hands or offering a comforting touch.

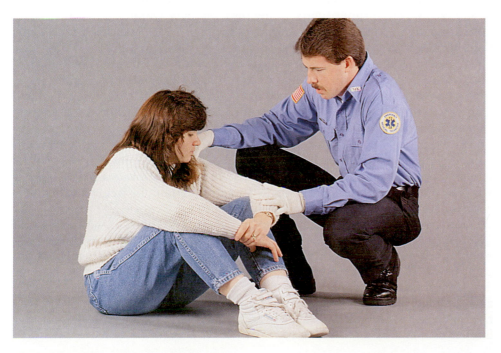

FIGURE 1-1   When you introduce yourself to your patient, shaking hands or offering a comforting touch will help build trust.

Unless your patient is critical, work efficiently but don't rush. As you ask questions, you can delegate other personnel to conduct a focused physical exam, take vital signs, place oxygen, set up an IV, and get the stretcher. Your role as interviewer is to establish patient contact and learn the history.

Be aware of your patient's comfort. If the setting does not lend itself to personal questions, move your patient to a more suitable location. For example, teenage girls usually will not truthfully answer questions about pregnancy with their parents nearby. Other patients may not reveal relevant items about their medical history with bystanders listening. Sometimes moving your patient to the ambulance offers the needed privacy. If your patient is in obvious distress, try to alleviate his pain or discomfort while you interview him. For example, you may control minor bleeding and cover a wound that causes your patient distress. You might also immobilize a painful fracture site while you conduct the interview. Watch also for subtle signs of discomfort such as squirming, grimacing, and wincing.

ASKING QUESTIONS

Remembering everything your patient tells you is impossible. Taking notes is acceptable, and most patients will not mind your doing so. If your patient becomes concerned about the notes, simply explain why you are taking them and reassure him that your interactions are confidential. Make sure you maintain contact with your patient. Avoid focusing so closely on the clipboard questionnaire that you ignore your patient, with whom you are trying to establish a caring rapport. Jot down pieces of information crucial to your verbal and written reports such as past history, medications, and vitals.

Asking questions in a way that elicits accurate information from your patients is an art. To gather the patient history, you can use a combination of open-ended and closed-ended questions. Paramedics must understand these two very different types of questions. **Open-ended questions** allow your patient to explain how he feels in detail, in his words, instead of giving "yes" or "no" answers. His responses are usually more accurate and complete. "Can you describe the pain in your chest?" or "Where do you hurt?" are open-ended questions. They deal in generalizations, allowing your patient to respond freely and without limits. Some patients may wander off course when answering open-ended questions, and occasionally you will need to refocus the interview.

Closed-ended questions elicit a short answer to a very direct question. They limit your patient's response to one or two words. They are appropriate when time or your patient's mental status or condition does not allow open-ended questions. For example, if your patient is gasping for breath while you are trying to determine the cause, phrase your questions for one-word answers or yes-no nods: "Does your pain radiate to the shoulder?" or "Do you take diuretics?" Closed-ended questions may be the most effective and efficient way to get your patients to describe their symptoms in exact terms. Their disadvantages are that you may inadvertently lead your patient toward certain answers and that they elicit only the limited information for which they ask.

Some patients have difficulty describing their symptoms. In these cases, ask questions with multiple-choice options. For example, "Is your pain sharp, dull, burning, pressure-like, stabbing, or like something else?" Other patients may become confused, especially when more than one person is asking them questions. Avoid this by limiting the interview to one person, asking one question at a time, and allowing time for your patient to answer. Do not rush. You can become an efficient history taker by knowing which questions will elicit the most important information and by maintaining your patient's attention.

To gather the patient history, you can use a combination of open-ended and closed-ended questions.

* **open-ended questions** questions that allow your patient to answer in detail.

* **closed-ended questions** questions that elicit a one- or two-word answer.

LANGUAGE AND COMMUNICATION

Use appropriate language. Nothing distances you from your patient more quickly than sophisticated medical terminology. "Have you ever had a heart attack?" is better than "Have you ever had an MI?" Effective communication means connecting with your patient. Most of your patients will not understand medical terms. Use an appropriate level of questions, but do not appear condescending. Other barriers to communication include cultural differences, language differences, deafness, speech impediments, and even blindness. When you encounter such obstacles, try to enlist someone who can communicate with your patient and act as an interpreter. An alternative is to adopt a conservative approach toward assessment, field diagnosis, and treatment.

Listening is an important part of the interview. The old saying, "Listen to your patient; he will tell you what is wrong," explains why it is crucial for a skilled clinician to be a good listener. Listen closely to what your patients tell you. Be careful not to develop tunnel vision from dispatch information. Begin your assessment without any preconceived notions about your patient's injuries or illnesses. Also watch for subtle clues that your patient may not be telling the truth. For example, your patient tells you that his chest pain went away, but his facial expressions and body language suggest otherwise. Developing good communication skills takes time and practice.

Avoid working your way in strict order down any prearranged list of questions (such as those in this chapter). Use these lists as a guide only. Listen to your patients and watch for clues to important signs, symptoms, emotions, or other factors. Then modify your questions to follow those clues. The following practices promote **active listening.**

✳ active listening the process of responding to your patient's statements with words or gestures that demonstrate your understanding.

Facilitation Maintain sincere eye contact, use concerned facial gestures, and lean forward while you listen. Cues such as "Mm-hmm," "Go on," or "I'm listening" all help your patient open up. Sometimes strategic silence is also helpful.

Reflection Repeat your patient's words. This encourages him to provide more details. Just make sure not to disturb his train of thought. For example:

Patient:	I can't breathe.
You:	You can't breathe?
Patient:	No, it feels like I can't take in a full breath because my chest hurts.
You:	Your chest hurts, too?
Patient:	Yes, it started this morning when I was working in the yard. I usually take a Nitro but I'm all out.

This simple reflection encouraged the patient to reveal facts about his history of heart disease. If the paramedic had merely investigated the chief complaint of dyspnea, discovering its true cause may have taken longer. Since the primary problem is not always the chief complaint, allowing your patient to take the lead is sometimes advantageous.

Clarification In crisis, patients often cannot clearly describe what they feel. They will use vague, general words. Do not hesitate to ask for clarification. For example:

You:	Do you have any allergies?
Patient:	Yes, the last time I took penicillin I had a bad reaction.
You:	Can you describe the reaction?
Patient:	Well, I got itchy all over with a rash.
You:	Did you have any difficulty breathing or feel like you were choking?
Patient:	Oh, no, just the itching and rash.

By asking for clarification you distinguish between a simple allergic reaction and life threatening anaphylaxis.

Content Review

ACTIVE LISTENING SKILLS
Facilitation
Reflection
Clarification
Empathy
Confrontation
Interpretation

Empathy Your patients may be telling you very personal and sometimes embarrassing information about themselves. They may feel frightened, ashamed, and upset to have to tell a stranger these things. Show empathy by responding with "I understand" or "That must have been very difficult" or "I can't imagine having open heart surgery." Sometimes just a gesture like handing someone a tissue or patting him on the shoulder conveys empathy.

Confrontation Sometimes patients will hide the truth or mask it with other symptoms. Often you will detect inconsistencies in your patient's story. In these cases, you should confront your patient with your observations. For example, "You say your chest doesn't hurt, but you keep rubbing it." Confrontation may help your patient bring his hidden feelings into the open.

Interpretation Interpretation takes confrontation a step further. Here you interpret your observations and question your patient about what you believe may be the problem. For example, "You say your chest doesn't hurt but you keep rubbing it. Are you afraid you are having a heart attack but don't want to admit it?" Interpretation can backfire if your patient feels you are unjustly accusing him; however, if your patient trusts you and you use interpretation cautiously, it can demonstrate empathy and enhance your rapport.

Asking about Feelings Your patients are people, not clinical subjects. Ask them how they feel about what they are experiencing. Let them know you are interested in them as people, not just as patients. Showing genuine interest in their problems may unlock the door to key information that they otherwise might not have shared with you.

TAKING A HISTORY ON SENSITIVE TOPICS

Paramedic students normally have difficulty questioning their patients about embarrassing, sensitive, or very personal topics such as sexual activities, death and dying, physical deformities, bodily functions, and domestic violence. Even though you may feel uneasy discussing these matters, you may learn important information about your patient's illness. To become more comfortable dealing with these subjects, watch experienced clinicians discuss them with their patients. Familiarize yourself with and practice some opening questions on sensitive topics that both put your patient at ease and encourage him to talk about it. If a particular area makes you most uncomfortable, attend a lecture or seminar and learn how professionals deal with this subject daily. Make the unfamiliar familiar and it will seem less imposing.

Let's look at two sensitive topics—physical violence and the sexual history. Your patient may not want to reveal a history of physical abuse. You should consider it when any of the following conditions are present:

- Injuries that are inconsistent with the story given
- Injuries that embarrass your patient
- A delay between the time of the injury and seeking help
- A past history of "accidents"
- Suspicious behavior of the supposed abuser

To earn your patient's trust, try to make him or her feel that the problem is not uncommon and that you understand the reasons for what has occurred. For example, you can ask your female patient, "Sometimes when husbands and wives argue a lot, it leads to physical fighting. I noticed you have some bruises on your arms and legs. Can you tell me what happened? Did someone hit you?" With active listening techniques, such questioning will help establish a rapport that encourages open communication.

Taking a sexual history can be the most embarrassing and uncomfortable topic for an inexperienced health care provider. The sexual history is normally taken later during the history but can be a part of the present illness or past history, depending on your patient's chief complaint. For example, if your patient complains of a genitourinary problem, the sexual history becomes important during the present illness questioning. If your patient has a history of sexually transmitted disease, then the sexual history is relevant to the past history. Whenever you begin the sexual history, it is helpful to prepare your patient with introductory statements and questions like, "Now I need to ask you some questions about your sexual health and activity. It may help me determine the cause of your problem and provide better care for you. This information will be strictly confidential. May I begin?" If your patient consents, proceed as follows: "Are you sexually active? Have you had sex with anyone in the last six months? Do you have more than one partner? Do you have sex with men, women, or both? Do you take precautions to avoid infection or unwanted pregnancy? Do you have any problems or concerns about your sexual function?" This may seem very uncomfortable for the beginning paramedic but with time and clinical experience you will develop a sense of where and when these questions are appropriate. It is critical that you remain calm, objective, and nonjudgmental regardless of how your patient answers.

THE COMPREHENSIVE PATIENT HISTORY

This section presents the components of a comprehensive patient history in a systematic order. In practice, you will ultimately select only those components that apply to your patient's situation and status. For example, if you conduct preemployment physical exams for a company, you may use the entire form. On the other hand, if you respond to a gasping patient in acute pulmonary edema, you will focus on the present illness. Common sense and clinical experience will determine how much of the following history to use.

Common sense and clinical experience will determine how much of the history to use.

PRELIMINARY DATA

For documentation, always record the date and time of the physical exam. Determine your patient's age, sex, race, birthplace, and occupation. This provides a starting point for the interview and establishes you as the interviewer. Who is the source of the information you receive about your patient? Is it the competent patient himself, his spouse, a friend, or a bystander? Are you receiving a report from a first responder, the police, or another health care worker? Do you have the medical record from a transferring facility? After you have gathered the information, you should establish its reliability, which will vary according to the source's knowledge, memory, trust, and motivation. Again, reconfirm the information with the patient, if possible. This is a judgment call based on your experience. For example, if the patient information you received from a particular EMT first responder has been accurate in the past, you probably will trust it again. On the other hand, if the nurse at a physician's office has repeatedly provided you with erroneous information, you probably will doubt her accuracy.

THE CHIEF COMPLAINT

The history begins with an open-ended question about your patient's chief complaint. The chief complaint is the pain, discomfort, or dysfunction that caused your patient to request help. In a medical case, it may be a woman's call for help because she has chest pain. In a trauma case, it may be a bystander's call for assistance to a "man down" or a police officer's reporting an injury in an auto

collision. Your patient may have called for more than one symptom. It is important to begin with a general question that allows your patient to respond freely.
For example, "Why did you call us today?" or "What seems to be the problem?"
Avoid the tunnel vision that often biases paramedics who focus on dispatch information that may or may not accurately describe the situation. As you interview and assess your patient, the chief complaint becomes more specific.

The chief complaint differs from the **primary problem.** While the chief complaint is a sign or symptom noticed by the patient or a bystander, the primary
problem is the principal medical cause of the complaint. For example, your patient's chief complaint may be leg pain, while the primary problem is a tibia fracture. When possible, report and record the chief complaint in your patient's own
words. For example, "I am having a hard time breathing" is better than "the patient has dyspnea." For the unconscious patient, the chief complaint becomes
what someone else identifies or what you observe as the primary problem. In
some trauma situations, for instance, the chief complaint might be the mechanism of injury such as "a gunshot to the chest," or "a fall from 25 feet."

THE PRESENT ILLNESS

Once you have determined the chief complaint, explore each of your patient's
complaints in greater detail. Be naturally inquisitive when exploring the events
surrounding these complaints. A practical template for exploring each complaint
follows the mnemonic OPQRST—ASPN, an acronym for *Onset, Provocation,
Quality, Region/Radiation, Severity, Time, Associated Symptoms,* and *Pertinent
Negatives.* This line of questioning provides a full, clear, chronological account
of your patient's symptoms.

Onset Did the problem develop suddenly or gradually? What was your patient
doing when the symptoms started? In medical emergencies, investigate your patient's activities at the time of, or shortly before, the signs or symptoms developed. In some cases, especially trauma, you may have to gather information from
a few weeks before the onset of symptoms. For example, the signs and symptoms
of a subdural hematoma may not appear until weeks following an injury. Was
the patient exercising or exerting himself, or at rest or sleeping? Was he eating or
drinking? If so, what? In trauma cases, assure that a medical problem did not
cause the accident. For example, the sudden onset of an illness such as a seizure
or syncope may have caused a fall.

Provocation/Palliation What provokes the symptom (makes it worse)? Does
anything palliate the symptom (make it better)? In many illnesses, certain factors
such as motion, pressure, and jarring may increase or decrease pain, discomfort,
or dysfunction. Does eating, movement, exertion, stress, or anything else pro-
voke the current problem. Positioning also may be a factor. Your patient may
wish to curl up and lie on his side to reduce abdominal pain. Your congestive
heart failure patients will sit bolt upright to ease respiration. They also may sleep
with several pillows raising their upper body to relieve paroxysmal nocturnal
dyspnea (PND), a sleep-disturbing breathing difficulty caused by fluid that ac-
cumulates in the lungs when they are supine. Ask your patient how breathing affects the discomfort. Deep breathing may increase the acute abdomen patient's
pain. A patient with pleuritic or rib-fracture pain will not breathe deeply, whereas
breathing may not affect the pain of angina. Any patient with respiratory pain
will breathe with shallower but more frequent breaths.

If your patient took a medication shortly before you arrived, its effect or lack
of effect may help determine the problem. Drugs such as bronchodilators, hypoglycemic agents, antihypertensives, and anticonvulsants are commonly prescribed and taken at home. Investigate any medication used to relieve a problem

and note its effectiveness. Ask about any activity, medication, or other circumstance that either alleviates or aggravates the chief complaint.

Quality How does your patient perceive the pain or discomfort? Ask him to explain how the symptom feels, and listen carefully to his answer. Does your patient call his pain crushing, tearing, oppressive, gnawing, crampy, sharp, dull, or otherwise? Quote his descriptors in your report.

Region/Radiation Where is the symptom? Does it move anywhere else? Identify the exact location and area of pain, discomfort, or dysfunction. Does your patient complain of pain "here," while holding a clenched fist over the sternum, or does he grasp the entire abdomen with both hands and moan? If your patient has not done so, ask him to point to the painful area. Identify the specific location, or the boundary of the pain if it is regional.

Determine if the pain is truly pain (occurring independently) or **tenderness** (pain on palpation). Also determine if the pain moves or radiates. Localized pain occurs in one specific area, while radiating pain travels away from the source, in one, many, or all directions. Evaluate moving pain's initial location and progression and any factors that affect its movement.

✱**tenderness** pain that is elicited through palpation.

Note any pain that may be referred from other parts of the body. **Referred pain** is felt in a part of the body away from the source of the disease or problem. The heart and diaphragm are two areas that most commonly produce referred pain. Cardiac problems such as myocardial infarction or anginal pain are usually referred to the left arm, with occasional referral to the neck, jaw, and back. Pain associated with irritation of the diaphragm (most commonly blood in the abdomen of the supine patient) generally is referred to the clavicular region.

✱**referred pain** pain that is felt at a location away from its source.

Severity How bad is the symptom? Severity is the intensity of pain or discomfort felt by your patient. Ask him how bad the pain feels, and then have him compare it to other painful problems he has experienced. Sometimes a patient can describe the severity of the pain on a scale from one to ten, with ten being the worst pain he has ever felt. Also notice the amount of discomfort your patient's condition causes. How easy is it to distract your patient from his concern over the pain? Is your patient very still and resistive to your touch? Is he writhing about? The answers should give you a good idea of the intensity of your patient's pain.

Time When did the symptoms begin? Is a symptom constant or intermittent? How long does it last? How long has this symptom affected your patient? For several days, hours, or just a few minutes or seconds? When did any previous episodes occur? How does this episode's length vary from earlier ones?

Associated Symptoms What other symptoms commonly associated with the chief complaint in certain diseases can help rule in your field diagnosis. For example, if the chief complaint is chest pain, ask, "Are you short of breath? Are you nauseous? Have you vomited? Are you dizzy or light-headed?" The presence of these symptoms would help support a field diagnosis of cardiac chest pain.

Pertinent Negatives Are any likely associated symptoms absent? Their absence is as important to the field diagnosis as their presence, because they help rule out a particular disease or injury. Note any element of the history or physical exam that does not support a suspected or possible field diagnosis. For example, it is significant if your patient who complains of chest pain denies shortness of breath, nausea, and lightheadedness.

THE PAST HISTORY

The past medical history may provide significant insights into your patient's chief complaint and your field diagnosis. Look in-depth at your patient's general state of health, childhood and adult diseases, psychiatric illnesses, accidents or

The past medical history may provide significant insights into your patient's chief complaint and your field diagnosis.

injuries, surgeries, and hospitalizations. They may reveal general or specific clues that will help you to correctly assess his current problem. Your patient's condition, the situation, and time constraints will determine how much information you can and should gather on the scene. For example, asking about childhood diseases may not be relevant for your acute cardiac or trauma patient.

General State of Health How does your patient perceive his general state of health?

Childhood Diseases What childhood diseases did your patient have? Did he have mumps, measles, rubella, whooping cough, chickenpox, rheumatic fever, scarlet fever, or polio? Again, this line of questioning's relevance depends on the patient and the situation.

Adult Diseases Is your patient a diabetic? Does he have a history of heart disease, breathing problems, high blood pressure, or similar conditions? A preexisting medical problem may contribute to your patient's current problem or influence his care during the next few hours. To discover significant preexisting medical problems, ask if your patient has recently seen a physician or been hospitalized. If so, for what conditions? If you discover a preexisting problem, investigate its effects on your patient. When did the problem last affect him? Is your patient on any special diets or prescribed medications or restricted in activity? Even with the trauma patient, do not forget that a medical problem may have led to an accident or may complicate the effects of trauma. Also, obtain the name of your patient's physician since it may be helpful to the emergency department staff.

Psychiatric Illnesses Does your patient have a history of mental illness? Has he ever been diagnosed with depression, mania, schizophrenia, or other problems? Is he being treated for a mental illness? If so, what medications is he taking? Has he ever had thoughts of suicide? Has he ever attempted suicide? Tailor these questions for patients you suspect of having a mental illness.

Accidents or Injuries Has your patient ever had a serious accident or injury requiring hospitalization? Has he had a previous injury that could be a factor in his current problem? For example, a seemingly minor head injury one week ago may present now as a subdural hematoma in your unconscious elderly patient. Keep this line of questioning to relevant information only. An old football injury or childhood aceration is probably not influencing your patient's chest pain and respiratory distress today. But his pneumonectomy (surgical removal of a lung) probably is the reason for the absence of lung sounds on his right side.

Surgeries or Hospitalizations Has your patient had any other hospitalizations or surgeries not already mentioned. Again, these may offer some insight into your suspected field diagnosis. For example, your patient is an 85-year-old man with a long history of congestive heart failure and no history of chronic lung disease. He suddenly presents with severe difficulty in breathing and audible wheezing. You should suspect the obvious—a cardiac problem. Don't look for the five-legged cat.

CURRENT HEALTH STATUS

The current health status assembles all the factors in your patient's present medical condition. Here, you try to gather information that completes the puzzle surrounding your patient's primary problem. Look for clues and correlations among the various sections of this part of the history. For example, your patient is a heavy smoker, has many allergies to inhaled particles, works in a coal mine, and frequently uses bronchodilating medications. He now complains of shortness of breath and expiratory wheezing. He is probably having an exacerbation of his chronic lung disease.

Current Medications Is your patient taking any medications? These include over-the-counter drugs, prescriptions, home remedies, vitamins, and minerals. If so, why? Your patient's explanation may not be medically accurate, but it may help to determine underlying conditions. For example, your 65-year-old patient tells you she takes a "water pill." You can safely assume she takes a **diuretic,** and has a history of renal or cardiac problems. A medication not taken as prescribed may be responsible for the current medical problem—possibly by under- or over-medication. A recently prescribed medication may cause an allergic or untoward (severe and unexpected) reaction. It also may be out of date and no longer effective. Even for trauma, emergency department personnel will need to know what medications your patient is taking. For example, if your patient takes warfarin, an anticoagulant, it would interfere with the normal clotting process and actually promote bleeding. If practical, bring your patient's medications to the hospital (Figure 1-2).

Allergies Does your patient have any known allergies, especially to penicillin, the "caine" family (local anesthetics), tetanus toxoid, and narcotics? These agents are occasionally given in emergency situations. What type of reaction did your patient have to the medication. For example, was it just a mild allergic reaction with a rash and itching or localized swelling or anaphylactic shock? Knowledge of your patient's allergies may prevent additional complications during the emergency department visit, especially if he becomes disoriented or unconscious during transport. If your patient is short of breath with wheezing, ask about environmental allergies. In cases of possible anaphylaxis, ask about allergies to drugs, to foods such as shellfish, nuts, and dairy products, and to insect bites and stings.

Tobacco Does your patient use tobacco? If so, how (cigarettes, cigars, pipe, smokeless, or other), how much, and for how long? To quantify his smoking history, multiply the number of packs smoked per day by the number of years he has smoked. The result is his pack/year history. For example, if your patient smoked two packs of cigarettes per day for 25 years, he is a 50 pack/year smoker. Anything over 30 pack/years is considered significant.

Alcohol, Drugs, and Related Substances Alcohol and drugs are often contributing factors in, if not the primary cause of, your patient's medical problems. Your job is not to pass judgment, but to gather data that will help direct your patient's medical treatment. Remaining nonjudgmental will aid you in your questioning. Start with a general question such as "How much alcohol do you drink?" If you suspect a drinking problem may be a factor, you can use the CAGE questionnaire (an alcoholism screening instrument) to determine the presence of alcoholism. Reserve this line of questioning for the chronic patient in a controlled setting. It would be inappropriate in a bar with an unruly, intoxicated patient.

The CAGE Questionnaire

Have you ever felt the need to *C*ut down on your drinking?

Have you ever felt *A*nnoyed by criticism of your drinking?

Have you ever had *G*uilty feelings about drinking?

Have you ever taken a drink first thing in the morning as an *E*ye-opener?

Two or more "yes" answers suggest alcoholism and further lines of inquiry.

Ask about blackouts, accidents, or injuries that happened while drinking. Also ask about alcohol-related job losses, marital problems, and arrests while under the influence of alcohol. Similarly, ask about drug use. For example, "Do you use marijuana, cocaine, heroin, sleeping pills, or painkillers? How much do you take? How do these drugs make you feel? Have you had any bad reactions?"

✷ **diuretic** a medication that stimulates the kidneys to excrete excess water.

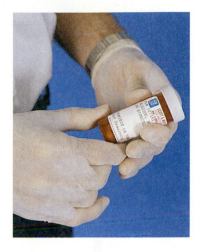

FIGURE 1-2 You should take your patient's medications with you to the hospital, when practical.

> **Content Review**
>
> ### CAGE QUESTIONNAIRE
>
> **C**ut down
> **A**nnoyed
> **G**uilty
> **E**ye-opener

As your patients realize you are not judging their substance abuse, they may feel more comfortable telling you about their patterns of use.

Diet Ask about your patient's normal daily intake of food and drink. Perhaps your 78-year-old retiree just moved to the Arizona desert and underestimated the increased fluid loss due to sweating. He does not realize he needs to increase his daily fluid intake, and now he presents weak and dizzy from dehydration. Are there any dietary restrictions or supplements? Ask specifically about his use of foods with stimulating effects such as coffee, tea, cola drinks, and other beverages containing caffeine. For example, your 23-year-old patient with a rapid heart beat (200 beats per minute) drinks continuous cups of coffee each morning at her highly stressful job.

Screening Tests Ask about certain screening tests that may have been done for your patient. Some examples include a purified protein derivative (PPD) test for suspected tuberculosis, Pap smears and mammograms for female problems, stool testing for occult blood, and cholesterol tests. Record the dates of the tests and their results.

Immunizations Ask your patient about his immunizations for diseases such as tetanus, pertussis, diphtheria, polio, measles, rubella, mumps, influenza, hepatitis B, and pneumococcal vaccine. For example, ask the parent of a child suspected of epiglottitis if he had the hemophilus influenza B vaccine. The H-flu is a common cause for epiglottitis in children.

Sleep Patterns Ask your patient what time he normally goes to bed and arises. Does he take daytime naps? Does he have problems falling asleep or staying asleep?

Exercise and Leisure Activities Does your patient exercise regularly or lead a sedentary existence? Sometimes your patient's lifestyle will support your field diagnosis.

Environmental Hazards Ask about possible hazards in the home, in school, and at the workplace. For example, your patient may live or work in an area with high levels of toxic substances. Many health problems can be traced to these environmental causes.

Use of Safety Measures In an auto accident, did your patient use a seat restraint system? Were all passengers belted in? Did the air bag deploy? Such information aids you and the emergency department staff in determining the extent of damage caused by a particular mechanism of injury. For bicycle, in-line skate, and skateboard injuries, ask about the use of helmets and knee and elbow pads.

Since many disease processes are hereditary, it is important to learn the medical history of immediate family members.

Family History Since many disease processes are hereditary, the medical history of immediate family members is important. In the nonemergency setting you may explore deep into the family tree and chart the medical history of grandparents, parents, aunts, and uncles. In the emergency setting, learning that your 45-year-old patient with chest pain had a father and brother who both died of heart attacks in their late forties is important information. Look for a family history of diabetes, heart disease, hypercholesterolemia, high blood pressure, stroke, kidney disease, tuberculosis, cancer, arthritis, anemia, allergies, asthma, headaches, epilepsy, mental illness, alcoholism, drug addiction, and any symptoms like your patient's.

Home Situation and Significant Others Who lives at home with your patient? Ask him about his home life—or lack of one. Ask about friends, family, support groups, loved ones. Find out if he has a support network and whom it includes. Who takes care of him when he needs help? Loneliness and isolation may complicate your patient's physical symptoms.

Daily Life Ask your patient to describe his typical day. When does he get up? What does he do first? Then what? Such questions reveal a lot about your patient's state of mind and general wellness. Is he busy, active, and motivated to get up in the morning? Does he merely exist from the time he awakens and go through life with no purpose or direction? Is he under high levels of stress from morning to night in a job that requires him to take his problems home with him? Find out what kind of life your patient leads. It may reveal a lot about his illness.

Important Experiences Ask about your patient's upbringing and home life growing up. How much schooling does he have? Was he in the military? What kinds of jobs has he held? What is his financial situation? Is he married, single, divorced, or widowed? What does he do for fun and relaxation? Is he retired or looking forward to retirement? Again, the answers give you a broader picture of your patient.

Religious Beliefs Some religions forbid certain treatments and have guidelines regarding the management of illness and injury. For example, some forbid whole blood transfusions. Knowing if your patient is guided by these beliefs can help you understand and care for him better. These questions require some expression of sensitivity, or it might be best to ask broadly if he has any limitations in medical care.

The Patient's Outlook Find out what your patient thinks and how he feels about the present and future.

REVIEW OF SYSTEMS

The **review of systems** is a series of questions designed to identify problems your patient has not already mentioned. It is a system-by-system list of questions that are more specific than those asked during the basic history. Again, the patient's chief complaint, condition, and clinical status determine how much, if any, of the review of systems you will use. For example, if your patient complains of chest pain, you may want to review the respiratory, cardiac, gastrointestinal, and hematological systems. If your patient complains of a headache, you may want to review the **HEENT** (head, eyes, ears, nose, and throat), neurologic, peripheral vascular, and psychiatric systems. Let your patient lead you through the history. The following sampling includes a few of the many questions that you might ask.

✱ **review of systems** a list of questions categorized by body system.

✱ **HEENT** head, eyes, ears, nose, and throat.

General What is your patient's usual weight, and have there been any recent weight changes? Has he had weakness, fatigue, or fever?

Skin Has your patient noticed any new rashes, lumps, sores, itching, dryness, color change, or changes in nails or hair? Could cosmetics or jewelry have caused these problems?

Head, Eyes, Ears, Nose, and Throat (HEENT) Has your patient had headaches or recent head trauma? How is his vision? Does he wear glasses or contact lenses? When was his last eye exam? Has he experienced any of the following: pain, redness, excessive tearing, double vision, blurred vision, spots, specks, flashing lights? Has he ever had glaucoma or cataracts? How is his hearing? Does he use hearing aids? Has he ever experienced ringing in the ears (**tinnitus**), vertigo, earaches, infection, or discharge? Does he have frequent colds, nasal stuffiness, nasal discharge, hay fever, nosebleeds, sinus problems? Does he

✱ **tinnitus** the sensation of ringing in the ears.

wear dentures? When was his last dental exam? Describe the condition of his teeth and gums. Do his gums bleed? Does he get a sore tongue, dry mouth, frequent sore throats, or hoarseness? Does he have lumps or swollen glands? Has he ever had a goiter, neck pain, difficulty swallowing, or stiffness?

Respiratory Has your patient ever had wheezing, coughing up blood (**hemoptysis**), asthma, bronchitis, emphysema, pneumonia, TB, or pleurisy? When was his last chest X-ray? Is he coughing now? If so, can you describe the sputum?

* **hemoptysis** coughing up blood.

Cardiac Has your patient ever had heart trouble, high blood pressure, rheumatic fever, heart murmurs, chest pain or discomfort, palpitations, shortness of breath (**dyspnea**), shortness of breath while lying flat (**orthopnea**), or peripheral edema? Has he ever been awakened from sleep with shortness of breath (**paroxysmal nocturnal dyspnea**)? Has he ever had an ECG or other heart tests?

* **dyspnea** the sensation of having difficulty in breathing.

* **orthopnea** difficulty in breathing while lying supine.

* **paroxysmal nocturnal dyspnea** sudden onset of shortness of breath at night.

Gastrointestinal Has your patient ever had trouble swallowing, heartburn, loss of appetite, nausea/vomiting, regurgitation, vomiting blood (**hematemesis**), indigestion? How often does he move his bowels? Describe the color and size of his stools. Have there been any changes in his bowel habits? Has he had rectal bleeding or black, tarry stools, hemorrhoids, constipation, diarrhea? Has he had abdominal pain, food intolerance, or excessive belching or passing of gas? Has he had jaundice, liver or gallbladder problems, or hepatitis?

* **hematemesis** vomiting blood.

Urinary How often does your patient urinate? Has he ever had excessive urination (**polyuria**), excessive urination at night (**nocturia**), burning or pain while urinating, blood in the urine (**hematuria**), urgency, reduced caliber or force of urine flow, hesitancy, dribbling, or incontinence? Has he ever had a urinary tract infection or stones?

* **polyuria** excessive urination.

* **nocturia** excessive urination at night.

* **hematuria** blood in the urine.

Male Genital Has your patient ever had a hernia, discharge from or sores on the penis, testicular pain or masses? Has he ever had a sexually transmitted disease? If so, how was it treated?

Female Genital At what age did your patient have her first menstrual period? Describe the regularity, frequency, duration, and amount of bleeding of her periods. When was her last menstrual period? Does she bleed between periods or after intercourse? Has she ever had difficulty with her period (**dysmenorrhea**) or premenstrual tension? At what age did she become menopausal? Were there symptoms or bleeding? Has she ever had any vaginal discharge, lumps, sores, or itching? Has she ever had a sexually transmitted disease? If so, how was it treated? How many times has she been pregnant? How many deliveries? Any abortions (spontaneous or induced)? Some health care personnel use the G-P-A-L system to document a patient's history of pregnancy:

* **dysmenorrhea** menstrual difficulties.

Gravida	How many times pregnant?
Para	How many viable births?
Abortions	How many abortions?
Living	How many living children?

Has she ever had complications of pregnancy? Does she use birth control? If so, what type? If postmenopausal, is she on hormone replacement therapy?

Peripheral Vascular Has your patient ever had intermittent calf pain while walking (**intermittent claudication**), leg cramps, varicose veins, or blood clots?

* **intermittent claudication** intermittent calf pain while walking that subsides with rest.

Musculoskeletal Has your patient ever experienced muscle or joint pain, stiffness, arthritis, gout, or backache? Describe the location or symptoms.

Neurologic Has your patient ever experienced any of the following: fainting, blackouts, seizures, speech difficulty, vertigo, weakness, paralysis, numbness or loss of sensation, tingling, "pins and needles," tremors, or other involuntary movements?

Hematologic Has your patient ever been anemic? Has he ever had a blood transfusion? If so did he have a reaction to it? Does he bruise or bleed easily?

Endocrine Has your patient ever had thyroid trouble? Did he ever experience heat or cold intolerance, or excessive sweating? Does he have diabetes? Has he ever had excessive thirst, hunger, or urge to urinate?

Psychiatric Is he nervous? Is he under much stress and tension? Has he ever been depressed? Has he ever thought of committing suicide?

SPECIAL CHALLENGES

No matter how long you practice as a paramedic, some patients will present with special circumstances that challenge your skills. Your ability to deal with them will improve with time and practice.

SILENCE

Silence can become very uncomfortable if you are impatient. Why has your patient suddenly become silent? This question has no single answer. His silence can have many meanings and many uses. It may result from an organic brain condition that prevents him from forming thoughts. Or it may be due to dysarthria (difficulty in speaking due to muscular impairment). Maybe he is just collecting his thoughts or trying to remember details. Or maybe he is deciding whether he trusts you. He might be clinically depressed, or perhaps, he simply deals with situations by being quiet.

What do you do during the silence? Stay calm and observe your patient's nonverbal clues. Is he in pain? Is he scared? Is he on the verge of becoming hysterical or combative, or is he about to cry? You can encourage him to continue speaking by confronting him with your perceptions. For example, "I see you are obviously very upset about this. Do you want to talk about it?" If you sense your patient is not responsive to your questions, perform a brief orientation exam. Speak to him in a loud voice and call him by name. Shake him gently if he does not respond. If this does not elicit a response, assume a neurological problem and proceed accordingly.

Sometimes your behavior might have caused the silence. Are you asking too many questions too quickly? Have you offended your patient? Have you frightened him? Have you been insensitive? Have you failed to respond to your patient's needs? If your patient suddenly becomes silent, try to determine why, what is happening, and what you should do about it.

OVERLY TALKATIVE PATIENTS

The patient who rambles on can be just as frustrating to deal with as the one who will not talk at all. Why is your patient talking so fast and so much? Some patients react to stress this way. Maybe he has a lot to say. Maybe he needs someone to talk to; some lonely patients will take any opportunity to communicate with another human being. What can you do in the emergency setting when time is scarce? This problem has no perfect solution. You can lower your goals and accept a less comprehensive history. You can briefly give your patient free reign. You can focus on the important areas and ask closed-ended questions about them. You can interrupt him frequently and summarize what he says. Above all, try not to become impatient.

PATIENTS WITH MULTIPLE SYMPTOMS

Patients often present with multiple complaints. For example, your elderly patient may present you with a barrage of symptoms from an extensive medical history. Your challenge is to discover the chief complaint and why she called you today. If she complains of symptoms that suggest multiple disease states, the challenge is compounded. In these types of cases, you must sort through a multitude of information quickly and recognize patterns that lead you to a correct field diagnosis.

Some patients will answer "Yes" to every question you ask. They have every symptom you mention; although possible, this phenomenon is not probable. Your patient might simply misunderstand or be trying hard to cooperate; more than likely he has an emotional problem and requires a psychosocial assessment. Document your findings on your prehospital care report and request a psychological referral. Asking the patient what single complaint led him to call for help today often helps.

ANXIOUS PATIENTS

Anxiety is a natural reaction to stress. People who face serious illness or injury can be expected to exhibit some degree of anxiety. Sometimes this manifests itself as simple nervousness, tenseness, sweating, or trembling. Some patients will fall silent, while others will ramble. Still others may exhibit anxiety attacks marked by a rapid heart rate, nausea and vomiting, chest pain, and shortness of breath. When you detect signs of anxiety, encourage your patient to speak freely about it. For example, you can say, "I see you are concerned about this. Do you want to talk about it?"

PATIENTS NEEDING REASSURANCE

Appropriate reassurance is a cornerstone of patient care. You must be careful, however, not to be overly reassuring or to prematurely reassure your anxious patient. It is natural to say, "Relax, everything is going to be all right. We are going to take care of you and get you to the hospital. Just relax and you will be all right." But your patient may have anxiety about something of which you are not aware. For instance, if your chest pain patient is anxious, you might naturally assume he is apprehensive about dying. In reality he may be anxious about something entirely different. He may be embarrassed about his anxieties, and instead of helping him deal with them, you have helped him cover them up. Now he may decide you are not interested in what is really bothering him and block further communication. Listen carefully to your patient before offering reassurance.

ANGER AND HOSTILITY

You will often encounter angry patients or their families. They might be angry for many reasons. Your patient is sick, perhaps dying. The family is anticipating their future loss. Often they will lash out at the easiest target—you. Sometimes you cannot do anything quickly enough or well enough for them. Understand that their anger is a natural part of the grieving process and they may be merely venting their frustration. Unfortunately you find yourself at the receiving end of their outbursts. Try to accept their feelings without getting defensive or angry in return.

INTOXICATION

Dealing with belligerent, intoxicated patients challenges even the most experienced paramedic. These patients are irrational, they disrupt your control of the scene, and they rarely allow you to examine them. First and foremost, make sure your environment is safe. If your patient acts violently, call for the police before attempting any interaction. As you approach your patient, introduce yourself and offer a handshake. Avoid any challenging body language or remarks. Appear friendly and nonjudgmental, but always stay alert for a potential violent outburst. If your patient is shouting or cursing, do not try to get him to stop or to lower his voice. Listen to what he says, not how he says it, and try to understand his situation before making a clinical judgment. Sometimes a genuine offer of a place to sit will help calm an agitated, intoxicated person. Then you can begin your assessment.

CRYING

Sometimes your patients will cry. This can make any paramedic uncomfortable. Crying is just another form of venting, an important clue to your patient's emotions. Accept it as a natural release and do not try to suppress it. Be patient, allow your patient to cry, and then offer a supportive remark. Quiet acceptance and supportive remarks will open the lines of communication once your patient composes himself.

DEPRESSION

Depression is a common problem in medicine. It is also commonly misdiagnosed or ignored. It often presents with symptoms such as insomnia, fatigue, weight loss, or mysterious aches and pains. Depression is potentially lethal, so you must recognize its signs and evaluate its severity just as you would chest pain or shortness of breath. Ask your patient if he has ever thought about committing suicide; if he is currently thinking about suicide; if he has the means to commit suicide; and if he has ever attempted it. The more exact and precise his suicide plan, the more apt he is to carry it out.

* **depression** a mood disorder characterized by hopelessness and malaise.

SEXUALLY ATTRACTIVE OR SEDUCTIVE PATIENTS

Occasionally you will encounter a patient who is attracted to you or to whom you are attracted. These feelings are natural. The key is not to allow these feelings to affect your behavior. Always keep your relationship professional. If necessary, clearly tell any patient who behaves seductively that you are there on a professional basis, not a personal one. Afterward, determine if how you dressed, what you did, or what you said helped your patient get the wrong impression about your relationship. Did you send the wrong signals? Whenever possible, always have a partner with you to avoid any accusations of improper behavior or touching.

CONFUSING BEHAVIORS OR HISTORIES

You may encounter a patient whose story you just cannot follow. No matter what you ask, the answers leave you confused and frustrated. You cannot seem to develop a clear picture about your patient's problems. In fact, his answers don't even seem to make any sense. For example, you ask, "When did your headache begin?" and he answers, "My head feels like a squirrel." In these cases, the problem is most likely psychotic (mental illness) or organic (**dementia** or **delirium**). Also consider head injury or other physiological conditions such as stroke.

Many psychotic patients live and function in their communities, with varying degrees of success. Some will provide an accurate past history, others will not.

* **dementia** a deterioration of mental status that is usually associated with structural neurological disease.

* **delirium** an acute alteration in mental functioning that is often reversible.

If your patient's behavior seems distant, aloof, inappropriate, or even bizarre, suspect a mental illness such as schizophrenia. It may be helpful to focus your assessment on this patient's mental status, with special emphasis on thought, perceptions, and mood.

Delirium and dementia are disorders relating to cognitive function. Delirium is common in the acutely ill or intoxicated patient; dementia occurs more frequently in the elderly. These patients often cannot provide clear, accurate histories. Their descriptions of their symptoms and their accounts of how things happened will be vague and inconsistent. They may appear inattentive to your questions and hesitant in their answers. They may even make up stories to fill in the gaps in their memories. In these cases, do not spend too much time trying to get a detailed history, because you will only become more frustrated. Focus on the mental status exam, with special emphasis on level of response, orientation, and memory. For a more detailed discussion of these problems, see the chapter on psychiatric and behavioral emergencies in *Paramedic Care: Principles and Practice,* Volume 3.

LIMITED INTELLIGENCE

You can usually obtain an adequate history from a patient with limited intelligence. Do not assume that he will not be able to provide accurate information concerning his current or past medical status. Also, do not overlook obvious omissions because your patient appears to be giving you a good story. Try to evaluate your patient's education and mental abilities. If you suspect severe mental retardation, obtain the patient's history from family or friends. Above all, show a genuine interest in your patient and try to establish a positive relationship. Then, communication can still happen.

LANGUAGE BARRIERS

Few things are more frustrating than responding to an automobile accident with several patients who speak a language you do not understand. It is almost impossible to get an accurate history of the event. In these cases, try to locate an interpreter. Sometimes a family member speaks both languages and is willing to translate for you. Often, however, family members cause more confusion by paraphrasing what the patient and you are saying. Instead of hearing your patient's exact words, you hear the translator's version, and the true meanings become vague. Do not waste time using your broken foreign language from high school, because you will invariably confuse everyone involved.

HEARING PROBLEMS

The challenge of communicating with a hearing-impaired person is much like that of overcoming a language barrier. Some options, however, afford a degree of flexibility. You can try handwritten questions, but they can be time consuming. Sign language is effective if the patient practices it and you find a proficient interpreter. If your patient reads lips, you must modify your communication techniques accordingly. Always face him directly in a well-lit setting, and speak slowly in a low-pitched voice. Avoid covering your mouth and trailing off the end of your sentences. If your patient has one good ear, use that to your advantage. If he wears a hearing aid, make sure it is working. If he has eyeglasses, make sure he wears them. Augment your speech with hand gestures and facial expressions.

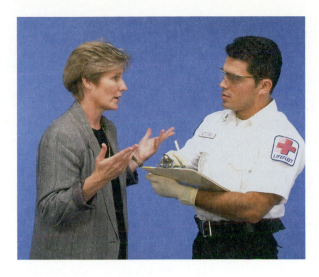

FIGURE 1-3 If the patient cannot provide useful information, gather it from family members or bystanders.

BLINDNESS

Blind patients present special problems. They need you to identify yourself immediately, since they cannot see your uniform. Always announce yourself and explain who you are and why you are there. If possible, take your patient's hand to establish a personal contact and to show him where you are. Remember that nonverbal communications such as hand gestures, facial expressions, and body language are useless in these cases. Your voice is your only tool for effective communication.

TALKING WITH FAMILIES OR FRIENDS

You will often encounter patients who cannot give you any useful information. In these cases, find a third party who can augment the patient history and offer a useful adjunct to the patient's answers (Figure 1-3). The typical case is the postictal patient who cannot describe his seizure activity to you. Another example is learning from his friend that your patient's wife died in an automobile accident just three weeks ago. Now you better understand why your patient appears depressed and suicidal. Make sure that patient confidentiality is a priority when you accept personal information from a family member, friend, or bystander. Patient assessment is a comprehensive history and physical exam process.

SUMMARY

This chapter dealt with taking a good history. While it presented the patient history in its entirety, common sense will determine which parts are appropriate for a given situation. Most of a paramedic's work is patient contact. It is making a connection with people in crisis. Patients most often comment on the attitudes of their paramedics. How well did they relate to them? Did they make them feel at ease? Did they care for them? Patients rarely comment on a paramedic's technical skills. Top-notch paramedics are technically skillful and treat all their patients with dignity and compassion. This begins with the history.

Good patient interaction can lead to good patient outcomes, improved patient satisfaction, and better adherence to treatment. As a paramedic you have the first opportunity to treat your patient when he enters the health care world. Let his first impression of the health care industry be your caring, compassionate, professional demeanor. Conducting effective and efficient interviews and communicating with your patient are essential to good medical practice. Medical interviewing is a basic clinical skill that must be learned and practiced, much like airway management.

YOU MAKE THE CALL

You are at lunch when the call comes in for chest pain at the baseball field. A large, midsummer crowd is at the multifield park complex. Upon arrival you meet Mr. George Harmon, a middle-aged man who sits in the bleachers in mild distress. You introduce yourself and begin an initial assessment. You rapidly assess mental status, airway patency, breathing, and circulation. His skin color, mental status, and ability to speak clearly in full sentences suggest he is hemodynamically stable. His strong, regular pulse and warm, dry skin confirm your initial impression. You are ready to elicit the history. Your patient complains of chest pain.

1. List some nonverbal communication techniques that will facilitate open discussion of your patient's problems.
2. Outline the components of the interview you would use for this patient in the following categories:
   a) History of Present Illness
   b) Past History
   c) Current Health Status
   d) Review of Systems

See Suggested Responses at the back of this book.

FURTHER READING

Bates, Barbara, Lynn S. Bickley, and Robert A. Hoekelman. *A Guide to Physical Examination and History Taking.* 6th ed. Philadelphia: J.B. Lippincott, 1995.

Coulehan, John L. and Marian R. Block. *The Medical Interview: Mastering Skills for Clinical Practice.* 3rd ed. Philadelphia: F.A. Davis, 1997.

Epstein, Owen, et al. *Clinical Examination.* St. Louis: Mosby, 1997.

Lipkin, Mack Jr., Samuel M. Putnam, and Aaron Lazare. *The Medical Interview: Clinical Care, Education, and Research.* New York: Springer, 1994.

Seidel Henry M. *Mosby's Guide to Physical Examination.* 3rd ed. St. Louis: Mosby, 1994.

Willms, Janice L., Henry Schniederman, and Paula S. Algranati. *Physical Diagnosis: Bedside Evaluation of Diagnosis and Function.* Baltimore: Williams & Wilkins, 1994.

ON THE WEB

Visit Brady's Paramedic Website at www.bradybooks.com/paramedic.

CHAPTER 2

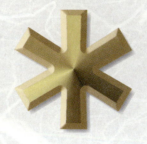

Physical Exam Techniques

Objectives

After reading this chapter, you should be able to:

1. Define and describe the techniques of inspection, palpation, percussion, auscultation. (pp. 29–33)
2. Describe the evaluation of mental status. (pp. 134–137)
3. Evaluate the importance of a general survey. (pp. 41–48)
4. Describe the examination of the following body regions, differentiate between normal and abnormal findings, and define the significance of abnormal findings:
   - skin, hair, and nails (pp. 49–57)
   - head, scalp, and skull (pp. 57–59, 62)

- eyes, ears, nose, mouth, and pharynx (pp. 59–74)
- neck (pp. 74–77)
- thorax (anterior and posterior) (pp. 77–83)
- arterial pulse including rate, rhythm, and amplitude (pp. 83–89)
- jugular venous pressure and pulsations (pp. 83–89)
- heart and blood vessels (pp. 83–89)
- abdomen (pp. 89–97)
- male and female genitalia (pp. 95–99)

Continued

Objectives Continued

- anus and rectum (pp. 99–100)
- peripheral vascular system (pp. 128–133)
- musculoskeletal system (pp. 100–128)
- nervous system (pp. 133–158)
- cranial nerves (pp. 137–147)

5. Describe the assessment of visual acuity. (pp. 60–61)
6. Explain the rationale for the use of an ophthalmoscope and otoscope. (pp. 39, 65–67)
7. Describe the survey of respiration. (pp. 34–36; 79–83)
8. Describe percussion of the chest. (pp. 79, 83)
9. Differentiate the percussion notes and their characteristics. (pp. 31–32)

10. Describe special examination techniques related to the assessment of the chest. (pp. 77–83)
11. Describe the auscultation of the chest, heart, and abdomen. (pp. 81, 83, 88–89, 94)
12. Distinguish between normal and abnormal auscultation findings of the chest, heart, and abdomen and explain their significance. (pp. 81, 83, 88–89, 94)
13. Describe special techniques of the cardiovascular examination. (pp. 83–89)
14. Describe the general guidelines of recording examination information. (pp. 164–168)
15. Discuss the examination considerations for an infant or child. (pp. 158–164)

CASE STUDY

The overnight crew at Station 51 tonight is paramedic Dale Monday and his EMT-basic partner, Pam True. Early into their shift they are called to a "man-down" at Cirrincione's, a popular Italian restaurant featuring Sicilian cuisine. Upon arrival they find Robert Dalton, an agitated male in his early 70s who just can't seem to stand up. Mr. Dalton is alert and oriented. He complains of general weakness and of being unable to stand without wobbling or to walk a straight line.

Dale begins to elicit a history from Mr. Dalton's wife. She claims he has been having these problems off and on for the past few days but that this is worse. Mr. Dalton denies any chest pain, shortness of breath, dizziness, or nausea. His past history includes coronary artery disease, hypertension, and congestive heart failure. He takes nitroglycerin as needed, furosemide, aspirin, digoxin, captopril, and a potassium supplement. He and his wife have not yet eaten tonight. Dale tells his partner to get the stretcher and continues his assessment, which includes a focused physical exam and vital signs.

Because they have a 35-minute ride to McGivern General Hospital, Dale decides to perform a detailed physical exam en route. His patient appears to be an otherwise healthy 72-year-old man. He is well-dressed and well-groomed. His vital signs are blood pressure—150/86; heart rate—88, strong and regular; respirations—18; skin—warm, dry, and pink. Dale finds no evidence of head

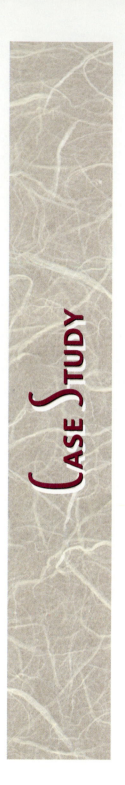
trauma. His patient's ears, nose, and throat are normal. He shows no facial drooping or slurred speech. His pupils are equal and reactive to light and accommodation. Visual acuity is normal. Extraocular muscles are intact. Dale notes nystagmus with his patient's left lateral gaze. He finds no palpable nodes. His patient's trachea is midline, and his chest and abdomen appear normal. His distal extremities are warm and pink. Deep tendon reflexes are 2+ in the upper extremities and 1+ in the lower. His peripheral pulses are strong.

Dale decides to conduct a complete neurological examination. His patient's mental status is normal. He is alert and oriented to person, place, and time. His responses are appropriate and timely, and he does not drift off the topic or lose interest. His posture is somewhat slumped, and he has trouble maintaining his balance when standing. He also complains of difficulty buttoning his shirt. He has no tremors or fasciculations. His facial expressions are appropriate for the situation. His speech is inflected, clear and strong, fluent and articulate, and he can vary his volume. He expresses his thoughts clearly and speaks spontaneously with a clear and distinct voice. His present state of uncoordinated movement and imbalance agitates him, yet he organizes his thoughts and speaks logically and coherently.

Satisfied that Mr. Dalton's mental status is normal, Dale continues with the motor function exam. Mr. Dalton's general posture is slumped to the left. He has no tremors except at the very end of fine motor movements. His overall muscle bulk, tone, and strength appear normal.

Dale then asks his patient to perform a series of tests aimed at evaluating coordination. First, he asks him to tap the distal joint of his thumb with the tip of his index finger as rapidly as possible. Next he asks him to place his hand palm-up on his thigh, quickly turn it over palm-down, and then repeat this movement as rapidly as possible for 15 seconds. Mr. Dalton cannot perform these tests with his left hand. Nor can he perform point-to-point testing on his left side, and he has tremors at the far point. Finally, he cannot perform the heel-to-shin movement on his left side.

Convinced that his patient is having a left cerebellar infarct, Dale contacts McGivern General Hospital and gives his report to Dr. Hunt, a very impressed emergency physician. Computed tomography and magnetic resonance imaging results confirm Dale's report.

Although patient assessment formally starts with the history, the physical examination actually begins when you first set eyes on your patient.

PHYSICAL EXAMINATION APPROACH AND OVERVIEW

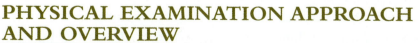

Although assessment of a medical patient formally starts with the history, the physical examination actually begins when you first set eyes on your patient. Upon meeting him you immediately assess his general appearance, level of consciousness, breathing effort, and skin color. If you initially use touch as a reassuring gesture, you can also assess skin condition and peripheral pulses. Your physical assessment continues throughout the history as you ask questions and observe your patient's body language, facial expressions, and general demeanor. Thus, you cannot draw an exact dividing line between the history and the physical exam. In emergency street medicine, the two usually occur simultaneously.

The purpose of the physical exam is to investigate areas that you suspect are involved in your patient's primary problem. As we covered the entire history in the previous chapter, we present the entire physical exam in this one. Again, if you practice in a setting other than the prehospital, such as conducting pre-employment physicals for a company, you might perform the entire physical examination outlined here. On an emergency run, you limit the exam to only those aspects that you decide are appropriate. Practice and clinical experience will dictate your ability to apply the skills you learn in this section to real situations.

The purpose of the physical exam is to investigate areas that you suspect are involved in your patient's primary problem.

EXAMINATION TECHNIQUES

Four techniques—inspection, palpation, auscultation, and percussion—are the foundation of the formal physical exam. Each can reveal information essential to a comprehensive patient assessment.

Inspection

Inspection is the process of informed observation (Figure 2-1). A simple, noninvasive technique that clinicians often take for granted, it is also one of their most valuable tools in appraising patient condition. With a keen eye, you can evaluate your patient's condition in great detail.

Inspection begins when you first meet your patient and continues while you take his history. Often, this first impression forms the basis for your history because you will judge your patient's clinical status immediately. Notice how he presents himself. Is he conscious and alert or unconscious and flaccid? Is he lying on the floor, sitting upright, or limping badly on one foot? Is he breathing normally or gasping for each breath? You can learn a great deal about your patient's

* **inspection** the process of informed observation.

Content Review

PHYSICAL EXAMINATION TECHNIQUES
- Inspection
- Palpation
- Percussion
- Auscultation

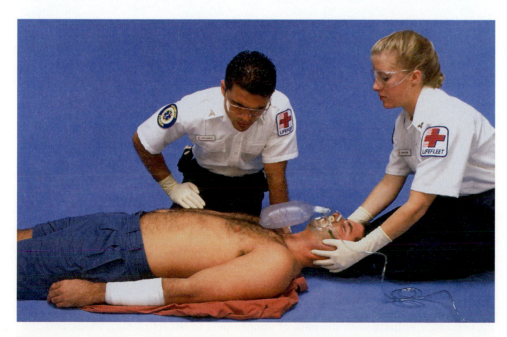

FIGURE 2-1   Inspect your patient's body for signs of injury or illness.

neurological, musculoskeletal, and respiratory systems just by careful observation. Watch for changes in his emotional and mental status throughout the history and physical exam.

During the formal physical exam, consciously evaluate each body area, looking for discoloration, unusual motion, or deformity. Pay special attention to areas where you most expect to find signs and where the patient complains of symptoms. For example, if your patient struck his chest against a bent steering wheel, you would expect to see chest wall abnormalities. Remember that you may not notice the skin color changes that follow a significant contusion until after your patient arrives at the emergency department.

Effective inspection depends on good lighting, adequate time, and a curiosity for looking beyond the obvious. During your inspection, draw on your past clinical experiences to identify the signs of illness and injury. Knowing what you are looking for is essential. Do not hurry. Give yourself enough time to inspect and then to process what you see. Inspection is an ongoing process that should not end until you transfer your patient to emergency department staff. Finally, while respecting your patient's modesty and dignity, never allow clothing to obstruct your examination.

Palpation

Palpation is usually the next step in assessing your patient, although sometimes you will inspect and palpate your patient simultaneously. **Palpation** involves using your sense of touch to gather information. With your hands and fingers you can determine a structure's size, shape, and position. You also can evaluate its temperature, moisture, texture, and movement. You can check for growths, swelling, tenderness, spasms, rigidity, pain, and crepitus. When you become skilled at this procedure, you can detect a distended bladder, an enlarged liver, a laterally pulsating abdominal aorta, or the position of a fetus.

Certain parts of your hands and fingers are better than others for specific types of palpation. For example, the pads of your fingers are more sensitive than the tips for detecting position, size, consistency, masses, fluid, and crepitus; there-

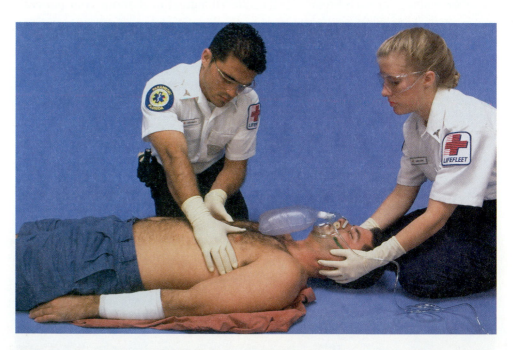

FIGURE 2-2 Palpate with the pads of your fingers to detect masses, fluids, and crepitus.

fore, you would use them to palpate lymph nodes or rib fractures (Figure 2-2). The palm of your hand is better for sensing vibrations such as fremitus. Because its skin is thinner and more sensitive, the back of your hand or fingers is better for evaluating temperature.

Palpation may be either deep or light. You control its depth by applying pressure with your hand and fingers. Since deep palpation may elicit tenderness or disrupt tissue or fluid, you should always perform light palpation first. Use light palpation to assess the skin and superficial structures. Press in approximately one centimeter. Apply the same gentle pressure you use to feel a pulse. Too much pressure dulls your sensitivity and can injure your patient.

To assess visceral organs such as those in the abdomen, use deep palpation. Apply pressure by placing the fingers of the opposite hand over the sensing fingers and gently pressing in about four centimeters. This will increase your sensitivity to any masses, guarding, or other abdominal pathology. Feel for areas of warmth that might reflect injury before significant edema or discoloration occur. Observe how your patient responds with facial expressions while you palpate tender areas. Even if he is unconscious, he may respond to pain with facial expressions or purposeful or purposeless motion.

Palpation begins your physical invasion of your patient. Three common sense tips will help make it therapeutic and respectful. Keep your hands warm, keep your fingernails short, and be gentle to avoid discomfort or injury to your patient.

To make palpation therapeutic and respectful, keep your hands warm, keep your fingernails short, and be gentle.

Percussion

Percussion is the production of sound waves by striking one object against another. In this technique, you strike a knuckle on one hand with the tip of a finger on the opposite hand. The impact causes vibrations that produce sound waves from four to six centimeters deep in the underlying body tissue. We hear these sound waves as percussion tones. The density of the tissue through which the sound must travel determines the degree of percussion. The denser the medium, the quieter the tone. The tone's resonance or lack of resonance indicates whether the underlying region is filled with air, air under pressure, fluid, or normal tissue. Listen to each sound and evaluate its meaning (Table 2-1).

Move across the area that you are percussing and compare sounds with what you know to be normal there. For example, in the chest you expect to hear the resonant sound of a healthy lung filled with air and tissue. In a pneumothorax or emphysema, however, you may hear the hyperressonant sound of air trapped in the chest. In a hemothorax, you may hear the dull sound of blood in the same area.

Percussion is simple. Place one hand on the area of the body you wish to percuss. Use a finger of that hand (usually the middle finger) as the striking surface. Sharply tap the distal knuckle of that finger with the tip of your other middle finger (Figure 2-3 on next page). The tap should come from snapping the wrist, not the forearm or shoulder. Snap the finger back quickly to avoid dampening the

✱ **percussion** the production of sound waves by striking one object against another.

Table 2-1	PERCUSSION SOUNDS				
Sound	Description	Intensity	Pitch	Duration	Location
Tympany	Drumlike	Loud	High	Medium	Stomach
Hyperresonance	Booming	Loud	Low	Long	Hyperinflated lung
Resonance	Hollow	Loud	Low	Long	Normal lung
Dull	Thud	Medium	Medium	Medium	Solid organs—liver
Flat	Extremely dull	Soft	High	Short	Muscle, atelectasis

FIGURE 2-3 Percuss your
patient to evaluate vibrations
and sounds.

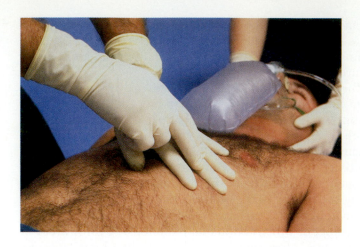

sound. When percussing the chest, make sure the finger lies between the ribs and
parallel to them. In this way you will percuss the tissue underneath the ribs, not
the ribs themselves.

*You must practice percussion
on healthy people in order to
recognize abnormalities in
sick or injured patients.*

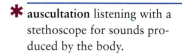

A wall in your home is a good place to practice your percussion skills. As you
percuss the air-filled area between studs, you will hear a hollow, resonant sound.
Wall spaces filled with insulation will sound less resonant. When you percuss
over a wall stud, you will notice a flatter, dull sound. You can apply this principle to the percussion of body cavities. Compare the sounds on the affected side
with those on the unaffected side. The key is knowing what is normal, so above
all you must practice percussion on healthy people in order to recognize abnormalities in sick or injured patients.

Unfortunately at most emergency scenes, especially those in the street, noise
prevents percussing your patient effectively. Your clinical experience and common sense will tell you when to use this valuable assessment technique.

Auscultation

* **auscultation** listening with a
stethoscope for sounds produced by the body.

Auscultation involves listening for sounds produced by the body, primarily the
lungs, the heart, the intestines, and major blood vessels. It is difficult to master. You
may hear some sounds clearly, such as stridor, the high-pitched squeal of a partially
obstructed upper airway. Most, however, require a stethoscope. You should perform auscultation in a quiet environment. Unfortunately, this is not always practical in emergency services. Hearing the low amplitude heart and lung sounds
against on-scene noise or in-transit background noise may be especially difficult.

For your patient's comfort, warm the end piece of your stethoscope with your
hands before auscultating. To auscultate, hold the end piece of your stethoscope between your second and third fingers and press the diaphragm firmly against your
patient's skin (Figure 2-4). If you are using the bell side, place it evenly and lightly
on the skin. Avoid touching the tubing with your hands or allowing it to rub any
surfaces. Make sure the earpieces point anteriorly before you put them in your ears.

Listen for the presence of sound and its intensity, pitch, duration, and quality. When reporting and recording lung sounds, always note abnormal sounds
(crackles, wheezes), their locations (bilateral, right lower lobe, bases), and their
timing during the respiratory cycle (inspiratory, end-expiratory). Sometimes,
closing your eyes helps you concentrate on the sounds by eliminating visual stimuli. Try to isolate and concentrate on one sound at a time. Generally, auscultate
after you have used other assessment techniques. The only exception is the abdomen, which you should auscultate before palpation and percussion. A para-

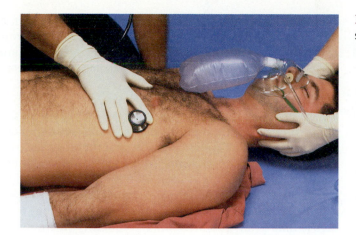

FIGURE 2-4 Auscultate body sounds with the stethoscope.

medic should be proficient in auscultating blood pressure, lung sounds, heart sounds, bowel sounds, and arterial bruits. As with any other physical assessment tool, you cannot detect abnormalities unless you know what is normal. Take every opportunity to auscultate lung, heart, and bowel sounds regularly.

Measurement of Vital Signs

The four basic vital signs in medicine are pulse, respiration, blood pressure, and body temperature. While any complete physical examination should include all four, the first three are most important in prehospital care. They are the primary indicators of your patient's health. Measure them early in the physical examination and, in emergency situations, repeat them often and look for trends. For example, in a serious head injury, watch for your patient's systolic blood pressure to rise, his pulse pressure to widen, and his pulse rate to fall. These trends suggest an increase in intracranial pressure, a serious medical emergency. Conversely, a falling blood pressure with an increasing pulse rate may indicate shock. As a paramedic you should become an expert at taking vital signs on patients of every age.

Measure vital signs early in the physical examination and, in emergency situations, repeat them often and look for trends.

Pulse As the heart ejects blood through the arteries, a pulse wave results. Each pulse beat corresponds to a cardiac contraction and results from the ejected blood's impact on the arterial walls. The pulse is a valuable indicator of circulatory function. Your patient's pulse rate, rhythm, and quality indicate his hemodynamic (circulatory) status and the critical nature of his condition. *Rate* refers to the number of pulsations felt in one minute. It can be slow (bradycardic), normal, or fast (tachycardic). *Rhythm* refers to the pulse's pattern and the equality of intervals between beats. It can be regular, regularly irregular, or irregularly irregular. *Quality* refers to the pulse's strength. Terms such as bounding or thready are used to describe the pulse's quality.

The normal pulse rate for an adult is 60–100 beats per minute. Rates below 60 are bradycardic; rates above 100 are tachycardic. **Bradycardia** may indicate an increase in parasympathetic nervous system stimulation. It might also be the result of a head injury, hypothermia, severe hypoxia, or drug overdose. Bradycardia is sometimes a normal finding in the well-conditioned athlete. Treat bradycardia only if it compromises your patient's cardiac output and general circulatory status. **Tachycardia** usually indicates an increase in sympathetic nervous system stimulation with which the body is compensating for another problem such as blood loss, fear, pain, fever, or hypoxia. It is an early indicator of shock and may indicate ventricular tachycardia, a life-threatening cardiac dysrhythmia.

＊ **pulse rate** number of pulses felt in one minute.

＊ **pulse rhythm** pattern and equality of intervals between beats.

＊ **pulse quality** strength, which can be weak, thready, strong, or bounding.

＊ **bradycardia** pulse rate lower than 60.

＊ **tachycardia** pulse rate higher than 100.

The pulse's rhythm, when present, may be regular, regularly irregular, irregularly irregular, or grossly chaotic. Irregular pulse rates may be due to extra beats, skipped beats, or pacemaker problems and usually indicate a cardiac abnormality. The rhythm's effect on cardiac output determines if intervention is necessary.

The pulse's quality can be weak, strong, or bounding. Weak, thready pulses indicate a decreased circulatory status such as shock. Strong, bounding pulses may indicate high blood pressure, heat stroke, or increasing intracranial pressure. The pulse location may be another indicator of your patient's clinical status. The presence of a carotid pulse generally means that his systolic blood pressure is at least 60 mmHg. The presence of peripheral pulses indicates a higher blood pressure; their absence suggests circulatory collapse. Practice locating each of the pulse locations (Figure 2-5). As with other vital signs, take your patient's pulse frequently in the emergency setting and note any trends.

Respiration Since oxygen and carbon dioxide exchange is essential to sustain life, **respiration** must occur continuously and must be effective. The lungs supply the arteries with oxygen and maintain the blood's pH by eliminating or retaining carbon dioxide. These two functions occur during respiration. Continuously observe your patient's respiratory rate, effort, and quality. Look for subtle signs of distress. Recognize when your patient requires rapid intervention such as aggressive airway management, positive pressure ventilation, and oxygenation. These interventions, some invasive, often will make the difference between life and death.

Content Review

NORMAL ADULT VITAL SIGNS

- Pulse rate: 60–100
- Respiratory rate: 12-20
- Systolic blood pressure ranges:
  Male: 120–150
  Female: 110–140 before menopause, 120–150 after menopause
- Body temperature: 98.6°F (37°C)

* **respiration** exchange of oxygen and carbon dioxide in the lungs and at the cellular level.

Recognizing when your patient's respiration requires rapid intervention often will make the difference between life and death.

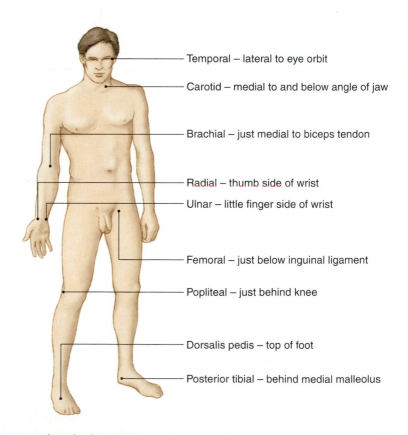

Temporal – lateral to eye orbit

Carotid – medial to and below angle of jaw

Brachial – just medial to biceps tendon

Radial – thumb side of wrist

Ulnar – little finger side of wrist

Femoral – just below inguinal ligament

Popliteal – just behind knee

Dorsalis pedis – top of foot

Posterior tibial – behind medial malleolus

FIGURE 2-5   Know each pulse location.

Your patient's **respiratory rate** is the number of times he breathes in one minute. In general the normal respiratory rate for a healthy adult at rest is 12 to 20 breaths per minute. Rapid breathing (**tachypnea**) can be the result of hypoxia, shock, head injury, or anxiety. Slow breathing (**bradypnea**) can be caused by drug overdose, severe hypoxia, or central nervous system insult. Very rapid or very slow breathing rates require rapid intervention to ensure that the adequate exchange of gases continues.

Your patient's **respiratory effort** is how hard he works to breathe. Normal inhalation involves using the respiratory muscles (diaphragm and intercostals) to increase the chest's inner diameter. It is an active process that requires energy. The increasing space creates negative pressure, like a vacuum, that draws air into the lungs. Exhalation is the passive process of the respiratory muscles' elastic recoil. This normally effortless process can become difficult with some respiratory conditions. For example, an airway obstruction may compromise inhalation. The resultant increased breathing effort is evident in accessory muscle use, retractions, and possibly abnormal breath sounds.

Diseases such as asthma and emphysema, where the smaller airways collapse and trap air in the distal airways, may obstruct exhalation. Exhalation then becomes an active process that leads to respiratory distress and failure. Some injuries can decrease the respiratory effort. Rib fractures, for example, will cause a decrease in chest wall expansion because it hurts to breathe. A pneumothorax decreases effective gas exchange because the air enters the pleural space instead of the alveoli. Children become tired and decrease their respiratory effort, making their condition even worse. Evaluating your patient's respiratory effort will provide invaluable information about his respiratory status.

The **quality of respiration** refers to its depth and pattern. The depth, or **tidal volume,** of respiration is the amount of air your patient moves in and out of his lungs in one breath. The normal depth for a healthy adult at rest should be approximately 500 ml, just enough to cause the chest to rise. The tidal volume may increase during exercise or anxiety. It may decrease in the presence of a rib injury when every breath hurts.

Assess your patient's respiratory depth by inspecting and palpating the chest wall for symmetrical chest expansion, by feeling and listening for air movement and noise from the nose and mouth, and by auscultating for lung sounds. The depth may be shallow, normal, or deep. Once again, to recognize inadequate respiratory depth, you must know what is normal. The respiratory pattern should be regular. Variations in respiratory pattern can be associated with specific diseases (Table 2-2 on next page). Some irregular patterns such as Cheyne-Stokes may indicate serious brain or brain stem problems.

Blood Pressure **Blood pressure** is the force of blood against the arteries' walls as the heart contracts and relaxes. It is equal to cardiac output times the systemic vascular resistance. Any alteration in the cardiac output or the vascular resistance will alter the blood pressure. An important indicator of your patient's condition, blood pressure is measured during both systole and diastole. **Systolic blood pressure** (the higher numeric value) measures the maximum force of blood against the arteries when the ventricles contract. **Diastolic blood pressure** (the lower numeric value) measures the pressure against the arteries when the ventricles relax and are filling with blood. The diastolic blood pressure is a measure of systemic vascular resistance and correlates well with changes in vessel size. The sounds of the blood hitting the arterial walls are called the **Korotkoff sounds.**

Many factors may influence your patient's blood pressure. Anxiety, for example, may cause it to rise. His position (sitting, lying, standing) also may affect the measurement. If your patient has recently been smoking, exercising, or eating, you must wait at least five to ten minutes to allow his blood pressure to return to

* **respiratory rate** number of times patient breathes in one minute.

* **tachypnea** rapid breathing.

* **bradypnea** slow breathing.

Very rapid or very slow breathing rates require rapid intervention to ensure that the adequate exchange of gases continues.

* **respiratory effort** how hard patient works to breathe.

* **quality of respiration** depth and pattern of breathing.

* **tidal volume** amount of air one breath moves in and out of lungs.

* **blood pressure** force of blood against arteries' walls as the heart contracts and relaxes.

* **systolic blood pressure** force of blood against arteries when ventricles contract.

* **diastolic blood pressure** force of blood against arteries when ventricles relax.

* **Korotkoff sounds** sounds of blood hitting arterial walls.

Table 2-2   BREATHING PATTERNS

	Condition	Description	Causes
	Eupnea	Normal breathing rate and pattern	
	Tachypnea	Increased respiratory rate	Fever, anxiety, exercise, shock
	Bradypnea	Decreased respiratory rate	Sleep, drugs, metabolic disorder, head injury, stroke
	Apnea	Absence of breathing	Deceased patient, head injury, stroke
	Hyperpnea	Normal rate, but deep respirations	Emotional stress, diabetic ketoacidosis
	Cheyne-Stokes	Gradual increases and decreases in respirations with periods of apnea	Increasing intracranial pressure, brain stem injury
	Biot's	Rapid, deep respirations (gasps) with short pauses between sets	Spinal meningitis, many CNS causes, head injury
	Kussmaul's	Tachypnea and hyperpnea	Renal failure, metabolic acidosis, diabetic ketoacidosis
	Apneustic	Prolonged inspiratory phase with shortened expiratory phase	Lesion in brain stem

Never use blood pressure as the single indicator of your patient's condition; always correlate it with his other clinical signs of end-organ perfusion.

* **perfusion** passage of blood through an organ or tissue.

* **pulse pressure** difference between systolic and diastolic pressures.

* **hypertension** blood pressure higher than normal.

* **hypotension** blood pressure lower than normal.

a resting level before you measure it. Because of these many intangibles, you should never use blood pressure as the single indicator of your patient's condition. Always correlate it with his other clinical signs of end-organ **perfusion** such as level of response, skin color, temperature, and condition, and peripheral pulses.

The average blood pressure in the healthy adult is 120/80. Females usually will have a lower blood pressure until menopause. **Pulse pressure** is the difference between the systolic and diastolic pressures. For example, a blood pressure of 120/80 represents a pulse pressure of 40 mmHg. A normal pulse pressure is generally 30–40 mmHg. In certain conditions, such as pericardial tamponade or tension pneumothorax, the pulse pressure will narrow. In others, such as increasing intracranial pressure or fever, the pulse pressure will widen. Again, take your physiologically unstable patient's blood pressure as often as every five minutes to chart trends.

What is normal? This question has no easy answer. Generally, systolic blood pressure in adults ranges from 100 to 135 mmHg, diastolic from 60 to 80 mmHg. **Hypertension** in adults is defined as a pressure higher than 140/90. A blood pressure of 130/70, however, may represent hypertension if a patient's usual pressure is 90/60 or **hypotension** if his usual pressure is 170/90. The numbers are not as important as detecting trends and assessing end-organ perfusion. Do not define hypotension by numbers but by whether perfusion is adequate to sustain life.

Hypertension can result from cardiovascular disease, kidney disease, stroke, or head injury, where it is a classic sign of increasing intracranial pressure. It may be a predisposing factor to, and preexist in, stroke or cardiovascular disease. Did the hypertension occur before or after the condition? Hypotension usually indicates shock due to cardiac insufficiency (cardiogenic shock), low blood volume (hypovolemic shock), or massive vasodilation (vasogenic shock). Orthostatic hypotension is a decrease in your patient's blood pressure when he stands or sits up.

If you suspect shock due to blood or fluid volume loss and you do not suspect a spinal injury, perform a tilt test. Take your patient's pulse and blood pressure while he is supine. Then have him sit up and dangle his feet, then stand. In 30–60 seconds retake his vital signs. The healthy patient's vital signs should not change. The tilt test is positive either if his pulse rate increases 10–20 beats per minute or if his systolic blood pressure drops 10–20 mmHg. (Research has found that an increase in heart rate is a more sensitive indicator of hypovolemia than a decrease in systolic blood pressure.) This finding is common in patients suspected of hypovolemia.

Body Temperature The body works hard to maintain a temperature of approximately 98.6°F (37°C). This temperature reflects the balance between heat production and heat loss through the skin and respiratory system. Even a slight variance can mean that significant events are happening within the body or on the body from environmental factors. Assess your patient's temperature to approximate his internal core temperature.

An increase in body temperature (**hyperthermia**) can result from environmental extremes, infections, drugs, or metabolic processes. Ordinarily the body's cooling mechanisms maintain a steady core temperature. In an extremely hot and humid environment or in cases like heat stroke, the cooling mechanisms can fail and the core temperature will rise despite an internal thermostat that wants to maintain a normal temperature. Fever, on the other hand, results when the body tries to make its internal environment inhospitable to invading organisms. It often presents with a history of illness. The skin is somewhat dry until the fever breaks and the body's cooling mechanisms begin to take effect. As the body temperature rises, it begins to threaten body processes, specifically those of the brain. A temperature of up to 102°F (38°C) increases metabolism markedly. As body temperature rises above 103°F (39°C), the neurons of the brain may denature. At temperatures above 105°F (41°C), brain cells die and seizures may occur.

Extreme cold also affects body temperature. When peripheral vasoconstriction and shivering mechanisms can no longer balance heat production and loss, core temperature drops (**hypothermia**). At a body temperature of 93°F (34°C), normal body warming mechanisms begin to fail. As the core temperature drops below 90°F (31°C), shivering stops, heart sounds diminish and cardiac irritability increases. If the temperature drops much below 70°F (22°C), your patient will present with a deathlike appearance and, possibly, irreversible asystole (absence of heartbeat).

A variety of methods can provide accurate temperature readings. You can use glass thermometers to take oral, rectal, or axillary temperatures. A rectal thermometer is the preferred device for children younger than six years old and for patients with an altered level of consciousness. An axillary temperature reading is the least accurate of the three methods.

EQUIPMENT

To conduct a comprehensive physical examination you will need a stethoscope, a sphygmomanometer, an ophthalmoscope, an otoscope, a scale, and other equipment. The ophthalmoscope, otoscope, and scale are not considered prehospital assessment tools.

Stethoscope The **stethoscope** is a basic paramedic tool used to auscultate most sounds (Figure 2-6 on next page). It transmits sound waves from the source through an end piece and along rubber tubes to the ear. One side of the end piece is a rigid diaphragm that best transmits high-pitched sounds such as heart sounds and blood pressure sounds. The diaphragm also screens out low-pitched sounds such as lung sounds and bowel sounds. The other side of the end piece is a bell that uses the skin as a diaphragm. The sounds that the bell transmits vary with the amount of pressure exerted. For example, with light pressure the bell picks up low-pitched sounds; with firm pressure it acts like the diaphragm and transmits high-pitched sounds. Whether you use the bell or the diaphragm depends on which sounds you are auscultating. To hear blood pressure or heart sounds, for instance, use the diaphragm; to hear lung or bowel sounds, use the bell side.

Even a slight variance in body temperature can mean that significant events are happening within the body.

✳ **hyperthermia** increase in body's core temperature.

✳ **hypothermia** decrease in body's core temperature.

✳ **stethoscope** tool used to auscultate most sounds.

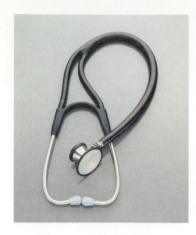

FIGURE 2-6 Use a stethoscope to auscultate most sounds.

Accurate auscultation depends in part on the quality of your instrument. Your stethoscope should have the following important characteristics:

- A rigid diaphragm cover
- Thick, heavy tubing that conducts sound better than thin, flexible tubing
- Short tubing (30–40 cm) to minimize distortion
- Earpieces that fit snugly—large enough to occlude the ear canal—and are angled toward the nose to project sound toward the eardrum
- A bell with a rubber-ring edge to ensure good contact with the skin

Sphygmomanometer The circumstances and the patient care setting determine what type of equipment you use to measure blood pressure (Figure 2-7). Intensive care unit staff commonly use intra-arterial pressure devices for critically ill patients who need continuous monitoring. When a noisy environment makes auscultation difficult or when the sounds are especially weak, a doppler device that amplifies the sounds is useful. You will see these devices in the emergency department, newborn nursery, emergency vehicles, and labor and delivery suites. The most familiar blood-pressure measuring device is the aneroid **sphygmomanometer.** You will use it with your stethoscope to auscultate the sounds of the blood moving through an artery, usually the brachial artery. Because your patient's blood pressure is important in evaluating his condition, you must be able to measure it accurately.

A sphygmomanometer includes a bulb, a cuff, and a manometer. The cuff has an airtight, flat, rubber bladder enclosed within a fabric cover. Cuffs are avail-

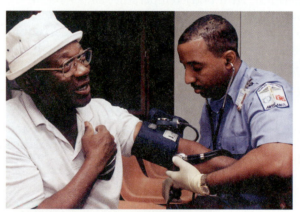

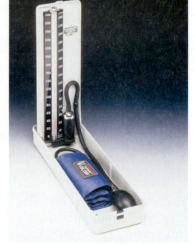

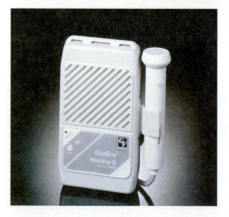

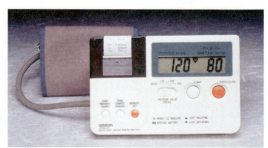

FIGURE 2-7 Use a blood pressure device suited to the circumstances. Clockwise from upper left: aneroid sphygmomanometer, mercury sphygmomanometer, digital electronic, and doppler device.

able in various sizes and designs. Flexible tubing attaches the rubber bulb to the cuff. Squeezing the bulb pumps air into the cuff's bladder. A control valve allows you to inflate and deflate the cuff. To inflate the cuff, close the valve by turning it clockwise; to deflate the cuff, open the valve by turning it counterclockwise.

The **manometer** is a pressure gauge with a scale calibrated in millimeters of mercury (mmHg). Each line represents 2 mmHg. The heavy lines are 10 mmHg of mercury apart. The aneroid manometer displays the scale on a circular dial. As the pressure in the bladder changes, the needle moves and indicates the pressure reading at a given moment. When you use an aneroid sphygmomanometer, keep the dial in plain sight. The aneroid types lose their calibration, so you will need to calibrate them periodically against a mercury-type device.

> * **manometer** pressure gauge with a scale calibrated in millimeters of mercury (mmHg).

The mercury sphygmomanometer displays the scale along a glass tube connected to a reservoir of mercury. As pressure in the cuff increases, the mercury in the tube rises. When using a mercury sphygmomanometer, keep the scale at eye level and vertical. Available as portable, wall-mounted, or floor units, mercury sphygmomanometers are more accurate than aneroid, but they are impractical for prehospital use.

Ophthalmoscope An **ophthalmoscope** allows you to examine the interior of your patient's eyes. It is a handheld device comprised of a light source and a series of lenses and mirrors (Figure 2-8).

> * **ophthalmoscope** handheld device used to examine interior of eye.

Otoscope To visualize the ear canal and tympanic membrane you will need an **otoscope**. The otoscope provides illumination for inspecting the ear canal and tympanic membrane (eardrum) and the internal nose. It has a light source, a speculum you insert into the ear canal, and a magnifying glass through which you visualize the inner structures of the ear (Figure 2-9).

> * **otoscope** handheld device used to examine interior of ears and nose.

Scale The standing platform scale measures weight and height (Figure 2-10). To measure weight it uses a system of counterbalanced weights that you calibrate before each use. Your patient simply stands on the scale, and you add or

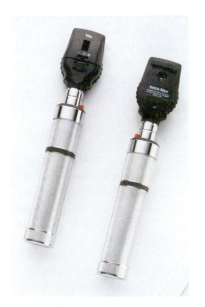

FIGURE 2-8 Visualize the interior of your patient's eyes with an ophthalmoscope.

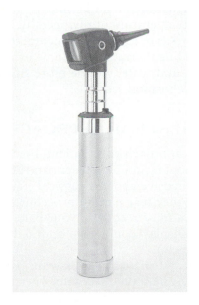

FIGURE 2-9 An otoscope enables you to inspect the ear canal and tympanic membrane.

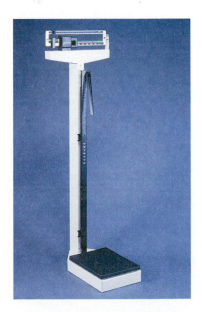

FIGURE 2-10 Use a platform scale to measure your patient's weight and height.

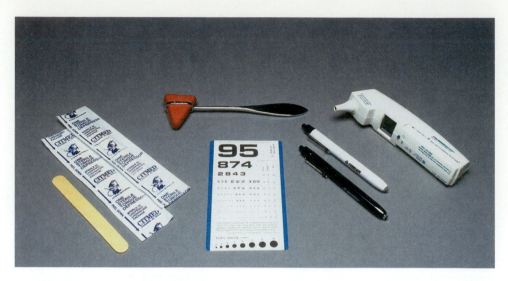

FIGURE 2-11   Essential assessment tools.

subtract weight in small increments until it balances. To measure your patient's height, pull up the height adjustment and position the head piece at his crown. Electronic scales are becoming more popular. They calculate your patient's weight electronically and display it as a digital readout. You also calibrate them before each use.

Additional Equipment   Besides the above items, you will need sterile tongue blades to inspect inside the mouth and to initiate a gag reflex; a penlight to test your patient's pupillary responses; a visual acuity chart or card to measure visual acuity; a reflex hammer to test deep tendon reflexes; and a thermometer to measure body temperature (Figure 2-11). The danger of breakage limits glass thermometers' usefulness in the prehospital setting, and their inability to record temperatures below 96°F (36°C) prevents them from helping you evaluate the hypothermic patient. Available battery-operated devices measure temperature orally, rectally, and in the ear canal. If your service operates in areas of low environmental temperatures, equip your ambulance with a low-reading thermometer. Some of these items, such as the ophthalmoscope, otoscope, and scale, will be more suited to a medical clinic setting than to a typical prehospital scene.

THE GENERAL APPROACH

How you approach your patient, both in the emergency setting and elsewhere, will set the stage for an efficient and effective patient assessment.

How you approach your patient, both in the emergency setting and elsewhere, will set the stage for an efficient and effective patient assessment. Most patients are apprehensive about a physical examination. They feel exposed and vulnerable, and they fear painful procedures. This anxiety is multiplied in an emergency. You must recognize your patient's apprehension and take steps to alleviate it. Display confidence and skill while you complete your history and physical exam.

If you systematically assess your patient's complaints and efficiently perform your duties, he should feel safe. Then add the personal touches of active listening, a reassuring voice, and gestures that convey your sincere compassion and interest. Most patients will respond favorably. Let your patient know that you are not just checking off items on a diagnostic list; you are conducting a personal examination of *his* problems.

Proficiency will come only with clinical practice. In time, you will become adept at focusing the exam on your patient's chief complaint and present illness. In the emergency setting, no matter how nervous and apprehensive you may be, never let your patient see anything but a calm, professional, confident demeanor. This will help alleviate his anxiety about disclosing personal information to, and being examined by, a nonphysician. Try to remain objective, even when confronted by alarming or disgusting information. A bad bedsore, a perverted sexual story, or black tarry stools (melena) can test even the most experienced clinician's composure. Simply thinking about how embarrassed your patient must be may help you keep your own poise.

OVERVIEW OF A COMPREHENSIVE EXAMINATION

This section gives an overview of the comprehensive physical exam. Later in the chapter we will discuss each component in detail. The key to an effective comprehensive exam is to integrate each individual section into a unified patient assessment. Chapter 3 provides a template for conducting a problem-oriented patient assessment on both medical and trauma patients.

As a paramedic, you will determine which elements of the comprehensive exam to use. You will base your decision on your patient's presenting problem and clinical status. For example, if you are conducting comprehensive physicals for your fire department, you may choose to use the entire examination. If you are assessing a child just struck by an automobile and lying unconscious in the street, you will narrow your focus to the child's injuries. A comprehensive examination should include a general survey and a detailed assessment of anatomical regions.

The key to an effective comprehensive exam is integrating each individual section into a unified patient assessment.

THE GENERAL SURVEY

A general survey is the first part of a comprehensive examination. It begins with noting your patient's appearance and goes on to include vital signs and other assessments.

Appearance

A thorough evaluation of your patient's appearance can provide a great deal of valuable information about his health. Note his level of consciousness, posture, and any obvious signs of distress, such as sitting upright gasping for each breath or slumped to one side. Is his motor activity normal or does he have noticeable tremors or paralysis? Observe his general state of health, his dress, grooming, and personal hygiene. Obvious odors can also furnish significant information.

Level of Consciousness Is your patient awake? Is he alert? Does he speak to you in a normal voice? Are his eyes open, and does he respond to you and others in the environment? If he is not apparently awake, speak to him in a loud voice. If he does not respond to your verbal cues, shake him gently. If he still does not respond, apply a painful stimulus such as pinching a tendon, rubbing his sternum, or rolling a pencil across a nail bed. Note his response.

Signs of Distress Is your patient in distress? For example, does he have a cardiac or respiratory problem, as evidenced by labored breathing, wheezing, or a cough? Is he in pain, as evidenced by wincing, sweating, or protecting the painful area? Is he anxious, as evidenced by his facial expression, cold moist palms, or nervous fidgeting?

Apparent State of Health Is your patient healthy, robust, and vigorous? Or is he frail, ill-looking, or feeble? Does he have an obvious abnormality? Base your evaluation of his general state of health on your observations throughout the interview and physical examination.

Vital Statistics Vital statistics, weight and height, are used widely in clinical medicine. Accurately measuring your patient's weight and height with a scale, however, is not a practical prehospital assessment procedure. You will occasionally estimate your patient's weight to administer medications of which the dose is weight dependent. You also may use a **Broselow Tape** to measure your infant patient's length. The Broselow tape provides information concerning drug dosages, airway management adjuncts, and intravenous calculations based on your patient's height.

Note your patient's general stature. Is he lanky and slender, short and stocky, muscular and symmetrical? Does he have any obvious deformities or disproportionate areas? Is he extremely thin or obese? If obese, is the fat evenly distributed or is it concentrated in his trunk? Has he gained or lost weight recently?

Sexual Development Is your patient's sexual maturity appropriate for his or her age and gender? Consider such indicators as voice, facial and body hair, and breast size.

Skin Color and Obvious Lesions Is your patient's skin pale, suggesting decreased blood flow or anemia? Does he have central (lips, oral mucosa) or peripheral (nail beds, hands) cyanosis, the bluish color resulting from decreased oxygenation of the tissues? Does he have the yellow color of jaundice or high carotene levels? Note any rashes, bruises, scars, or discoloration.

Posture, Gait, and Motor Activity Observe your patient's posture and presentation. Is he sitting straight up and forward, bracing his arms (tripodding)? This suggests a serious breathing problem such as acute pulmonary edema or airway obstruction. Does one side of his body droop and seem immobile, suggesting a stroke? Does he sit quietly or does he seem restless? Does he have tremors or other involuntary movements?

Dress, Grooming, and Personal Hygiene Does your patient dress appropriately for the climate and situation? Are his clothes clean and properly fastened? Are they conventional for his age and social group? Abnormalities in dress might suggest the cold intolerance of hypothyroidism or the hiding of a skin rash or needle marks, or they might simply reflect personal preference. Look at his shoes. Are they clean? Do they have holes, slits, open laces, or other alterations to accommodate painful foot conditions such as gout, bunions, or edema? Does he wear a slipper, or slippers, instead of shoes? Is he wearing unusual jewelry such as a copper bracelet for arthritis or a medical information tag? Do his grooming and hygiene seem appropriate for his age, lifestyle, occupation, and social status? Does his lack of concern over appearance (overgrown nails and hair, for instance) suggest a long illness or depression?

Odors of Breath or Body Does your patient have any unusual or striking body or breath odors? The acetone breath of a diabetic, the bitter-almond breath of a cyanide poisoning, the putrid smell of bacterial infection, or the obvious smell of alcohol may give important clues to the underlying problem. Avoid tunnel-vision when you smell alcohol, which often masks other serious illnesses such as liver failure or injuries such as a subdural hematoma.

Facial Expression Watch your patient's facial expressions throughout your interaction. His face should reflect his emotions during the interview and physical exam. The patient with hyperthyroidism may stare intently. The Parkinson's patient's face may appear immobile.

Vital Signs

Take a complete set of vital signs to include pulse, respiration, blood pressure, and temperature.

Pulse To take the pulse of a conscious adult or large child, the most accessible and commonly used location is the radial artery. With the pads of your first two or three fingers, compress the radial artery onto the radius, just below the wrist on the thumb side (Procedure 2-1a on next page). In the unconscious patient, begin by checking his carotid pulse. To locate the carotid pulse, palpate medial to and just below the angle of the jaw. Locate the thyroid cartilage (Adam's apple) and slide your fingers laterally until they are between the thyroid cartilage and the large muscle in the neck (sternocleidomastoid). In infants and small children, use the brachial artery or auscultate for an apical pulse. Remember that auscultating an apical pulse does not provide information about your patient's hemodynamic status. To locate the brachial artery, feel just medial to the biceps tendon. Auscultate the apical pulse just below the left nipple. First, note your patient's pulse rate by counting the number of beats in one minute. If his pulse is regular, you can count the beats in fifteen seconds and multiply that number by four. If his pulse is irregular, you must count it for a full minute to obtain an accurate total. Note also the pulse's rhythm and quality.

Respiration To measure your patient's respiratory rate, place one hand on your patient's chest and count the breaths he takes in thirty seconds (Procedure 2-1b). Multiply that number by two. Because your patient may consciously or subconsciously control his breathing, try to evaluate it without his knowing. Also assess his respiratory effort and quality of respiration.

Blood pressure To measure your patient's blood pressure, first choose the arm you will use. Remove any clothing that covers the upper arm; do not take the blood pressure over clothing, if possible. Look for a dialysis shunt in patients with renal failure. Do not take a blood pressure in that arm. Place the arm in a slightly flexed position, palm up and fingers relaxed. Support the upper arm at the level of your patient's heart.

Use the correct size cuff to obtain an accurate measurement. Its width should be one half to one third the circumference of your patient's arm. For most adults, unless they are obese or extremely slim, the large size cuff (15 cm wide) will suffice. If your patient has an obese arm, use a larger cuff. If the larger cuff is still too small, use your patient's forearm and place your stethoscope over the radial artery. For all patients, use a cuff that covers approximately two thirds of his upper arm or thigh. Using a cuff that is too wide, too narrow, too long, or too short will result in an inaccurate measurement.

Turn the control valve counterclockwise to open it; squeeze all the air out of the bladder before applying the cuff. Locate the brachial artery by palpating on the medial side of the antecubital space until you feel a pulse. Place the lower edge of the cuff one inch above the antecubital space. Find the center of the bladder (usually marked on the cuff with an arrow), and place it directly over the artery. Fasten the cuff so it is smooth and fits tightly enough to obtain an accurate reading. If you have difficulty inserting a finger between the cuff and your patient's arm, it is snug enough. Also make sure the rubber tubing is clear of the cuff. Check the placement of the manometer so you can see it easily.

Now palpate the radial artery. With your other hand, turn the control valve completely clockwise and squeeze the bulb rapidly to inflate the cuff to approximately 30 mmHg over the point where the radial pulse disappears. Place your stethoscope directly over the brachial artery and hold it firmly in place without pressing on the artery (Procedure 2-1c). Turn the control valve counterclockwise slowly and steadily to deflate the cuff at a rate of 2–3 mmHg per heart beat. Deflating too slowly or too rapidly will cause an inaccurate reading.

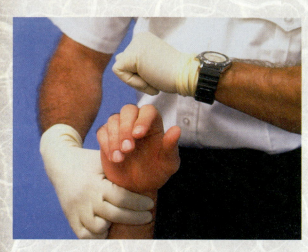

2-1a   Assess the pulse as an indicator of circulatory function.

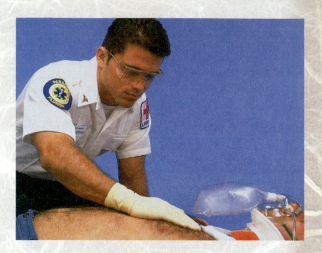

2-1b   Count your patient's respirations.

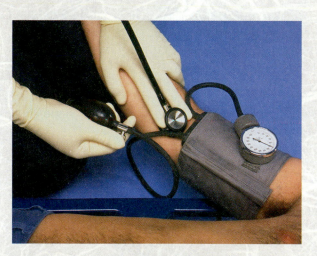

2-1c   Assess blood pressure with a sphygmomanometer and stethoscope.

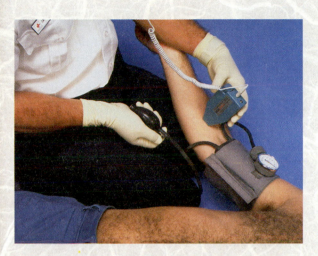

2-1d   If you cannot hear blood pressure with a stethoscope, use an ultrasonic Doppler.

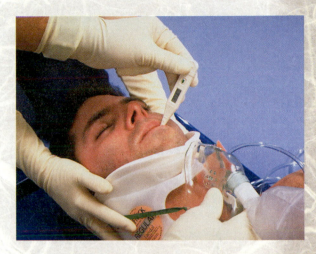

2-1e   Use a battery-operated oral thermometer to take your patient's temperature.

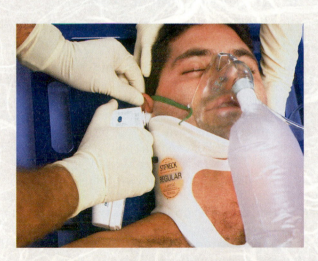

2-1f   Use a specially designed, battery-operated thermometer to measure temperature inside the ear.

As you slowly deflate the cuff, watch the manometer and listen for the Korotkoff sounds. When you hear the first pulse beat, note the reading on the manometer dial or mercury column. This is the systolic pressure. Continue deflating the cuff until the pulsations diminish or become muffled. This is the diastolic pressure.

If you do not obtain a reading, wait 30 seconds to allow the blood pressure to normalize before inflating the cuff again. Sometimes you can palpate the artery during the deflation. The point at which you feel the pulse return marks the systolic reading. You cannot evaluate the diastolic pressure with the palpation method. To take your patient's blood pressure with a Doppler, follow the same procedure as for the palpation method, but instead of palpating for the return of the pulse, place the Doppler device over the palpated artery and listen for the "whooosh" of flowing blood indicating the systolic measurement (Procedure 2-1d). Record the blood pressure on your patient's chart. Include the systolic and diastolic pressures (for instance, 134/78), the arm used (right/left), and your patient's position (lying, sitting, standing).

Temperature The type of glass thermometer you use determines how long you must leave it in place to get an accurate reading. To take your patient's temperature orally with a glass thermometer, place the thermometer under his tongue for at least 3–4 minutes. It may provide a false reading if your patient has swallowed liquid or smoked within 15–30 minutes. To use a rectal thermometer, lubricate it well and then insert it 1.5 inches into the rectum; leave it in place for at least 2-3 minutes. If you use an axillary thermometer, it must remain under your patient's armpit at least 10 minutes. If your service uses battery operated devices, become familiar with them and follow the manufacturer's instructions for their use (Procedure 2-1e). For example, when using the tympanic membrane device, place the speculum into the ear canal, push the button and hold it for two to three seconds, then remove the device (Procedure 2-1f). The temperature is then displayed on a digital readout.

Additional Assessment Techniques

Additional assessment techniques include pulse oximetry, cardiac monitoring, and blood glucose determination.

Pulse Oximetry The **pulse oximeter** is a noninvasive device that measures the oxygen saturation of your patient's blood. It can reliably indicate your patient's cardiorespiratory status because it may tell you how well he is oxygenating the most peripheral vessels of his circulatory system. It also quantifies the effectiveness of your interventions such as oxygen therapy, medications, suctioning, and ventilatory assistance. For example, on room air, your patient's reading is 92%; after two minutes of high-flow oxygen therapy, it is 99%, showing a definite improvement.

The pulse oximeter has a probe-sensor and a monitoring unit with digital readouts. Attach the probe-sensor clip to your patient's finger, toe, or earlobe (Figure 2-12). The probe directs two lights (one red and one infrared) through a small area of tissue. The lights penetrate the tissue and are absorbed. Since saturated and desaturated hemoglobin absorb the lights differently, the sensors can determine their individual concentrations. The result is a measurement of your patient's oxygen saturation, or SaO_2.

Normal oxygen saturation at sea level should be between 96% and 100%. Generally, if the reading is below 95%, suspect shock, hypoxia, or respiratory compromise. Provide your patient with the appropriate airway management and supplemental oxygen and watch him carefully for further changes. Any reading below 90% requires aggressive airway management, positive pressure ventilation, or oxygen administration. The unresponsive patient may require invasive airway management and positive pressure ventilation.

✳ pulse oximeter noninvasive device that measures the oxygen saturation of blood.

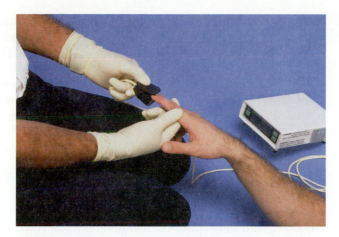

FIGURE 2-12 Pulse oximetry allows you quickly and accurately to determine your patient's oxygenation status.

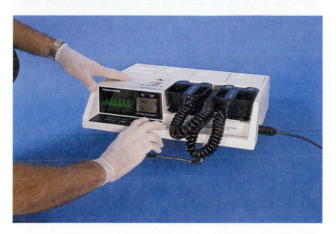

FIGURE 2-13 The cardiac monitor is essential to managing advanced cardiac life support.

Several factors affect the accuracy of a pulse oximetry reading. The sensors can accurately measure the oxygen saturation only if blood flow through the tissue is adequate. Most pulse oximeters display a digital readout of the pulse rate; others display a pulsation wave. In either case, if the display does not match your patient's actual pulse, the SaO_2 reading will be erratic. If your patient has decreased blood flow through the tissue, as in hypovolemia or hypothermia, you will obtain a false reading.

In cases of carbon monoxide (CO) poisoning, your saturation readings will be high while your patient's tissues are severely ischemic. This is because the CO molecule saturates the hemoglobin molecule 200 times more easily than does oxygen and the pulse oximetry probe cannot distinguish between hemoglobin that is bound to carbon monoxide and hemoglobin that is bound to oxygen. Your patient's hemoglobin is in fact saturated, but with carbon monoxide, not oxygen. Other than these limitations, the pulse oximeter, when teamed with other patient assessment techniques, can be a useful tool in the prehospital setting.

Cardiac Monitoring The **cardiac monitor** is essential in assessing and managing the patient who requires advanced cardiac life support (ACLS) (Figure 2-13). The most simple prehospital machines monitor the electrical activity of the heart in three "leads" or positions. These "limb leads" adequately identify life-threatening cardiac rhythms. Also available for prehospital use are 12-lead ECGs. They are essential in gathering data to confirm a myocardial infarction.

Other features of cardiac monitors include pacing capabilities and the "quick-look" paddles and the "hands-off" defibrillation pads used in cardiac arrest. The paddles, which you place on your patient's chest, allow you to check

✱ **cardiac monitor** machine that displays and records the electrical activity of the heart.

the cardiac rhythm and deliver a rapid electrical countershock. The hands-off defibrillation pads have two large electrodes that you attach to the chest wall. These replace the paddles and allow you to deliver a countershock without fear of injuring yourself.

All monitor-defibrillators can deliver a synchronized countershock in the presence of an unstable tachycardia. Most have a transcutaneous pacemaker that is placed externally on the chest and provides an electrical impulse to stimulate cardiac contraction in cases of bradycardia and heart blocks. This is a temporary measure until a permanent pacemaker can be implanted. Finally, some ECG machines have a "code summary" feature that prints out the electrical record of events and their times. This helps you document your patient's progress while in your care.

The cardiac monitor is a useful tool for measuring electrical activity, but it has one major disadvantage. It cannot tell you if the heart is pumping efficiently, effectively, or at all. The ECG reading does not necessarily correlate with the mechanical function of the heart. Electrical activity can exist with no mechanical contraction. Always assess your patient and compare what you see on the monitor with the rate and quality of the pulse.

Blood Glucose Determination In cases of altered mental status due to diabetic emergencies, seizures, and strokes, you will want to measure your patient's blood glucose level. The arrival of inexpensive, handheld **glucometers** makes this test easy to perform in the field. Most diabetic patients do it several times each day at home by themselves.

To perform this procedure you will need a glucometer with test strips, a finger stick device with sterile lancets, alcohol wipe, and tissue or gauze pads. Simply place a drop of your patient's capillary blood from a finger stick onto a chemical reagent strip (Figure 2-14). Following the manufacturer's instructions, place the test strip in the glucometer and wait for the reading to appear. This procedure takes less than one minute to perform.

Since all glucometers work differently, you must read the manufacturer's instructions carefully. The slightest mistake can alter the measurement's accuracy. For example, make sure the code numbers on the test strips match those on the digital reading. Also make sure you do not allow alcohol to contaminate the blood. Glucometers are moderately accurate when used properly and calibrated daily.

Always compare what you see on a cardiac monitor with what you feel for a pulse.

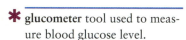

* **glucometer** tool used to measure blood glucose level.

FIGURE 2-14   Use a glucometer to determine your patient's blood glucose.

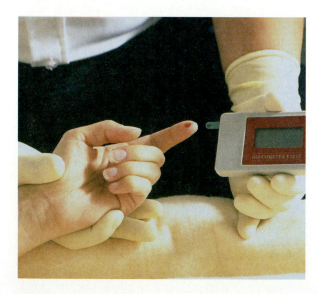

ANATOMICAL REGIONS

After you complete the general survey, you will examine the body regions and systems in more detail. Again, the specific situation and your experience and common sense will determine whether you conduct a thorough examination, as you would when performing physicals for an insurance company, or narrow the focus of your examination, as you might in an emergency setting.

THE SKIN

The skin is the largest organ in the human body, making up 15% of our total body weight. The skin performs many important functions. It protects the body against foreign substance invasion and minor physical trauma. It provides a watertight barrier to keep body fluids in and environmental fluids out. It excretes sweat, urea, and lactic acid and regulates body temperature through radiation, conduction, convection, and evaporation. It provides sensory perception through nerve endings and specialized receptors. It helps regulate blood pressure by constricting skin blood vessels, and it repairs surface wounds by exaggerating the normal process of cell replacement.

The skin consists of two layers that lie atop the subcutaneous fat—the epidermis and the dermis (Figure 2-15). The thickness of each layer varies with age and body site. The outer layer, the epidermis, is comprised mostly of dying and dead cells that are shed constantly and replaced from beneath by new cells. It is avascular (has no blood vessels), so blood vessels from the underlying dermis must

Content Review

ANATOMICAL REGIONS
- Skin
- Head, eyes, ears, nose, throat
- Neck
- Chest
- Abdomen
- Extremities
- Posterior body
- Neurological

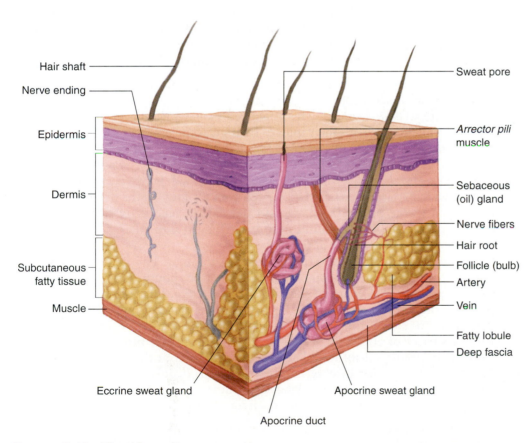

FIGURE 2-15   The skin.

supply its nutrition. The dermis is rich in blood supply and nerve endings. It also contains some hair follicles and sebaceous glands that secrete an oil called sebum. This oil lubricates the epidermis and helps make the watertight seal. The subcutaneous tissue under the dermis contains fat, sweat glands, and hair follicles.

The two types of sweat glands are eccrine glands and apocrine glands. Eccrine glands, also known as merocrine glands, open onto the skin surface and help control body temperature through water excretion. They are widely distributed but are most heavily concentrated in the axilla and genital areas. Apocrine glands are found exclusively in the armpits and genital region, and they open into hair follicles. These glands respond to emotional stress. During adolescence, the apocrine glands enlarge and actively increase the axillary sweating that causes adult body odor. Also during this period, the sebaceous glands increase their activity, giving the skin an oily appearance. This predisposes the teenager to acne problems.

As we age, sebaceous and sweat gland activity decreases. As a result, the skin becomes drier and produces less perspiration. The epidermis thins and flattens, and the dermis loses some of its vascularity. The skin wrinkles as it loses turgor. In warmer climates, the skin can become thickened, yellowed, and furrowed and take on a weather-beaten appearance. Elderly people develop a variety of spots on the thin skin of the backs of their hands and forearms. Whitish, depigmented marks are known as pseudoscars. Purple spots (purpura) caused by minor capillary bleeding may appear and fade after a few weeks.

Although you will observe your patient's skin throughout your assessment, a comprehensive physical exam must also include a concentrated inspection of all areas of the skin. The skin provides data on a variety of systemic problems in addition to skin-related disorders. Examining the skin requires good light and a keen eye. The characteristics of normal skin vary with your patients' racial, ethnic, and familial backgrounds. Evaluate its color, moisture, temperature, texture, mobility and turgor, and any lesions. Always wear protective gloves if your patient has any areas of open skin, exudative lesions, or rashes.

Color Normal skin color in light-skinned people is pink, indicating adequate cardiorespiratory function and vascular integrity. This means that the capillaries in the skin are well-oxygenated. The bright red oxyhemoglobin in the oxygen-rich blood circulating through the capillary beds gives the epidermis its pink appearance. A pale color suggests decreased blood flow through the skin. This is typical in hypothermia, hypovolemia, and compensatory shock, where blood flow through the distal capillary beds is severely diminished. It also is common in anemia, in which your patient's red blood cell count is low. As the hemoglobin loses its oxygen to the tissues, it changes to the darker, blue deoxyhemoglobin. Increased deoxyhemoglobin causes cyanosis, a bluish skin color. Cyanosis means that less oxygen is available at the tissue level.

Evaluate skin color where the epidermis is thinnest. This includes the fingernails and lips and the mucous membranes of the mouth and conjunctiva. In dark-skinned people, evaluate the sclera, conjunctiva, lips, nail beds, soles, and palms. Note any discoloration caused by vascular changes underneath the skin. Petechiae are small, round, flat, purplish spots caused by capillary bleeding from a variety of etiologies. Ecchymosis is a blue-black bruise resulting from trauma or bleeding disorders. Jaundice first appears in the sclera and then, in the late stages of liver disease, all over the skin. If only your patient's palms, soles, and face are yellow, he may have carotanemia, a harmless nutritional condition caused by eating a diet high in carrots and yellow vegetables or fruits.

Moisture Inspect and palpate the skin for dryness, increased sweating, and excessive oiliness. Dry skin, common during the cold winter months and in the elderly, may be the result of other conditions. Excessive oiliness, especially where the sebaceous glands are concentrated in the face, neck, back, chest, and buttocks, may suggest acne or hyperthyroidism. Increased sweating may indicate a sympathetic nervous system response to anxiety, fear, or exertion.

Temperature Use the backs of your fingers to feel the skin temperature in several different locations. Compare symmetrical body areas. Generalized warming or cooling suggests an environmental, infectious, or thyroid problem. Localized warmth may indicate bleeding or swelling.

Texture Feel your patient's skin. Is it rough or smooth? Are there large patches or small areas of scaling? Observe the skin's thickness. Thin and fragile skin is a sign of debilitating disease in the elderly. Thick skin often occurs with eczema and psoriasis. Inspect the palms and soles for calluses.

Mobility and Turgor Test the skin's **turgor** and elasticity by picking up a fold of skin over a bony prominence and then releasing it. Normal skin immediately returns to its original state. Poor turgor (tenting) results from dehydration. Test the skin's mobility by moving it over the bony prominence. Decreased mobility suggests edema or scleroderma, a progressive skin disease.

✱ **turgor** normal tension in the skin.

Lesions A skin **lesion** is any disruption in normal tissue. Skin lesions are classified as vascular, involving a blood vessel (Figure 2-16); primary, arising from previously

✱ **lesion** any disruption in normal tissue.

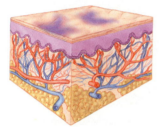

Purpura – Reddish-purple blotches, diameter more than 0.5 cm

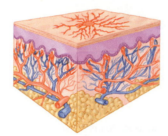

Spider angioma – Reddish legs radiate from red spot

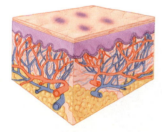

Petechiae – Reddish-purple spots, diameter less than 0.5 cm

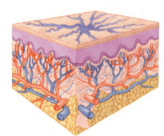

Venous star – Bluish legs radiate from blue center

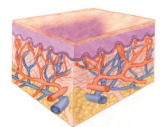

Ecchymoses – Reddish-purple blotch, size varies

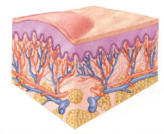

Capillary hemangioma – Irregular red spots

FIGURE 2-16 Vascular skin lesions.

normal skin (Figure 2-17); or secondary, resulting from changes in primary lesions (Figure 2-18). Skin lesions can take any shape, color, or arrangement. Note their anatomical location and distribution. Are they generalized or localized? Do they involve exposed surfaces or areas that fold over? Do they relate to possible irritants such as wristbands, bracelets, necklaces? Are they linear, clustered, circular, or dermatomal (following a sensory nerve pathway)? What type are they? Inspect and feel all skin lesions carefully. Skin tumors are another variety of skin lesion. These include basal cell and squamous cell carcinomas, malignant melanomas, Kaposi's sarcoma in AIDS, actinic keratosis, and seborrheic keratosis.

When you detect a skin lesion, use anatomical landmarks to describe its exact location on the skin's surface. Describe its shape in terms such as oval, spherical, irregular, or tubular. Sometimes sketching an outline of the lesion is helpful. Record the size of the mass in centimeters, carefully measuring its length, width, and depth. Describe the consistency of the mass exactly as it feels to you (for instance, soft, firm, edematous, cystic, or nodular). Of particular concern is its mobility. If the mass is affixed to a specific structure, suspect a malignancy. Note any pain or tenderness surrounding the mass upon palpation. Pulsation in the mass is another significant finding. For example, a mass that pulsates in all directions suggests an aneurysm.

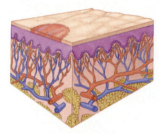

Macule – Flat spot, color varies from white to brown or from red to purple, diameter less than 1 cm

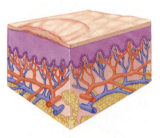

Plaque – Superficial papule, diameter more than 1 cm, rough texture

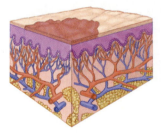

Patch – Irregular flat macule, diameter greater than 1 cm

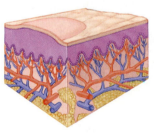

Wheal – Pink, irregular spot varying in size and shape

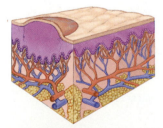

Papule – Elevated firm spot, color varies from brown to red or from pink to purplish red, diameter less than 1 cm

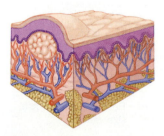

Nodule – Elevated firm spot, diameter 1–2 cm

FIGURE 2-17   Primary skin lesions.

THE HAIR

Hair is a tactile sensory organ, while also playing a role in sexual stimulation and attraction. It covers the entire body except the palms, soles, and parts of the sex organs. Hair develops from the base of the hair follicle, where it is nourished by the papilla, a vast capillary network. An involuntary arrector pili muscle fiber attaches to the base of the hair shaft. When these arrectores pilorum contract, the hair stands erect and goose bumps appear on the skin.

The two types of hair are vellus and terminal. Vellus hair is short, fine, and lacking pigment (similar to "peach fuzz"). Terminal hair is coarser, thicker, and pigmented. It appears on the eyebrows and scalp, in the armpits and groin of both sexes, and on the faces and bodies of males.

With aging the hair turns gray from a decrease in pigmentation and its growth declines. A transition from terminal to vellus hair on the scalp causes baldness in both men and women. The opposite occurs in the nares and ears of men, where terminal hair replaces vellus hair. Both genders generally experience a decrease in body hair as they age. Loss of the lateral third of the eyebrow is also normal in the elderly.

Inspect and palpate the hair, noting its color, quality, distribution, quantity, and texture. Is there hair loss? Is there a pattern to the loss? Patients undergoing

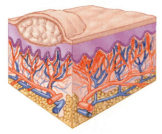

Tumor – Elevated solid, diameter more than 2 cm, may be same color as skin

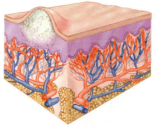

Pustule – Elevated area, diameter less than 1 cm, contains purulent fluid

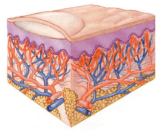

Vesicle – Elevated area, diameter less than 1 cm, contains serous fluid

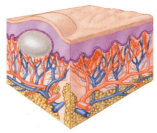

Cyst – Elevated, palpable area containing liquid or viscous matter

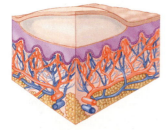

Bulla – Vesicle with diameter more than 1 cm

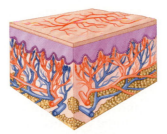

Telangiectasia – Red, threadlike line

FIGURE 2-17 (CONTINUED)   Primary skin lesions.

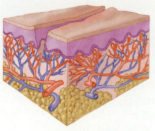

Fissure – Linear red crack ranging into dermis

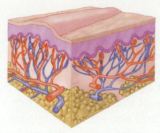

Scar – Fibrous, depth varies, color ranges from white to red

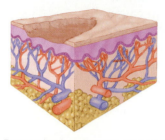

Erosion – Depression in epidermis, caused by tissue loss

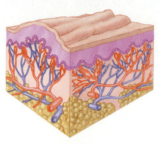

Keloid – Elevated scar, irregular shape, larger than original wound

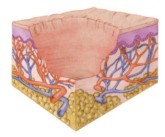

Ulcer – Red or purplish depression ranging into dermis, caused by tissue loss

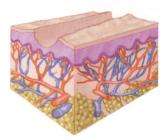

Excoriation – Linear, may be hollow or crusted, caused by loss of epidermis leaving dermis exposed

FIGURE 2-18   Secondary skin lesions.

chemotherapy for cancer may experience generalized hair loss. Failure to develop normal hair growth during puberty may indicate a pituitary or hormonal problem. Abnormal facial hair growth in women (hirsutism) also may indicate a hormonal imbalance. Part the hair in several places and palpate the scalp (Figure 2-19). A normal scalp is clean with no scaling, lesions, redness, lumps, or tenderness. Dandruff is characterized by mild flaking, psoriasis by heavy scaling, and seborrheic dermatitis by a greasy scaling. Try to differentiate the flaking of dandruff from the nits (eggs) of lice. Dandruff flakes off the hair easily, while nits firmly attach themselves to the hair shaft.

Feel the hair texture. In white people a soft hair texture is normal; in black people a coarser texture is normal. Very dry, brittle, or fragile hair is abnormal. Inspect and palpate the eyebrows. Note the quality and distribution of the hair and any scaling of the underlying skin. When assessing hair remember that the normal quantity and distribution of hair is related to gender and racial group. For instance, men have more trunk and body hair than women. Native American men have less facial and body hair than white men. In addition, Caucasians have more abundant and coarser body hair than Asians.

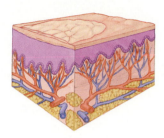

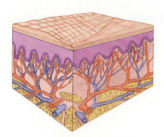

Scale – Elevated area of excessive exfoliation, varies in thickness, shape, and dryness, and ranges in color from white to silver or tan

Lichenification – Thickening and hardening of epidermis with emphasized lines in skin, resembles lichen

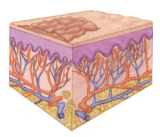

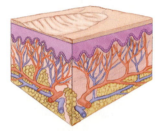

Crust – Reddish, brown, black, tan, or yellowish dried blood, serum, or pus

Atrophy – Skin surface thins and markings disappear, semitransparent parchment-like appearance

FIGURE 2-18 (CONTINUED)   Secondary skin lesions.

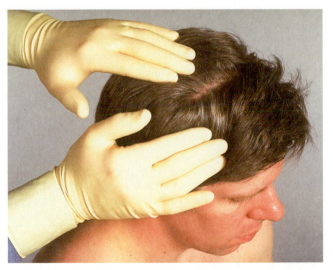

FIGURE 2-19   Inspect and palpate your patient's hair and scalp.

THE NAILS

Nails are found at the most distal ends of fingers and toes and are primarily for protection. Nails are strong yet flexible and provide a sharp edge for scratching, scraping, and clawing. They are made up of the nail plate, the nail bed, the proximal nail fold, and the nail root (Figure 2-20). The angle between the proximal nail fold and the nail plate should be less than 180°. Fingernails grow approximately 0.1 mm daily, slightly faster in the summertime. The nail plate lies on a highly vascular nail bed that gives the nail a pink appearance. Nail edges should

FIGURE 2-20 The nail.

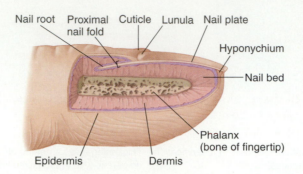

Nail root · Proximal nail fold · Cuticle · Lunula · Nail plate · Hyponychium · Nail bed · Phalanx (bone of fingertip) · Epidermis · Dermis

Table 2-3	ABNORMAL NAIL FINDINGS
Condition	**Description**
Clubbing	Clubbing occurs when normal connective tissue and capillaries increase the angle between the plate and proximal nail to greater than 180 degrees. The distal phalanx of each finger is rounded and bulbous. The proximal nail feels spongy. This is caused by the chronic hypoxia found in cardiopulmonary diseases and lung cancer.
Paronychia	This is an inflammation of the proximal and lateral nail folds. It may be acute or chronic. The folds appear red and swollen, and tender. The cuticle may not be visible. People who frequently immerse their hands in water are susceptible.
Onycholysis	The nail bed separates from the nail plate. It begins distally and enlarges the free edge of the nail. There are many causes, including hyperthyroidism.
Terry's nails	These appear as a mostly whitish nail with a band of reddish-brown at the distal nail tip. This may be seen in aging and with people suffering from liver cirrhosis, congestive heart failure, and diabetes.
White spots	Trauma to the nail often results in white spots that grow out with the nail. They often follow the curvature of the cuticle and can be the result of overzealous manicuring.
Transverse white lines	These are lines that parallel the lunula, rather than the cuticle. They may appear following a severe illness. They appear from under the proximal nail folds and grow out with the nail.
Psoriasis	These appear as small pits in the nails and may be an early sign of psoriasis.
Beau's lines	These are transverse depressions in the nails and are associated with severe illness. As with the Transverse white lines, they form under the nail fold and grow out with the nail. You may be able to estimate the timing or length of an illness by the location of the line.

be smooth and rounded. The nail plates should be smooth, flat, or slightly curved and should feel hard and uniformly thick. As we age, nail growth diminishes because of decreased peripheral circulation. The nails, especially the toenails, become hard, thick, brittle, and yellowish.

Inspect and palpate the fingernails and toenails. Observe the color beneath the transparent nail. Normally it is pink in Caucasians and black or brown in blacks. Note if the nails appear blue-black or purple, brown, or yellow-gray. Look for lesions, ridging, grooves, depressions, and pitting (Table 2-3). Depressions that appear in all nails are usually caused by a systemic disease. Gently squeeze the nail between your thumb and forefinger to test for adherence to the nail bed. A boggy nail suggests the clubbing seen in systemic cardiorespiratory diseases. The condition of the fingernails also can provide important insight into your patient's self care and hygiene. Check the toenails for any deformity or injury such as being ingrown.

THE HEAD

The scalp consists of five layers of tissue: <u>S</u>kin, <u>C</u>onnective tissue, <u>A</u>poneurosis, <u>L</u>oose tissue, and <u>P</u>eriosteum. You can remember their names with the convenient acronym, SCALP. The scalp is extremely vascular, as it protects and insulates the skull and sensitive brain tissue. When injured, it can bleed profusely.

The skull consists of the cranium and the face. The cranium comprises the frontal, parietal, temporal, occipital, ethmoid, and sphenoid bones and is covered by the scalp (Figure 2-21). The bones of the skull fuse at their sutures. The face includes the nasal bones, maxillary bones, lacrimal bones, zygomatic bones, the palate, the inferior nasal concha, and the vomer (Figure 2-22). The facial bones have air-filled compartments called sinuses and have cavities for the eyes, mouth, and nose (Figure 2-23). The movable mandible joins the skull at the temporomandibular joint (TMJ). The TMJ is in the depression just in front of the ear. It allows you to open and close your mouth and to jut your jaw forward. A variety of muscles gives the face its contour and general shape. Although facial characteristics vary according to race, gender, and body build, the skull and face should appear symmetrical.

You can also examine the skull when you inspect and palpate the scalp and hair. Look for any wounds or active bleeding. Observe the general size and contour of

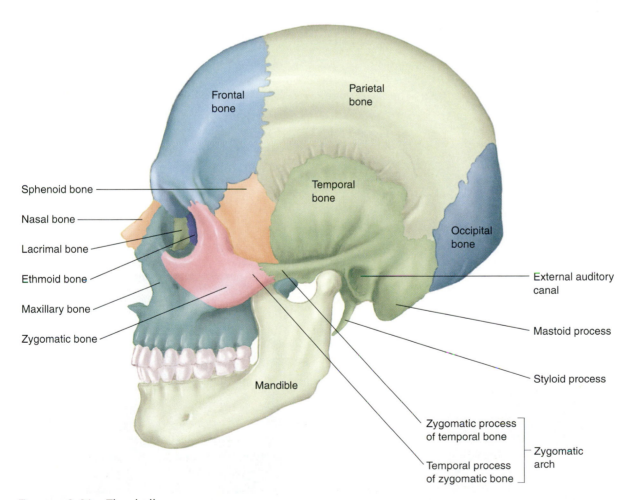

FIGURE 2-21   The skull.

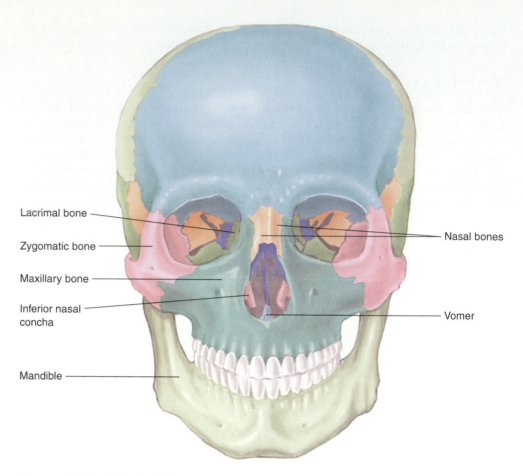

FIGURE 2-22 The facial bones.

Lacrimal bone

Zygomatic bone

Maxillary bone

Inferior nasal concha

Mandible

Nasal bones

Vomer

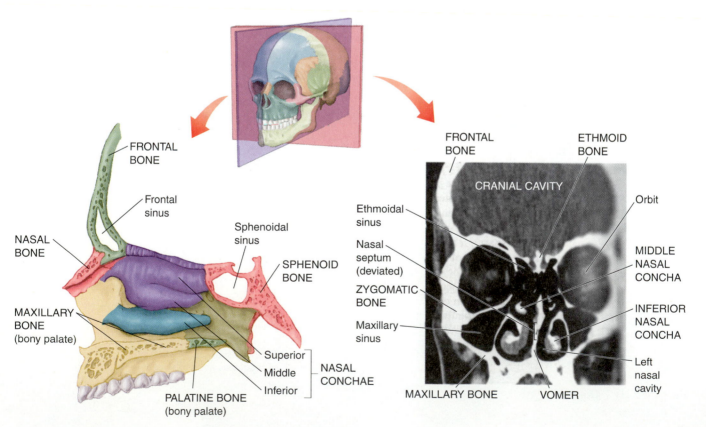

FRONTAL BONE

Frontal sinus

NASAL BONE

MAXILLARY BONE (bony palate)

Sphenoidal sinus

SPHENOID BONE

Superior

Middle

Inferior

NASAL CONCHAE

PALATINE BONE (bony palate)

FRONTAL BONE

ETHMOID BONE

CRANIAL CAVITY

Ethmoidal sinus

Nasal septum (deviated)

ZYGOMATIC BONE

Maxillary sinus

MAXILLARY BONE

VOMER

Orbit

MIDDLE NASAL CONCHA

INFERIOR NASAL CONCHA

Left nasal cavity

FIGURE 2-23 The sinuses.

the skull. Palpate the cranium from front to back (Procedure 2-2a on page 62). It should be symmetrical and smooth. Note any tenderness or deformities (depressions or protrusions). An indentation in the skull may suggest a depressed skull fracture. Note any areas of unusual warmth.

Inspect the face. Is it symmetrical? Are there any involuntary movements? Note any masses or edema. Observe the bony orbits of the eye for periorbital ecchymosis, a bluish discoloration also known as "raccoon eyes." Also check the mastoid process for discoloration (Procedure 2-2b). These are classic signs of a basilar skull fracture. They normally will not appear on the scene but will present hours after the injury occurs. Palpate the facial bones for stability and note any crepitus or loose fragments (Procedure 2-2c). Note whether your patient's facial expressions change appropriately with his mood.

Evaluate the TMJ. Place the tip of your index finger into the depression in front of the tragus (the cartilaginous projection just in front of the ear's outer opening) and ask your patient to open his mouth (Procedure 2-2d). The tips of your fingers should drop into the joint space. Palpate the joint for tenderness, swelling, and range of motion. Sometimes, you may hear a clicking or snapping. This is neither unusual nor problematic unless it is accompanied by pain, swelling, and crepitus. Test for range of motion by asking your patient to open and close his mouth, jut and retract his jaw, and move it from side to side. Finally, assess the skin of the face for color, pigmentation, texture, thickness, hair distribution, and lesions.

THE EYES

The eyes comprise external and internal parts. The external eye consists of the eyelid, conjunctiva, lacrimal gland, ocular muscles, and the bony skull orbit (Figure 2-24). The lacrimal glands, in the temporal region of the superior eyelid, produce tears that moisten the eye. The eyelids distribute the tears over the eye's surface. They also regulate the amount of light entering the eye and protect it from foreign bodies. The eyelashes extend from the eyelid's border. The conjunctiva is a thin membrane that covers the anterior surface of the eye and the inside of the eyelid. It protects the eye from foreign bodies. The ocular muscles control eye movement and are innervated by three cranial nerves: the oculomotor (CN-III), trochlear (CN-IV), and abducens (CN-VI) (Figure 2-25).

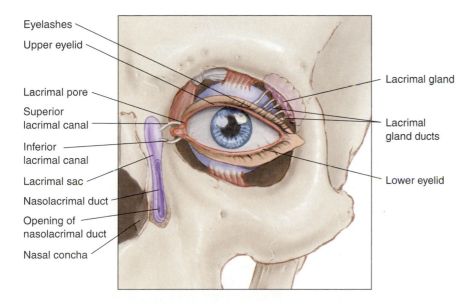

FIGURE 2-24   The external eye.

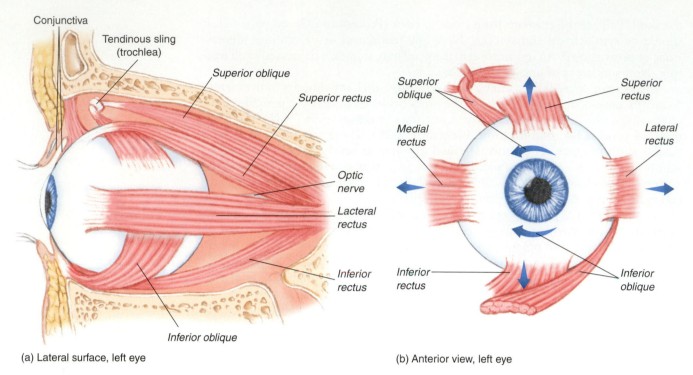

Conjunctiva

Tendinous sling (trochlea)

Superior oblique

Superior rectus

Optic nerve

Lacteral rectus

Inferior rectus

Inferior oblique

(a) Lateral surface, left eye

Superior oblique

Medial rectus

Inferior rectus

Superior rectus

Lateral rectus

Inferior oblique

(b) Anterior view, left eye

FIGURE 2-25   The extraocular muscles.

The internal eye consists of the sclera, cornea, iris, lens, and retina (Figure 2-26). The sclera, the white of the eye, is a dense, avascular structure that gives physical shape to the eyeball. The cornea separates the watery fluid in the anterior chamber from the external environment. It also permits light to enter the lens and reach the retina. The iris is a circular, contractile muscle; its pigment produces the color of the eye. The opening in the center of the iris is the pupil. The iris controls the amount of light reaching the retina by constricting and dilating. It is innervated by the optic nerve (CN-II), which senses light, and by the oculomotor nerve (CN-III), which constricts the pupil. The lens is a cellular structure immediately behind the iris. It is convex and transparent, allowing images to focus onto the retina. The retina is the sensory network of the eye. It transforms light rays into electrical impulses that the optic nerve transmits to the brain. Besides the optic nerve, the ophthalmic artery and vein provide necessary circulation to and from the eye. Accurate vision depends on these components' functioning effectively.

The ideal environment for an eye exam is a quiet room, free from distractions, in which you can control the lighting and make your patient comfortable. First, test for visual acuity. Place your patient 20 feet from a **visual acuity wall chart** or have him hold a **visual acuity card** 14 inches from his face. Ask him to cover one eye with a card and begin reading the lines (Procedure 2-3a on page 62). Record the visual acuity grade next to the smallest line in which he can read at least one half of the letters. The result is written as a fraction. The first number represents the distance away from the chart. The second number is the distance from which a normal eye could read the line. Normal is 20/20. A result of 20/70 means that a normal eye could read the line from 70 feet away but your patient could only read it from 20 feet. If no chart is available, you can have your patient count your raised fingers, read from a distance something you have printed, or distinguish light from dark. This type of exam is routinely conducted as part of a comprehensive physical exam in a clinic setting.

Test the visual fields by confrontation. Sit directly in front of your patient. Have him cover his left eye while you cover your right eye. Ask him to look at your nose. Extend your left arm to the side and slowly bring it toward you. Ask your patient to say when he first sees your finger. Use your own peripheral vision

✱ **visual acuity wall chart/card** wall chart or handheld card with lines of letters used to test vision.

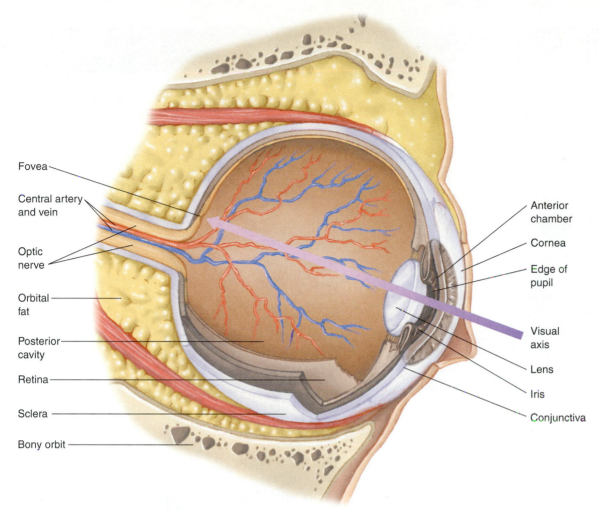

Fovea

Central artery and vein

Optic nerve

Orbital fat

Posterior cavity

Retina

Sclera

Bony orbit

Anterior chamber

Cornea

Edge of pupil

Visual axis

Lens

Iris

Conjunctiva

FIGURE 2-26   The internal eye.

VISUAL FIELD ABNORMALITIES

Horizontal defect

Blind eye

Bitemporal hemianopsia

Homonymous hemianopsia

Homonymous quadrantic defect

Left   Right

FIGURE 2-27   Visual field abnormalities.

as a guide. If he sees your finger when you do, his visual field is grossly normal in that direction. Do this test in all four quadrants (left and right, up and down). Then perform the same test with the other eye (Procedure 2-3b). Any abnormalities suggest a defect in peripheral vision. Some common abnormalities include a horizontal defect (loss of vision in the upper or lower half of an eye), a blind eye, bitemporal hemianopsia (loss of vision in the outside half of each eye), left or right homonymous hemianopsia (loss of vision in the right half of both eyes or the left half of both eyes), or homonymous quadrantic defect (loss of vision in the same quadrant of both eyes). Record the area of defect as illustrated in Figure 2-27.

Procedure 2-2   Examining the Head

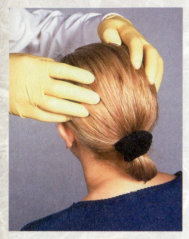

2–2a   Palpate the cranium from front to back.

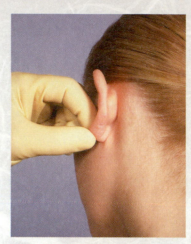

2–2b   Inspect the mastoid process.

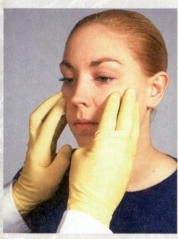

2–2c   Palpate the facial bones.

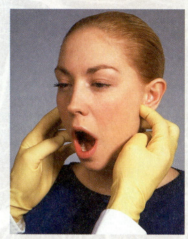

2–2d   Palpate the TMJ.

Procedure 2-3   Examining the Eyes

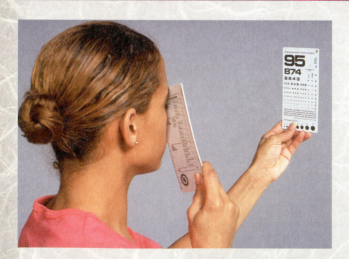

2-3a   Use a visual acuity chart to test visual acuity.

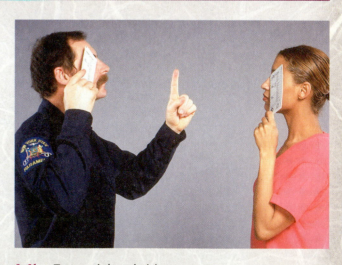

2-3b   Test peripheral vision.

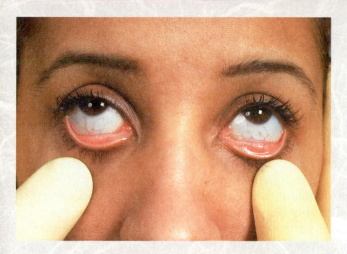

2-3c   Inspect the external eye.

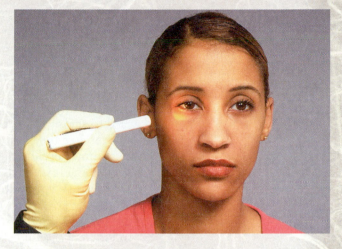

2-3d   Test the pupil's reaction to light.

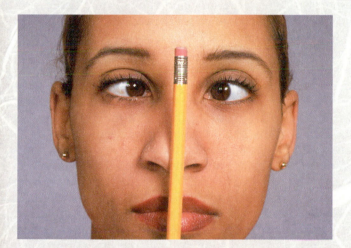

2-3e   Test for accommodation.

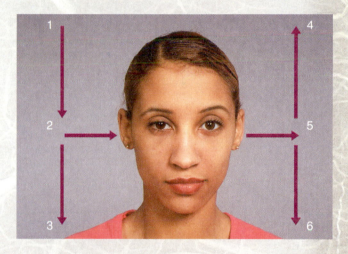

2-3f   Move your finger in an *H* pattern to test your patient's extraocular muscles.

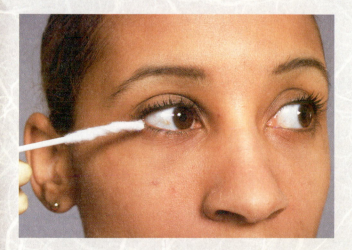

2-3g   Check the corneal reflex.

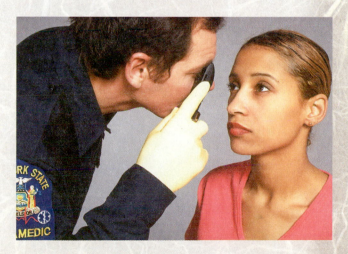

2-3h   Visualize the interior eye with an ophthalmoscope.

Now examine the external eyes. Place yourself directly in front of your patient. Inspect his eyes for symmetry in size, shape, and contour. Do they look alike? Do they protrude (proptosis)? Are they properly aligned? Note the eyelids' position relative to the eyeballs. They should cover the upper quarter of the iris. Are the eyes totally exposed or do the eyelids droop (ptosis)? Have your patient close his eyes. Do they close completely? Do you see any edema, inflammation, or mass? Note the eyelid's color. It should be pink, indicating good central oxygenation. If the lid is pale, your patient could be in shock or anemic. If cyanotic, he could have central hypoxemia. Are there any lesions?

Carefully observe the lids' shape and inspect their contours for any growths. If you see any drainage, note its color and consistency. Do the eyelashes turn inward to scrape against the eyeball or outward to prevent the complete closure of the eye? Are they clean and free from debris? Is there a stye (reddened swelling of the inner eyelid)? Quickly assess the regions of the lacrimal sacs and glands for swelling, excessive tearing, or dryness of the eyes.

Now ask your patient to look up while you pull down both lower eyelids to inspect the sclera and conjunctiva (Procedure 2-3c). Be careful not to put pressure on the eyeball. Ask your patient to look left and right, up and down. The conjunctiva should be clear and transparent, with no redness or cloudiness. Redness or a cobblestone appearance suggests an allergic or infectious conjunctivitis. Bright red blood in a sharply defined area surrounded by normal tissue, not extending into the iris, indicates a hemorrhage under the conjunctiva. Look for any nodules, swelling, or discharge. The normal sclera is white. A yellow sclera suggests the jaundice of liver disease.

With an oblique light source, inspect each cornea for opacities. Also check the lens for opacities that you may see through the pupil. Inspect the iris when you inspect the cornea. Shine the light directly from the lateral side and look for a crescent-shaped shadow on the medial side of the iris. Since the iris is flat, the light should cast no shadow. A shadow could suggest glaucoma, caused by a blockage that restricts aqueous humor from leaving the anterior chamber. This increases intraocular pressure and threatens your patient's eyesight.

Inspect the size, shape, and symmetry of the pupils. Are they unusually large (excessive dilation) or unusually small (excessive constriction)? Are they equal? Some patients (20%) have unequal pupils, a condition known as anisocoria; if the difference in the pupil's size is less than two millimeters and they react normally to light, anisocoria is benign. To test the pupils, first shine a light into one eye and observe that eye's reaction (Procedure 2-3d). This tests the eye's direct response. The pupil should constrict. Repeat this test for the other eye. Now shine a light into one eye and observe the other eye's reaction. This tests the eye's consensual response. Both eyes should react simultaneously to the light. Repeat this test for the other eye.

Normal pupils react to light briskly. A sluggish pupil suggests pressure on the oculomotor nerve (CN-III) from increased intracranial pressure. Bilateral sluggishness may indicate global hypoxia to the brain tissue or an adverse drug reaction. Constricted pupils suggest an opiate overdose, whereas fixed and dilated pupils usually mean brain death.

Now have your patient focus on an object in the distance. Then, ask him to focus on an object right in front of him. As he focuses on the near object, his pupils should constrict (near response). Now have your patient follow your finger or a pen, pencil, or similar object as you move it from a distance to the bridge of his nose (Procedure 2-3e). His eyes should converge on the object as the pupils constrict (accommodation). Finally, have your patient follow your finger as you move it in an *H* pattern in front of him (Procedure 2-3f). This tests the integrity of the extraocular muscles. Normal eye movements to follow your finger will be conjugate (together). Nystagmus is a fine jerking of the eyes; it may be normal if noted at the far extremes of the test. Check the corneal reflex by touching the eye gently with a strand of cotton and watch for your patient to blink (Procedure 2-3g).

Using an ophthalmoscope, visualize the eye's anterior chamber for cells, blood (hyphema), and pus (hypopyon) (Procedure 2-3h). Also visualize the retina, blood vessels, and optic nerve. Look for foreign bodies under the eyelid or in the cornea, check the cornea for lacerations, abrasions, and infection, and examine the vitreous humor. Look also for cataracts, papilledema caused by increased intracranial pressure, arterial and venous occlusions, and retinal hemorrhages, common clinical conditions you can visualize with an ophthalmoscope. Examining the eye's interior with an ophthalmoscope is a detailed process that is very difficult to master; it requires skill and practice.

Examining the eye's interior with an ophthalmoscope is a detailed process that is very difficult to master and requires skill and practice.

THE EARS

The ear has three components: the outer ear, the middle ear, and the inner ear (Figure 2-28). The outer ear consists of the auricle, the ear canal (external acoustic meatus), and the lateral surface of the tympanic membrane (eardrum). The auricle is the visible, skin-covered cartilage that extends outward from the skull. It comprises the helix (the prominent outer rim), the antihelix, (the inner rim) the lobe (which contains no cartilage), the concha (the deep cavity containing the opening to the ear canal), and the tragus (the protuberance that lies just in front of the concha).

Behind the ear lies the mastoid process of the temporal bone. It functions as an attachment for the sternocleidomastoid muscle and is palpable just behind the earlobe. The mastoid bone contains air-filled cells that are continuous with the middle ear. This is why an inner ear infection (otitis) often presents with tenderness in the mastoid area. The ear canal opens behind the tragus and is approximately 2-3 cm long in adults. Hair and sebaceous glands that produce wax (cerumen) line the distal third of the canal. At the end of the ear canal, the translucent tympanic membrane separates the ear canal from the middle ear.

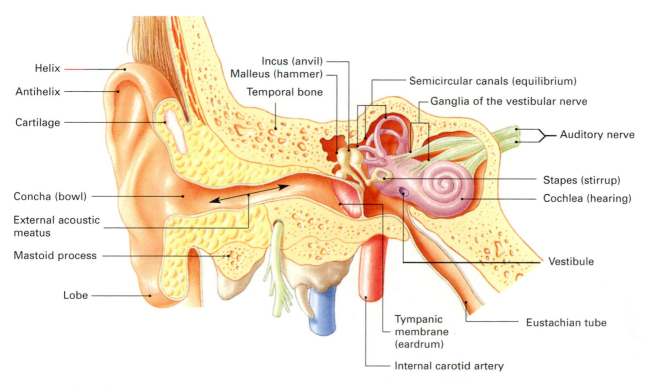

FIGURE 2-28 The ear.

The middle ear, an air-filled cavity in the temporal bone, begins with the medial surface of the tympanic membrane. It contains three small bones known as ossicles (the malleus, the incus, and the stapes) that transmit and amplify sound from the tympanic membrane to the inner ear. The irregularly shaped malleus connects directly to the medial surface of the tympanic membrane at the umbo. It pulls the eardrum inward, making it concave. A "cone of light" is visible here during otoscopy. A light shined on the translucent eardrum makes the middle ear somewhat visible. The eustachian tubes help move mucous from the middle ear to the nasopharynx. They also help equalize the pressure between the outside air and the middle ear during swallowing, sneezing, and yawning.

The inner ear cavity contains the vestibule, the semicircular canals, and the cochlea. The cochlea is a coiled structure that transmits sound to the acoustic nerve (CN-VIII). Hearing involves air conduction of vibrations from the environment to the tympanic membrane. These vibrations are transmitted through the eardrum to the ossicles and to the cochlea, which translates them into nerve impulses. The acoustic nerve transmits these nerve impulses to the brain. The labyrinth within the inner ear helps us maintain our balance by sensing the position and movement of our head. It also is innervated by the acoustic nerve.

Begin examining the external ears from in front of your patient. Are they symmetrical? Then examine each ear separately. Inspect the auricles for size, shape, symmetry, landmarks, color, and position on the head. Observe the surrounding area for deformities, lumps, skin lesions, tenderness, and erythema (redness). Pull the helix upward and outward and note any tenderness or discomfort (Procedure 2-4a on page 68). Press on the tragus and on the mastoid process (Procedure 2-4b). Pain or tenderness in any of these areas suggests infection such as otitis or mastoiditis. Discoloration in this area is known as Battle's sign, a common, but late, finding in a basilar skull fracture. An earache may arise from the ear itself or be referred from another place through adjoining and shared sensory nerve pathways. Sources of referred pain may include sinus problems, a bad tooth, temporomandibular joint pain, the common cold, a sore throat, and the cervical spine.

Inspect for discharge (otorrhea) from the ear canal (Procedure 2-4c). The discharge may contain mucus, pus, blood, or cerebrospinal fluid that may have leaked from the skull through a fracture in its base. Injuries to the ear itself can result from blunt trauma to the side of the head, causing temporary or permanent damage to the outer or middle ear. A ruptured eardrum can result from sticking a sharp object into the ear canal or from a pressure wave caused by an explosion.

Check hearing acuity by having your patient close one ear. Test the open ear by whispering, then speaking, in its direction (Procedure 2-4d). Repeat this test for the other ear. Hearing loss can result from many causes. These include trauma, accumulation of debris (particularly cerumen, or "wax") in the ear canal, tympanic membrane rupture, certain drugs, previous surgery, or even prolonged exposure to loud noise. Tinnitus is the perception of abnormal noise in the ear. It usually presents as a buzzing or ringing and is associated with some degree of hearing loss.

Visualize the inner ear canal and tympanic membrane using an otoscope. Attach to the otoscope the largest speculum that will fit into your patient's ear canal. Hold the otoscope either upward or downward. To enter the canal, first tilt your patient's head slightly away from you. Grasp the auricle gently and pull slightly up and backward to straighten the external canal (Procedure 2-4e). Insert the speculum gently and examine the ear canal for cerumen, discharge, redness, lesions, perforations, and foreign bodies.

Now focus farther back on the eardrum itself and note its color. The tympanic membrane should be a pearly, translucent gray. A change in color suggests a middle ear or tympanic membrane abnormality such as fluid or infection behind the eardrum. Observe the landmarks of the drum. You will need to move the scope around to visualize the drum's entirety. Begin with the light reflection

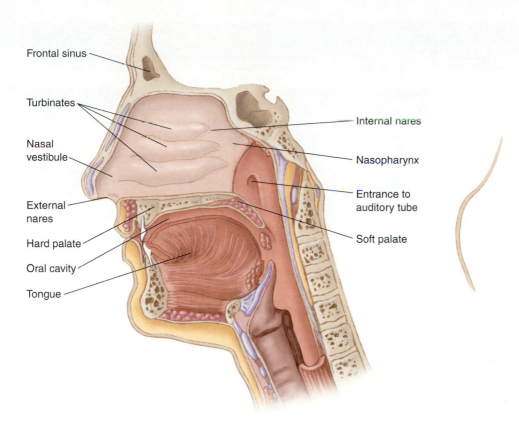

Frontal sinus

Turbinates

Nasal vestibule

External nares

Hard palate

Oral cavity

Tongue

Internal nares

Nasopharynx

Entrance to auditory tube

Soft palate

FIGURE 2-29   The nose.

in the anterior inferior quadrant. It should be sharp and bright. Then, check the center of the drum for bulging or protractions. Note the long process of the malleus. Finally move to the rim of the drum. Follow along the drum's perimeter and look for perforations from a ruptured tympanic membrane.

THE NOSE

The external nose comprises the nasal bones and cartilage covered by skin. The nares are the anterior openings in the nose. A cartilaginous bony septum divides the left and right nasal cavities. The turbinates, or conchae, are bony ridges on the medial surface of the nose (Figure 2-29). They create a turbulence to help clean, warm, and humidify the inspired air. Coarse nose hair, the turbinates, and the highly vascular and mucus-producing membrane make up the respiratory system's initial filtration system. The mucous membrane is comprised of mucus-producing glands and cells that moisten the inner respiratory tract.

The paranasal sinuses are air-filled extensions of the nasal cavities in the frontal, maxillary, ethmoid, and sphenoid bones (Figure 2-30). They are lined with mucous membranes and with cilia, fine hairlike projections that move secretions along pathways opening into the oral and nasal cavities. The sinuses help insulate the sensitive brain and provide the vocal resonance that is conspicuously absent during a bad head cold.

Check your patient's nose from the front and from the side and note any deviation in shape or color. Also note any nasal flaring, an indication of respiratory distress. Palpate the external nose for depressions, deformities, and tenderness (Procedure 2-5a on page 69).

To inspect the nose's internal structures, tilt your patient's head back slightly. Insert the speculum of your otoscope and check the nasal septum for deviation and

Procedure 2-4   Examining the Ears

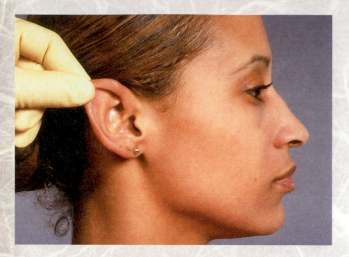

2-4a   Examine the external ear.

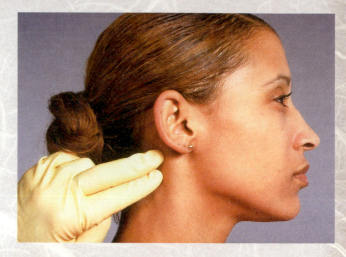

2-4b   Press on the mastoid process.

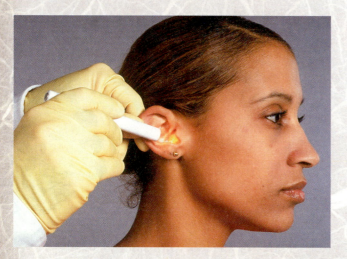

2-4c   Inspect the ear canal for drainage.

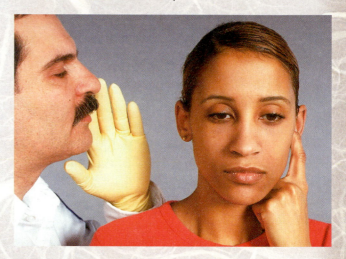

2-4d   Whisper in your patient's ear.

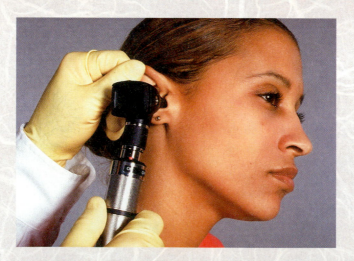

2-4e   Visualize the inner ear canal and tympanic membrane.

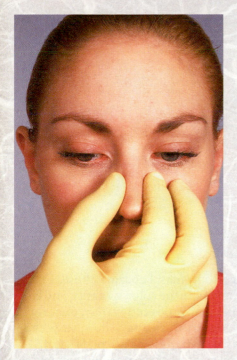

2-5a   Palpate the external nose.

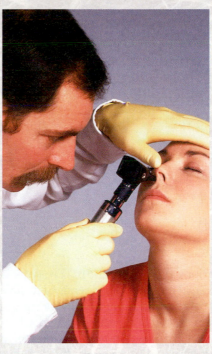

2-5b   Inspect the internal nose with an otoscope.

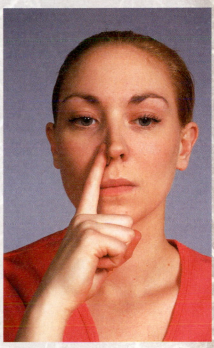

2-5c   Inspect the nose for nasal obstruction.

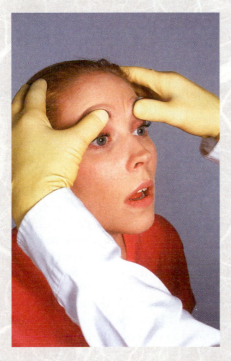

2-5d   Palpate the frontal sinus.

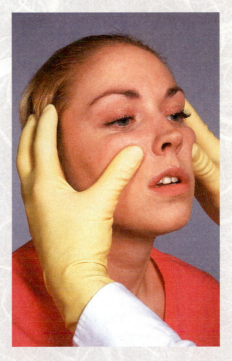

2-5e   Palpate the maxillary sinus.

FIGURE 2-30   The paranasal sinuses.

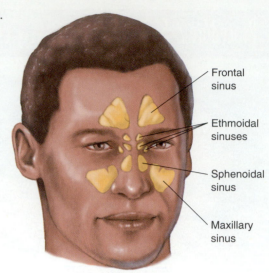

Frontal sinus

Ethmoidal sinuses

Sphenoidal sinus

Maxillary sinus

perforations (Procedure 2-5b). Erosions suggest intranasal cocaine abuse. Examine the nasal mucosa for evidence of drainage and note the color, quantity, and consistency of the discharge. Rhinitis (a runny nose) may produce a watery, clear fluid, as seen in seasonal allergies. If the discharge appears thick and yellow, suspect an infection. Epistaxis (a nosebleed) may be caused by trauma or a septal defect.

Test for nasal obstruction by occluding one side of the nose and having your patient breathe through the other side (Procedure 2-5c). It is normal for one side to be more patent than the other. A deviated septum, foreign body, excessive secretions, or mucosal edema may cause abnormal obstructions.

Inspect and palpate the frontal and maxillary sinuses for swelling and tenderness. To palpate the frontal sinus, press your thumbs upward, deep under the orbital ridges (Procedure 2-5d); to palpate the maxillary sinuses, press up under the zygomatic arches (cheeks) (Procedure 2-5e). You also can tap on each area for similar symptoms. Swelling or tenderness suggests a sinus infection or obstruction.

THE MOUTH

The lips mark the entrance to the mouth and play a role in the articulation of speech. The mouth houses the tongue, the gums (gingiva), and the teeth (Figure 2-31). The roof of the mouth is formed by the hard palate and the soft palate. The uvula is the peninsular extension of the soft palate that hangs in the back of the mouth. The oral cavity, lined with buccal (cheek/mouth) mucosa, is rich in mucous membranes. The parotid glands, just in front of the ears, and the submandibular glands, just beneath the mandible, secrete digestive enzymes and saliva into the oral cavity (Figure 2-32). The sublingual glands secrete enzymes just beneath the tongue. You can easily palpate these glands under the chin.

The tongue, a large, mobile muscle covered by mucous membranes, has many functions. It helps in chewing by keeping food on the teeth, and it assists in swallowing by moving the food into the oropharynx. It also contains the taste buds and is essential in forming words when we speak.

A highly vascular mucosa lines the gingiva, giving it a pink color. The teeth are anchored in bony sockets; only their white enamel-covered crowns are visible.

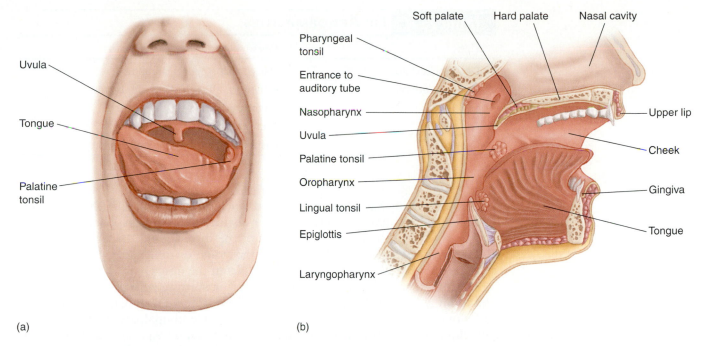

(a)

(b)

FIGURE 2-31 The mouth.

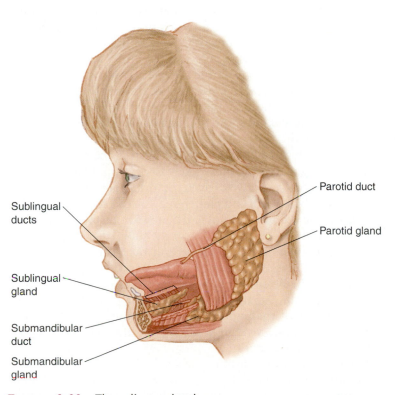

FIGURE 2-32 The salivary glands.

Table 2-4	LIP ABNORMALITIES
Lips	**Cause**
Dry, cracked lips	Dehydration, wind damage
Swelling/edema	Infection, allergic reaction, burns
Lesions	Infection, irritation, skin cancer
Pallor	Anemia, shock
Cyanosis	Respiratory or cardiac insufficiency

An adult normally has 32 permanent teeth, including incisors, canines, premolars, and molars. The pharynx consists of three distinct areas: the nasopharynx (behind the nasal cavity), the oropharynx (back of the throat), and the laryngopharynx (just above the epiglottis). At the back of the throat on either side, the tonsils help separate the oropharynx (food processing) from the nasopharynx (air passage).

Assess the mouth from anterior to posterior, starting with the lips. Note their condition and color. They should be pink, smooth, and symmetrical and devoid of lesions, swelling, lumps, cracks, or scaliness. Gently palpate the lips with the jaw closed and note any lesions, nodules, or fissures, especially at the corners (Procedure 2-6a on next page). Observe the undersurfaces of the upper and lower lips (Procedure 2-6b). They should be wet and smooth. Look for any of the lip abnormalities in Table 2-4.

To examine the mouth you will need a bright light and a tongue blade. Holding the tongue blade like a chopstick will give you good downward leverage. Examine the oral mucosa for color, ulcers, white patches, and nodules. The oral mucosa should appear pinkish-red, smooth, and moist. Note the color of the gums and teeth. The gums should be pink with a clearly defined margin surrounding each tooth. Inspect the teeth for color, shape, and position. Are any missing or loose? Suspect periodontal disease if the gums are swollen, bleed easily, and are separated from the teeth by large crevices that trap food. Use a tongue blade to move the lateral lip to one side while you examine the buccal mucosa and parotid glands (Procedure 2-6c). Note the buccal mucosa's color and texture.

Ask your patient to stick his tongue straight out and then to move it from side to side. Coating of the tongue indicates dehydration. Note its color and normally velvety surface. Hold the tongue with a 2″ × 2″ gauze pad and a gloved hand to manipulate it for inspection (Procedure 2-6d). Make sure to inspect the sides and bottom of the tongue because malignancies are more likely to develop there, especially in patients over age 50 who smoke, chew tobacco, or drink alcohol (Procedure 2-6e). The undersurface should be smooth and pink; often you can see the bluish discoloration of dilated veins or the yellowish tint of early jaundice. Inspect the floor of the mouth, the submandibular ducts, and the fold over the sublingual gland.

Now examine the normally white hard palate and the normally pink soft palate (Procedure 2-6f). Check them for texture and lesions. Observe the posterior pharyngeal wall. Press the blade down on the middle third of the tongue and have your patient say "aaaaahhhh." Examine the posterior pharynx, the palatine tonsils, and the movement of the uvula. Inspect the tonsils for color and symmetry. Look for exudate (pus), swelling, ulcers, or drainage. The uvula should move straight up with no deviation.

Note any odors from your patient's mouth. The smell of alcohol, feces (bowel obstruction), acetone (diabetic ketoacidosis), gastric contents, or the bitter-almond smell of cyanide poisoning may all provide important clues to your patient's problem. Also look for any fluids or unusual matter in your patient's mouth. For example, coffee-grounds-like material suggests an upper gastrointestinal (GI) bleed. Pink-tinged sputum indicates acute pulmonary edema, whereas a green or yellow

Pay special attention to anything in your patient's mouth that can eventually obstruct his upper airway.

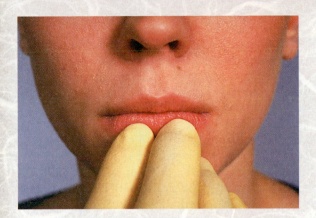

2-6a   Palpate the lips.

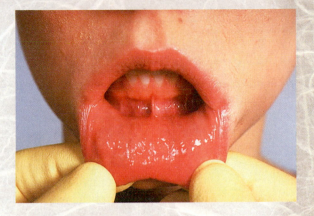

2-6b   Inspect the lips' undersurfaces.

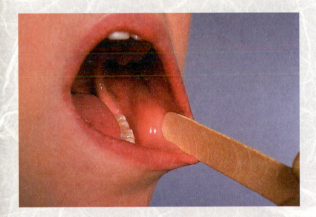

2-6c   Examine the buccal mucosa.

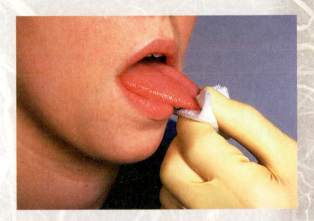

2-6d   Inspect the tongue using a gauze pad and a gloved hand.

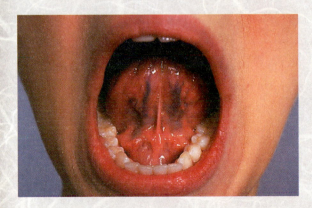

2-6e   Inspect under the tongue.

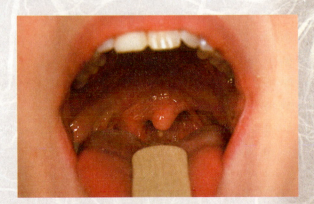

2-6f   Have your patient say "aaahhh" while you examine the soft palate and uvula.

phlegm suggests a respiratory infection. Pay special attention to anything in your patient's mouth that can eventually obstruct his upper airway, including dentures or missing teeth.

THE NECK

The neck houses many life-sustaining structures. It contains the spinal cord, blood vessels delivering blood to (carotid arteries) and from (jugular veins) the brain, and the conduits for air passage (larynx/trachea) into the lungs and food passage (esophagus) into the stomach. Any major disruption of these vital structures can cause rapid deterioration or immediate death. Especially during an emergency, examining the neck can be a critical part of your patient assessment.

From anterior to posterior, the thyroid gland, larynx and trachea, esophagus, and spinal column lie in the midline. The thyroid cartilage is the visible and palpable Adam's apple in the anterior neck midline (Figure 2-33). Just below it lie the cricoid cartilage and the rings of the trachea. The thyroid gland sits on both sides of the trachea, with its isthmus crossing the trachea. Between the thyroid cartilage and the large sternocleidomastoid muscles, the common carotid arteries extend toward the brain. The internal jugular veins are next to the carotids and are not visible. The external jugular veins extend diagonally across the surface of the sternocleidomastoid muscles and are clearly visible when they are distended or the patient is lying down. The lymph system helps drain fluid from the head and face and assists in fighting infection. A long chain of lymph nodes runs along the side of the neck, behind the ears, and under the chin (Figure 2-34). The nodes are palpable only when inflamed.

Briefly inspect your patient's neck for general symmetry and visible masses. Note any obvious deformity, deviation, tugging, masses, surgical scars, gland enlargement, or visible lymph nodes. Examine any penetrating injuries to the neck closely for damage to the trachea or major blood vessels; handle gently to avoid

Especially during an emergency, examining the neck can be a critical part of your patient assessment.

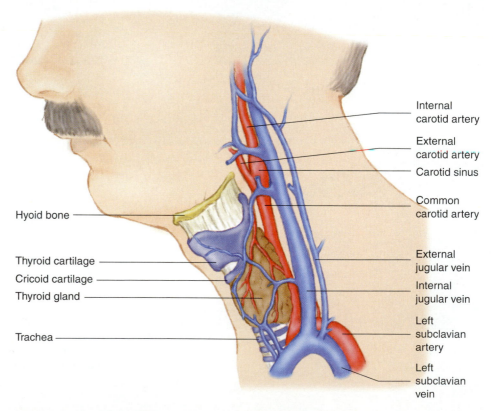

FIGURE 2-33   The neck.

Internal carotid artery

External carotid artery

Carotid sinus

Common carotid artery

External jugular vein

Internal jugular vein

Left subclavian artery

Left subclavian vein

Hyoid bone

Thyroid cartilage

Cricoid cartilage

Thyroid gland

Trachea

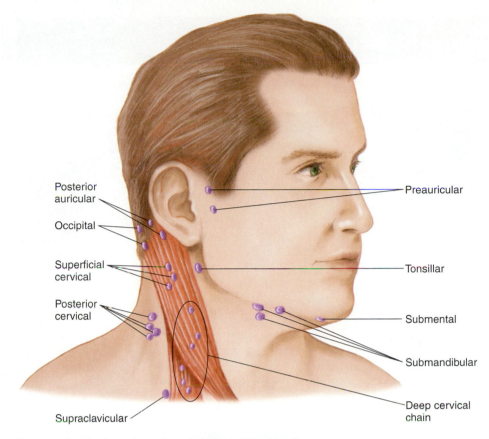

Posterior
auricular

Occipital

Superficial
cervical

Posterior
cervical

Supraclavicular

Preauricular

Tonsillar

Submental

Submandibular

Deep cervical
chain

FIGURE 2-34   Lymph nodes of the head and neck.

dislodging a clot that has halted bleeding. Immediately cover any open wounds
with an occlusive dressing to prevent air from entering a lacerated jugular vein
during inspiration. Look for jugular vein distention while your patient is sitting
upright and at a 45° degree incline.

Palpate the trachea for midline position (Procedure 2-7a on next page). Then
gently palpate the carotid arteries and note their rate and quality of their pulses.
(Procedure 2-7b). Now palpate the butterfly-shaped thyroid gland from behind
your patient. Rest your thumbs on his trapezius muscles and place two fingers of
each hand on the sides of the trachea just beneath the cricoid cartilage (Procedure 2-7c). Have your patient swallow and feel for the movement of the gland.
If you can feel it, it should be small, smooth, and free of nodules. Examining the
lymph nodes requires a systematic approach (Table 2-5). Using the pads of your

Table 2-5	LYMPH NODE EXAM
Node	**Exam**
Preauricular	Press on the tragus and "milk" anteriorly
Postauricular	Palpate on or under the mastoid process
Occipital	Palpate at the base of the skull lateral to the thick bands of muscle
Submental	Palpate at the base of the mandible under the chin
Submaxillary	Palpate along the underside of the jawline
Anterior cervical	Palpate anterior to the sternocleidomastoid muscle
Posterior cervical	Palpate posterior to the sternocleidomastoid muscle
Deep cervical	Encircle and palpate the sternocleidomastoid muscle
Supraclavicular	Palpate just above the clavicle in the deep groove

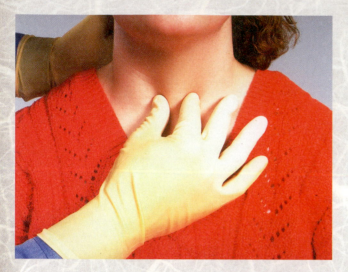

2-7a   Assess the trachea for midline position.

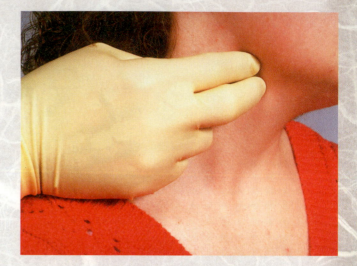

2-7b   Palpate the carotid arteries.

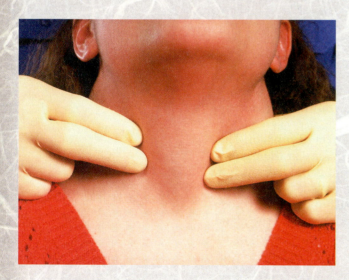

2-7c   Palpate the thyroid gland.

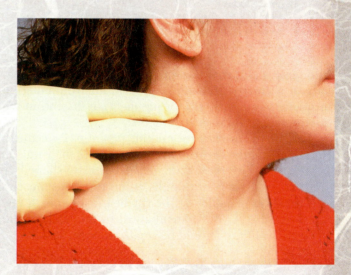

2-7d   Palpate the lymph nodes.

fingers palpate the nodes by moving the skin over the underlying tissues in each area (Procedure 2-7d). When swollen, the nodes are palpable, sometimes even visible. Note their size, shape, mobility, consistency, and tenderness. Tender, swollen, and mobile nodes suggest inflammation, usually from infection. Hard or fixed nodes suggest a malignancy. Inspect and palpate for subcutaneous emphysema, the presence of air just below the skin. This generally suggests a tear in the tracheo-bronchial tree or a pneumothorax.

THE CHEST AND LUNGS

The chest is a protective cage of bones, muscles, and cartilage (Figure 2-35). The bony cage comprises the three bones of the sternum (manubrium, body, and xiphoid process), the 12 pairs of ribs and their cartilaginous attachments, and the spinal column. In most adults, the transverse (side-to-side) diameter exceeds the anterior-posterior (front-to-back) diameter. The chest is divided into three cavities, the mediastinum, the right pleural cavity, and the left pleural cavity. The right chest contains three lung lobes (upper, middle, lower), while the left contains only two (upper, lower), to make room for the heart. The mediastinum contains the heart, the great vessels (vena cava, aorta, and pulmonary arteries and veins), the trachea, and the esophagus.

The chest wall can expand to create a vacuum that draws air into the lungs and helps return blood to the heart. The primary muscles of respiration are the diaphragm and external intercostals. During inhalation, the diaphragm contracts and moves downward while the external intercostals pull the chest wall upward and outward. The lungs, attached to the inner chest wall by a membrane called the pleura, expand also. The pleura consists of a parietal layer (lining the inner chest wall) and a visceral layer (covering the lungs) that glide over each other during breathing. A small amount of liquid between the layers helps create the vacuum for inhaling and acts as a lubricant. In cases of airway obstruction, a variety of accessory muscles in the neck and chest help lift the chest wall. Exhalation is primarily

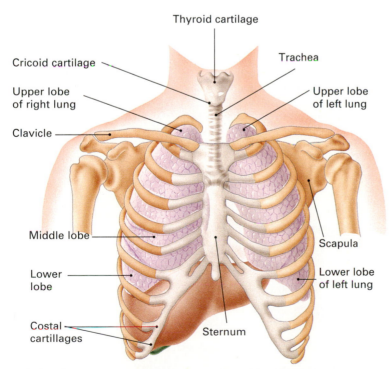

FIGURE 2-35   The thorax.

a passive process of muscle relaxation unless disease or injury forces the use of accessory muscles in the chest and abdomen to help expel air from the lungs.

A neurochemical process controls normal breathing. Specialized chemoreceptors monitor the blood for increases in carbon dioxide, decreases in oxygen, and changes in pH. The brain sends signals to the primary respiratory muscles to begin inspiration. The phrenic nerve, arising from cervical nerves 3, 4, and 5, innervates the diaphragm, while the thoracic spinal nerves innervate their respective intercostal muscles.

To assess the chest and thorax you will need a stethoscope with a bell and diaphragm, a marking pen, and a centimeter ruler. Have your patient sit upright, if possible, and expose his entire chest. At the same time, try to maintain your female patient's dignity when assessing her thorax and lungs by keeping her breasts covered. Perform your exam in the standard sequence—inspect, palpate, percuss, auscultate—and compare the findings from side to side. Always try to visualize the underlying lobes of the lungs during your exam.

Observe your patient's breathing. Look for signs of acute respiratory distress. Now count the respiratory rate and note his breathing pattern. Obviously-prolonged inhalation or exhalation indicates difficulty moving air in or out of the lungs. Do you hear sounds of an upper airway obstruction (inspiratory stridor) or a lower airway obstruction (expiratory wheezing, rhonchi)? Any gross abnormalities in the respiratory rate or pattern require rapid emergency intervention.

Inspect the anterior chest wall and assess its symmetry. Funnel chest (pectus excavatum) is a condition in which the lower portion of the sternum is depressed (Figure 2-36). With a pigeon chest (pectus carinatum), the sternum curves outward. Do both sides of your patient's chest wall rise in unison? Note whether he is using neck muscles during inhalation or abdominal muscles during exhalation. If his skin retracts in the area above his clavicles (supraclavicular), at the notch above his sternum (suprasternal), and between his ribs (intercostal), suspect a ventilation problem. If multiple ribs are fractured, creating a "floating segment" or "traumatic flail chest," you may find paradoxical (opposite) movement of that part of the chest wall during breathing.

Now look at his chest from the side. Normally an adult's thorax is twice as wide as it is deep. That is, the transverse diameter of the chest wall is usually twice the antero-posterior diameter. In infants, the elderly, or patients with chronic pulmonary disease, however, the antero-posterior diameter is increased, giving them a barrel chest appearance.

Any gross abnormalities in the respiratory rate or pattern require rapid emergency intervention.

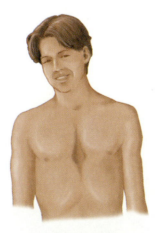
Funnel chest

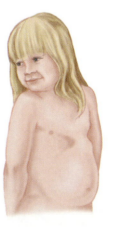
Pigeon chest

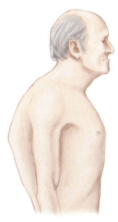
Barrel chest

FIGURE 2-36 Chest wall abnormalities.

POSTERIOR CHEST EXAMINATION

Next examine the posterior chest. Ask your patient to fold his arms across his chest and breathe normally during the exam. This moves his scapulae out of the way and allows you more access to his posterior lung fields. Inspect his posterior chest for deformities and symmetrical movement as he breathes. Some patients may exhibit thoracic kyphoscoliosis, an abnormal spinal curvature that deforms the chest and makes your lung exam more challenging. Inspect the intercostal spaces for retractions or bulging; both are abnormal. Retractions may appear when airflow is impeded during inspiration. Bulging may appear when airflow is impeded during exhalation. Respiratory movement should be smooth and effortless. When it is not, suspect underlying respiratory disease or structural impairment.

Palpate the rib cage for rigidity. Feel for tenderness, deformities, depressions, loose segments, asymmetry, and crepitus. Then evaluate for equal expansion. First, locate the level of the posterior 10th rib. To do this, find the lowest rib and simply move up two more ribs. An alternate method for locating the posterior 10th rib is to palpate the spinous processes. Ask your patient to touch his chin to his chest. The most prominent spinous process is the 7th cervical vertebra. Locate it and count down to T-10 in the midline. Now place your hands parallel to the 10th rib on your patient's back with your fingers spread. Lightly grasp his lateral rib cage with your spread hands (Procedure 2-8a on next page). Ask him to inhale deeply. Normally the distance between your thumbs will increase symmetrically by three to five centimeters during deep inspiration. If you detect decreased thoracic expansion or feel unilateral delay, suspect a disorder of the underlying lung, pleura, or diaphragm.

When your patient speaks, you can feel vibrations on his chest wall. This is known as tactile fremitus. Place the palm of your hand on your patient's chest wall and have him say "ninety-nine or one-on-one." As he does, palpate the posterior chest; feel the vibrations in different areas of the chest wall and compare symmetrical areas of the lungs (Procedure 2-8b). Identify and note any areas of increased, decreased, or absent vibrations. You will feel increased fremitus when sound transmission is enhanced through areas of consolidated lung tissue such as in a tumor, pneumonia, or pulmonary fibrosis. You will feel decreased or absent fremitus when sound transmission is diminished in a certain area, as may occur with a pleural effusion, emphysema, or pneumothorax.

Percuss your patient's posterior chest to determine whether the underlying tissues are air-filled, fluid-filled, or solid. Also percuss to determine the position and boundaries of the diaphragm and underlying organs. Percuss both sides of the chest symmetrically from the apex to the base at five-centimeter intervals, avoiding bony areas such as the scapulae (Procedure 2-8c). Percuss at least twice in each area and compare both sides of the thorax. Identify and note any area of abnormal percussion. For example, a hyperresonant sound in the right chest may indicate a pneumothorax, whereas a dull sound in the same area may indicate a hemothorax. Assess the percussion sounds according to their quality, intensity, pitch, and duration. Practice percussing the chest so that you will become familiar with the normal resonance of the lungs and be able to identify abnormal sounds.

Next assess for diaphragmatic excursion. Identify the level of the diaphragm during quiet breathing by percussing for dullness as the diaphragm moves during the respiratory cycle. Percuss at the lower rib margin on one side and note when dullness (muscle) replaces resonance (air). With a pen mark the location of the diaphragm at the end of inhalation and at the end of exhalation. The distance between the marks is the diaphragmatic excursion. In the normal healthy adult

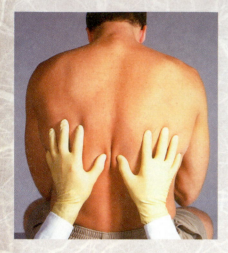

2-8a   Palpate the posterior chest for excursion.

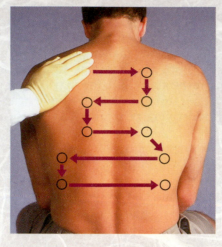

2-8b   Palpate the posterior chest for tactile fremitus.

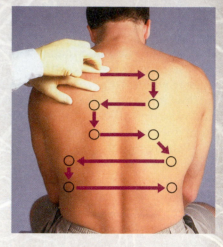

2-8c   Percuss the posterior chest.

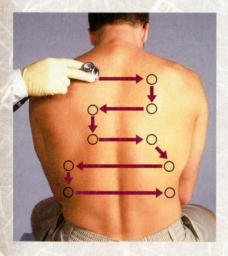

2-8d   Auscultate the posterior chest.

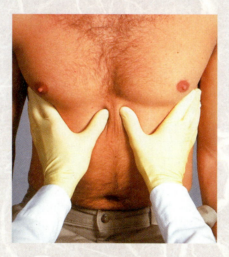

2-8e   Palpate the anterior chest for excursion.

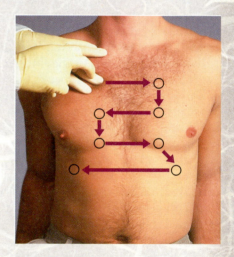

2-8f   Percuss the anterior chest.

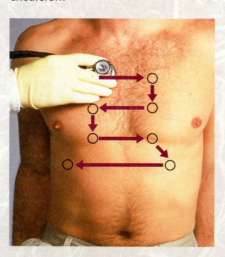

2-8g   Auscultate the anterior chest.

Table 2-6 NORMAL BREATH SOUNDS

Sound	Description	Location	Duration
Tracheal	Very loud, harsh	Over the trachea	Nearly equal inspiratory and expiratory phases
Bronchial	Loud, high pitch, hollow	Over the manubrium	Prolonged expiratory phase
Bronchovesicular	Soft, breezy, lower pitch	Between the scapulae / 2nd—3rd ICS lateral to the sternum	Approximately equal inspiratory and expiratory phases
Vesicular	Soft, swishy, lowest pitch	Lung periphery	Prolonged inspiratory phase

at rest, the diaphragmatic excursion should be approximately six centimeters. Now measure diaphragmatic excursion on the opposite side and compare the marks. If you find asymmetrical diaphragmatic levels, a paralyzed phrenic nerve may be the problem. Here, reevaluate your patient's respiratory depth for adequacy and provide the appropriate intervention as needed.

Auscultate your patient's chest for normal breath sounds, adventitious breath sounds, and voice sounds. Auscultate all lung fields and compare side-to-side. Evaluate the normal breath sounds produced by airflow through the upper and lower airways. These include tracheal, bronchial, bronchovesicular, and vesicular breath sounds (Table 2-6).

Besides the normal breath sounds already mentioned you also may hear adventitious sounds. These include crackles, wheezes, rhonchi, stridor, and pleural rubs.

Also known as "rales," **crackles** are light crackling, popping, nonmusical sounds heard usually during inspiration. They are produced by air passing through moisture in the broncho-alveolar system or from the abrupt opening of closed alveoli. Early inspiratory crackles, associated with chronic bronchitis and heart failure, begin shortly after inspiration starts, and they stop soon thereafter. These are coarse crackles—loud, low pitched, and long, similar to the sound of water boiling. They are often audible at the mouth.

Late inspiratory crackles, associated with congestive heart failure and interstitial lung diseases, begin in the first half of the inspiratory phase and continue into late inspiration. They are fine crackles—soft, high pitched, and very brief, similar to the sound of Rice Krispies crackling. They commonly appear first at the base of the lungs and move upward as your patient's condition worsens. Usually, you can expect them to shift to dependent regions with changes in your patient's position. For example, if your heart failure patient is sitting up, expect to hear crackles first in the bases. If he is bedridden, expect to hear crackles first in the back.

Wheezes are continuous, high-pitched musical sounds similar to a whistle. They result when air moves through partially obstructed smaller airways. Their causes include asthma, bronchospasm, and foreign bodies. You may hear them without a stethoscope or by auscultating the chest during any or all phases of the respiratory cycle. They often originate in the small bronchioles and first appear at the end of exhalation. The closer to inspiration they appear, the worse your patient's condition.

Rhonchi are continuous sounds with a lower pitch and a snoring quality. They are caused by secretions in the larger airways, a common finding in bronchitis (diffuse) and pneumonia (localized). Rhonchi usually appear in early exhalation but may occur in early inspiration as well.

Content Review

ADVENTITIOUS BREATH SOUNDS

- Crackles
- Wheezes
- Rhonchi
- Stridor
- Pleural rubs

✱ crackles light crackling, popping, nonmusical sounds heard usually during inspiration.

✱ wheezes continuous, high-pitched musical sounds similar to a whistle.

✱ rhonchi continuous sounds with a lower pitch and a snoring quality.

✻ stridor predominantly inspiratory wheeze associated with laryngeal obstruction.

✻ pleural friction rub the squeaking or grating sound of the pleural linings rubbing together.

Stridor is a predominantly high pitched inspiratory sound. It indicates a partial obstruction of the larynx or trachea.

Pleural friction rubs are the squeaking or grating sounds of the pleural linings rubbing together. They occur where the pleural layers are inflamed and have lost their lubrication. Pleural rubs are common in pneumonia and pleurisy (inflammation of the pleura). Because these sounds occur whenever your patient's chest wall moves, they appear during the entire respiratory cycle.

You may hear no breath sounds in some areas. This may result from effusion (fluid in the pleural space causing a decrease in functional lung tissue) or consolidation (infectious pus causing collapsed alveoli). In either case, note the area's size and intervene appropriately to ensure adequate ventilation and oxygenation of your patient.

Auscultate the posterior chest systematically. Have your patient fold his arms across his chest and breathe through his mouth more deeply and slowly than usual. Auscultate the same areas you percussed and compare the bilateral findings (Procedure 2-8d). Listen for at least one full breath at each location. Be alert for patient discomfort or hyperventilation. Note the pitch, intensity, and duration of each inspiratory and expiratory sound. If the sounds are decreased, suspect impaired airflow or poor sound transmission. If the sounds are absent, suspect no airflow. Note whether you hear sounds where you normally should. For example, when you auscultate over the peripheral lung fields, you should not hear tracheal, bronchial, or bronchovesicular breath sounds. Listen carefully and note what you hear, where you hear it, and when you hear it during the respiratory cycle. Also note whether the sounds change when your patient coughs or changes position.

If you hear abnormally located tracheal, bronchial, or bronchovesicular breath sounds, assess your patient's transmitted voice sounds. Ask him to repeat the words "ninety-nine" as you auscultate his chest wall. Normally you should hear muffled, indistinct sounds. Hearing the words clearly is an abnormal finding known as **bronchophony.** Bronchophony occurs when fluid (water, blood) or consolidated tissue (pus, tumor) replaces the normally air-filled lung. After you check your patient for bronchophony, assess him for **whispered pectoriloquy** and **egophony.** For pectoriloquy, ask your patient to whisper "ninety-nine" while you auscultate. As with bronchophony, the words will be clear and distinct if sound transmission through an area is abnormally enhanced. For egophony, ask him to repeat the long *e* sound while you auscultate. You should hear a muffled, long *e*. If vocal resonance is abnormally increased, you will hear an *a* sound instead. This is known as "*e* to *a* egophony."

✻ bronchophony abnormal clarity of patient's transmitted voice sounds.

✻ whispered pectoriloquy abnormal clarity of patient's transmitted whispers.

✻ egophony abnormal change in tone of patient's transmitted voice sounds.

Anterior Chest Examination

Your examination of the anterior chest will be similar to your examination of the posterior chest. Begin by having your patient lie supine with his arms relaxed but slightly abducted at his sides. Look for any gross deformities or asymmetrical movements. Does the chest wall rise symmetrically? Is there accessory muscle use? Look for abnormal retractions in the suprasternal, supraclavicular, and intercostal areas. Also check for callused elbows from tripodding (leaning with elbows on a table or chair arms), and finger clubbing—both common signs of chronic lung disease. Is the trachea midline or deviated; does it tug during inhalation? In cases of tension pneumothorax the trachea will deviate away from the affected side. In cases of pulmonary fibrosis and atelectasis it will tug toward the affected side during inhalation.

Palpate the anterior chest for deformities and areas of tenderness. Check for chest expansion by placing your thumbs along the costal margins on both sides and gently grasping the lateral rib cage (Procedure 2-8e). Ask your patient to inhale deeply. Normally your thumbs will separate symmetrically and the distance between them will increase from three to five centimeters. If you detect decreased thoracic expansion or feel unilateral delay, suspect a disorder of the underlying lung, pleura, or diaphragm.

As with the posterior chest, test for tactile fremitus, bronchophony, whispered pectoriloquy, and egophony if you detect abnormal breath sounds.

Percuss your patient's anterior chest to help determine whether the underlying tissues are air-filled, fluid-filled, or solid and to determine the position and boundaries of the diaphragm and underlying organs. Percuss each side of your patient's anterior chest from its apex to its base at five centimeter intervals at the mid-clavicular lines (Procedure 2-8f). Percuss at least twice in each area and compare both sides of the thorax. Identify and note any area of abnormal percussion. Remember that when percussing the right chest, you will hear dullness at the upper border of the liver. On the left side, you will hear the normal resonance of the lung change to tympany when you reach the stomach. You also will percuss an area of cardiac dullness from the 3rd to the 5th intercostal spaces.

Finally, auscultate the anterior and lateral thorax systematically. Have your patient breathe through his mouth more deeply and slowly than usual. Auscultate the same areas you percussed and compare symmetrical areas (Procedure 2-8g). Listen for at least one full breath at each location. Be alert for patient discomfort or hyperventilation. As with posterior chest auscultation, note the pitch, intensity, and duration of each inspiratory and expiratory sound and whether you heard sounds where you should normally expect them. Listen for adventitious sounds. If you hear abnormally located tracheal, bronchial, or bronchovesicular breath sounds, assess for bronchophony, whispered pectoriloquy, and egophony.

THE CARDIOVASCULAR SYSTEM

Mentally picture the heart and great vessels as you inspect the chest (Figure 2-37). The heart sits just behind the sternum between the 3rd and 6th costal cartilages and rotated to the left. Its most anterior surface, therefore, is the right

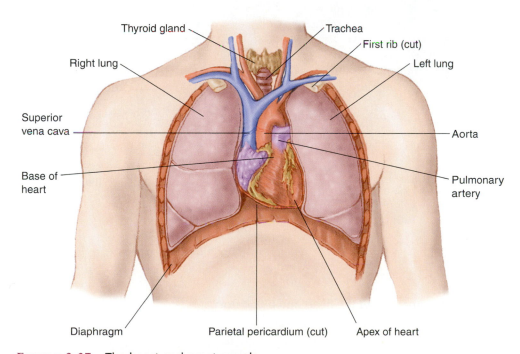

FIGURE 2-37 The heart and great vessels.

ventricle. The pulmonary artery, which carries deoxygenated blood to the lungs, leaves the right ventricle at the 3rd costal cartilage, close to the sternum. The left ventricle sits behind the right ventricle and a little to its left. It forms the left border of the heart and produces the apical impulse at the 5th intercostal space, near the mid-clavicular line. This is the point of maximum impulse (PMI). The aorta curves upward from the left ventricle to the level of the sternal angle (second costal cartilage), arches backward, and then turns back downward. To the right of the aorta, the superior vena cava returns blood to the right atrium.

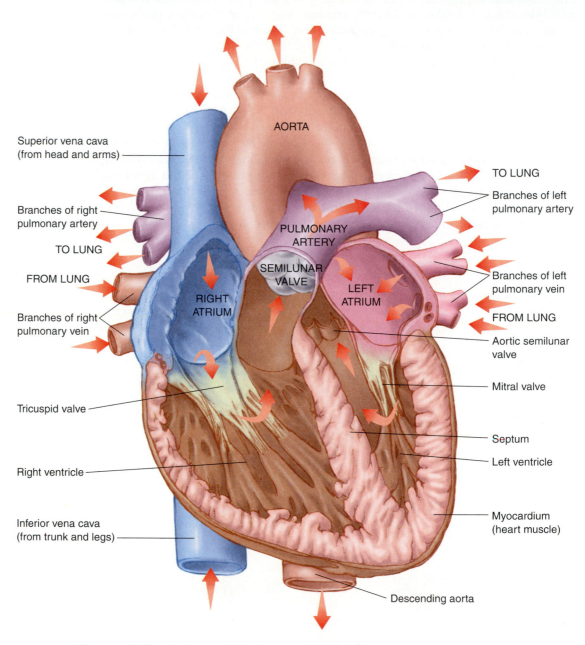

FIGURE 2-38   Anatomy of the heart and blood flow.

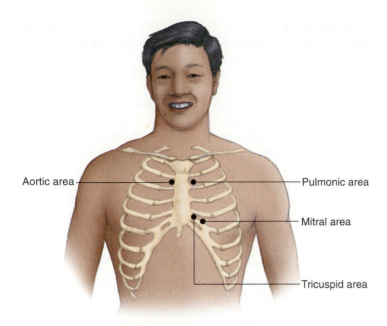

Aortic area

Pulmonic area

Mitral area

Tricuspid area

FIGURE 2-39   Sites for cardiac auscultation.

To assess cardiac function, you must understand the cardiac cycle (Figure 2-38). During **diastole,** the heart's resting period, the ventricles relax. The pressure in the atria is greater than the pressure in the ventricles. This opens the tricuspid valve on the right side and the mitral valve on the left, allowing blood from the atria to fill the ventricles. During **systole** the ventricles contract and the tricuspid and mitral valves close, preventing backflow into the atria. The vibrations of these valves' closings generate the first heart sound—S_1, or the "lub." The increased pressure in the right ventricle opens the pulmonic semilunar valve, sending deoxygenated blood to the lungs. The increased pressure in the left ventricle opens the aortic semilunar valve, sending freshly oxygenated blood to the body. At the end of systole, as pressure in the ventricles falls, the pulmonic and aortic semilunar valves close tightly to prevent backflow. These vibrations generate the second heart sound—S_2, or the "dub." This cycle repeats approximately 60–100 times per minute in the healthy adult at rest. Extra sounds known as heart murmurs result when valves do not fully open or close, causing turbulent flow that an experienced clinician can detect.

You must auscultate for heart sounds at the proper places on the chest wall (Figure 2-39). Always listen downstream. For example, since the tricuspid and mitral valves direct blood flow to the ventricles, which are toward your patient's feet, listen for S_1 at the apex of the heart. This is found near the lower left sternal border. Since the aortic and pulmonic valves direct blood flow to the lungs and aorta, which are toward your patient's head, listen for S_2 at the base of the heart. This is found at the 2nd intercostal space near the sternum.

The heart is an electrical-mechanical pump. Its job is to begin the movement of blood through the circulatory system. Its effectiveness is measured by **cardiac output.** Cardiac output is the amount of blood the heart ejects each minute, measured

* **diastole** phase of cardiac cycle when ventricles relax.

* **systole** phase of cardiac cycle when the ventricles contract.

Content Review

HEART SOUNDS
- S_1—"lub"
- S_2—"dub"
- Split S_1—"la-lub"
- Split S_2—"da-dub"
- S_3—"lub-dub-dee" (Kentucky)
- S_4—"dee-lub-dub" (Tennessee)
- Click
- Snap
- Pericardial friction rub
- Murmur

* **cardiac output** the amount of blood the heart ejects each minute, measured in ml.

* **stroke volume** the amount of blood the heart ejects in one beat.

in liters per minute. It is the product of the heart rate and the stroke volume. **Stroke volume** is the amount of blood the heart ejects in one beat. Changes in any of these components may severely affect cardiac output. For example, if your patient's heart rate falls to 30 beats per minute, or if a massive heart attack destroys 30–40% of his left ventricle, the cardiac output will greatly decrease.

Three factors determine stroke volume: preload, contractile force, and afterload. Preload, also known as end-diastolic pressure, is the amount of blood returned to the heart from the body. The greater the preload, the more the cardiac muscles will stretch, the harder they will contract, and the more blood the heart will eject. Contractile force refers to how forcefully the heart muscle contracts. It is regulated by the autonomic nervous system and the body's needs. Afterload refers to the resistance in the vessels that the heart must overcome to eject blood. It is determined mostly in the medium sized arterioles.

With each contraction of your patient's heart, you should feel an arterial pulse. Blood pressure is a measurable estimate of the pressure in the circulatory system during systole and diastole. Arterial blood pressure is affected by the stroke volume (left ventricular effectiveness), the condition of the aorta and large arteries, the peripheral vascular resistance (condition of the arterioles), and the circulating blood volume. Changes in any of these components can severely affect your patient's blood pressure. For example, if your patient loses 30–40% of his blood volume or experiences massive vasodilation, his blood pressure will drop drastically.

Venous pressure, on the other hand, is much lower than arterial pressure. It will remain so unless something restricts blood flow through the heart. For example, in congestive heart failure, a weakened heart cannot effectively move all the blood it receives from the body or the lungs. The resulting backup eventually raises venous pressure. Cardiac tamponade and tension pneumothorax inhibit venous return, causing a dramatic rise in venous pressure. You can easily observe and measure increases in venous pressure in the external jugular veins.

Several changes occur with aging. Since most patients with cardiac complaints are older, an understanding of these changes is essential. Changes in chest wall diameter make it more difficult to find the apical pulse. Extra heart sounds are more common. Many older patients will have heart murmurs, especially affecting the aortic valve that becomes stenotic over time. The aorta and large arteries stiffen from atherosclerosis, raising blood pressure. Older patients often develop mitral valve murmurs and regurgitation (backflow leakage into the left atrium during ventricular systole).

Begin your cardiovascular assessment by inspecting for signs of arterial insufficiency or occlusion in your patient's trunk and extremities. Look for skin pallor and other signs of decreased perfusion. Now assess the arterial pulses. Inspect the carotid arteries for visible pulsations just medial to the sternocleidomastoid muscles. Palpate the carotid arteries at the level of the cricoid cartilage to avoid pressing on the carotid sinus (Procedure 2-9a on next page). Never palpate both carotids simultaneously; doing so may decrease cerebral blood flow. Assess the carotid pulse for rate, rhythm, and quality. Does its quality vary? Do the variations correspond to respiration? For example, in pulsus paradoxus, the amplitude of the pulse diminishes with inspiration and increases with exhalation. Do you feel a vibration or humming (**thrills**) when you palpate the carotid artery? If so, auscultate the area with your stethoscope for **bruits,** the sounds of turbulent blood flow around a partial obstruction (Procedure 2-9b).

* **thrill** vibration or humming felt when palpating the pulse.

* **bruit** sound of turbulent blood flow around a partial obstruction.

If you have not already taken your patient's blood pressure, do so now. Also check for jugular venous pressure, which approximates your patient's right atrial pressure. Position your patient supine, with his head elevated to about 30°. Turning your patient's head away from the side you are assessing, identify the external jugular veins on both sides and locate the pulsations of the internal jugular veins. Look for the pulsation in the area around the suprasternal notch and where the sternocleidomastoid muscle inserts on the clavicle and manubrium.

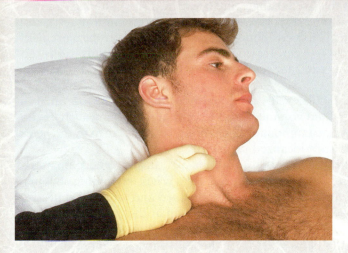

2-9a   Assess the carotid pulse.

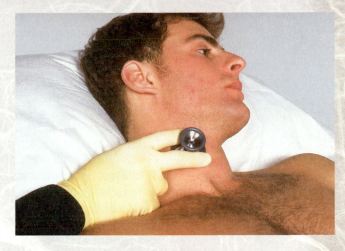

2-9b   Auscultate for bruits.

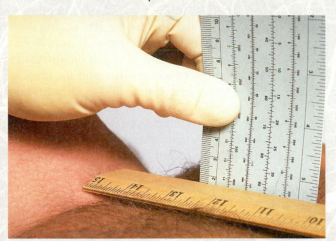

2-9c   Measure jugular venous pressure.

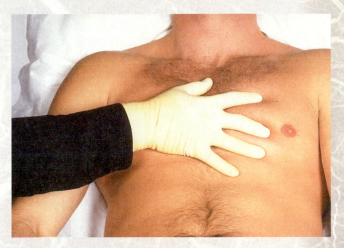

2-9d   Palpate for the apical impulse (PMI).

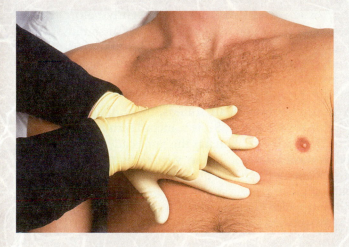

2-9e   Percuss for the PMI.

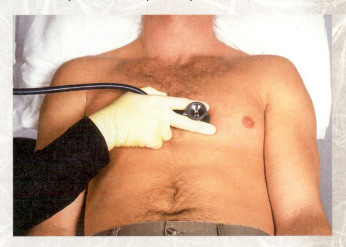

2-9f   Auscultate for heart sounds.

Now identify the internal jugular vein's highest point of pulsation (the point where the pulse diminishes) and measure its vertical distance from the sternal angle (midline at the 2nd costal cartilage). To do this, place a ruler perpendicular to the chest at the sternal angle and position a straightedge at a right angle to the ruler (Procedure 2-9c). Lower the straightedge until it rests atop the jugular vein pulsation. The corresponding ruler mark is your measurement. Normal venous pressure is 1–2 cm. If you cannot visualize the pulsations, observe the point where the external jugular veins collapse and use the same measuring parameters.

Examine the external jugular veins for equality of distention. Abnormal bilateral distention indicates fluid volume overload or that something such as congestive heart failure or cardiac tamponade is blocking venous return to the heart. Unilateral distention suggests a localized problem.

With your patient's head still raised to about 30°, inspect and palpate the chest for the apical impulse, or PMI (Procedure 2-9d). When examining a woman with large breasts, gently displace the left breast upward and laterally, if needed, or ask her to do this for you. First, look for a pulsation at the cardiac apex, normally at the 5th intercostal space just medial to the mid-clavicular line. This pulsation represents the PMI. It helps you locate the left ventricle's apex.

If you cannot see the pulsation, ask your patient to exhale and stop breathing for a few seconds. Lateral displacement of the PMI indicates an enlarged right ventricle. The PMI may be displaced upward and to the left in pregnant women. If your patient is obese or has a very muscular chest wall or a barrel chest you may not detect the PMI. Percussion may help if you have difficulty palpating the PMI. Start lateral and work your way toward the midline (Procedure 2-9e). When you hear a change from resonance (lung) to dull (heart), you have located the PMI.

Using the diaphragm of your stethoscope, auscultate your patient's anterior chest for normal heart sounds and for abnormal or extra heart sounds (Procedure 2-9f). Listen for the high-pitched sounds of S_1 at the 5th intercostal space at the left sternal border (tricuspid valve) and at the PMI (mitral valve) using the diaphragm of your stethoscope. Listen for the high-pitched sounds of S_2 at the 2nd intercostal space at the right sternal border (aortic valve) and 2nd intercostal space at the left sternal border (pulmonic valve). For a comprehensive auscultation of heart sounds, you should also listen at the 3rd and 4th intercostal spaces. Although nothing is specifically behind those spaces, you may hear something there that you will not hear in the other places if the heart is not anatomically perfect.

Because the mitral and aortic valves (left side) close slightly before the tricuspid and pulmonic valves (right side), you may hear two sets of sounds instead of one. This is known as splitting. A split S_1 sounds like "la-lub," a split S_2 like "da-dub." Instead of "lub-dub" you will hear "la-lub—da-dub." Splitting of S_2 during inspiration is normal in healthy children and young adults. Expiratory or persistent splitting suggests an abnormality.

You also may hear extra or abnormal heart sounds, depending on your patient's age and condition. A third heart sound, S_3, is sometimes called the ventricular gallop. It is the "dee" of "lub-dub-dee" and has the same cadence as the word "Kentucky." This extra heart sound develops from vibrations that result when blood fills a dilated ventricle. Commonly heard in children and young adults, an S_3 is usually considered pathologic in patients over age 30. It generally develops with ventricular failure and ventricular volume overload and disappears when the problem is resolved. S_3 is a low-pitched sound heard in early to mid-diastole. Listen for S_3 at the apex using the bell of your stethoscope with your patient lying on his left side.

Atrial gallop is the fourth heart sound, S_4. It is the "dee" of "dee-lub-dub" and has the same cadence as the word "Tennessee." An S_4 develops from vibrations produced in late diastole when atrial contraction forces blood into a ventricle that has decreased compliance or that resists filling and causes volume overload. It usually disappears when the problem is resolved. Listen for the low-pitched S_4 at the apex using the bell of your stethoscope with your patient lying on his left side.

Experienced cardiologists can also detect clicks, snaps, friction rubs, and murmurs. An ejection click results from a stiff or stuck valve. An opening snap results when a stenotic mitral or tricuspid valve's leaflets recoil abruptly after ventricular diastole. A pericardial friction rub occurs when inflammation causes the heart's visceral and parietal surfaces to rub together at each heartbeat. A murmur is a rumbling or vibrating noise that results from turbulent blood flow through the heart valves, a large artery, or a septal defect.

THE ABDOMEN

The key to evaluating the abdomen is visualizing the organs in the region you are examining. The abdominal cavity is divided into four quadrants: the right upper (RUQ), right lower (RLQ), left upper (LUQ), and left lower (LLQ). Their dividing lines intersect at the umbilicus (Figure 2-40). Age changes in the abdomen include increased fat storage around the midsection and hips and weakened abdominal musculature. The result is the "beer belly" appearance. Decreased sensation may diminish the normal signs and symptoms of serious disease. The classic signs and symptoms of abdominal diseases are often missing in the elderly.

The key to evaluating the abdomen is visualizing the organs in the region you are examining.

FIGURE 2-40   The abdominal quadrants.

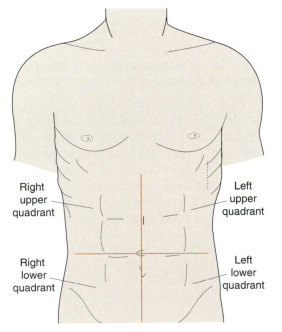

Right upper quadrant

Left upper quadrant

Right lower quadrant

Left lower quadrant

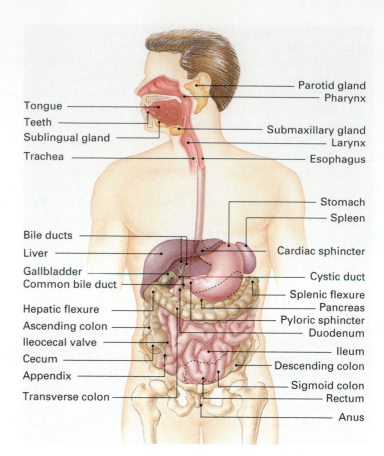

Labels on the figure:
Tongue
Teeth
Sublingual gland
Trachea
Parotid gland
Pharynx
Submaxillary gland
Larynx
Esophagus
Bile ducts
Liver
Gallbladder
Common bile duct
Hepatic flexure
Ascending colon
Ileocecal valve
Cecum
Appendix
Transverse colon
Stomach
Spleen
Cardiac sphincter
Cystic duct
Splenic flexure
Pancreas
Pyloric sphincter
Duodenum
Ileum
Descending colon
Sigmoid colon
Rectum
Anus

FIGURE 2-41   The digestive system.

ABDOMINAL ORGANS

Major organs of the digestive, urinary, reproductive, cardiovascular, and lymphatic systems lie in the abdomen. The peritoneum, a protective membrane, covers most of them.

Digestive Food travels down the esophagus to the stomach (in the LUQ) (Figure 2-41). It then passes into the first section of the small intestine, the duodenum, where digestive enzymes from the pancreas (just behind the stomach) and gallbladder (just behind the liver in the RUQ) help digestion. Food then begins its journey through the remainder of the long small intestine (the jejuneum and ileum), where the mesentery veins absorb nutrients from the food. Blood travels from the mesentery veins to the liver (RUQ) for processing and detoxification before it returns to the right heart. At the point where the small intestine turns into the large intestine lies the appendix (RLQ). The large intestine, or colon, has three distinct sections: the ascending colon (RLQ to RUQ), the transverse colon (RUQ to LUQ), and the descending colon (LUQ to LLQ). The large intestine is responsible for absorbing water from the feces and returning it to the general circulation. The remaining waste continues through the sigmoid colon (LLQ), rectum (midline), and anus.

Urinary The kidneys are pear-shaped solid organs imbedded in fat in the retroperitoneal space (RUQ, LUQ) (Figure 2-42). They receive blood from the

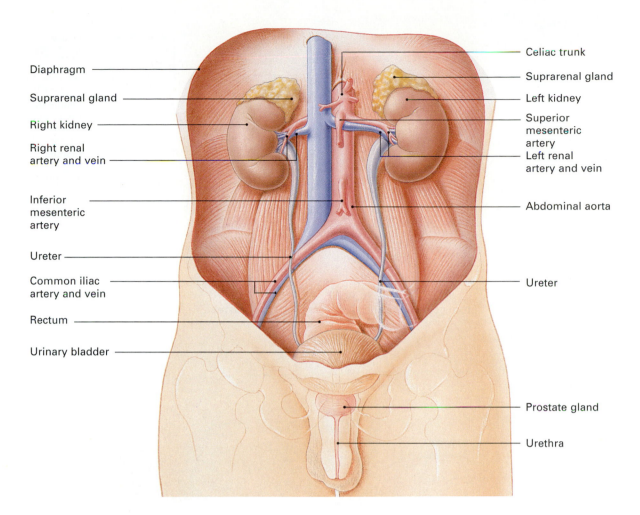

Diaphragm

Suprarenal gland

Right kidney

Right renal
artery and vein

Inferior
mesenteric
artery

Ureter

Common iliac
artery and vein

Rectum

Urinary bladder

Celiac trunk

Suprarenal gland

Left kidney

Superior
mesenteric
artery

Left renal
artery and vein

Abdominal aorta

Ureter

Prostate gland

Urethra

FIGURE 2-42   The urinary system.

renal arteries, which branch off the abdominal aorta. The kidneys filter blood and excrete impurities, acids, and electrolytes from the blood before returning it to the general circulation. The waste product is called urine. Ureters bring the urine to the bladder, just behind the pubic bone in the midline. The urethra connects the urinary bladder to the outside.

Female Reproductive   The ovaries (RLQ, LLQ) are walnut-sized organs that manufacture and produce the ova for fertilization (Figure 2-43). The fallopian tubes transport the ova toward the uterus (midline just above the urinary bladder). Fertilization occurs in the tubes. The fertilized ovum travels and implants in the uterus. The cervix is the opening to the uterus. The vagina is the birth canal.

Male Reproductive   The testes are located in the scrotal sac and produce reproductive sperm (Figure 2-44). The sperm collects in a small reservoir called the epididymis, which can become inflamed. During sex, the sperm travels via the vas deferens (RLQ, LLQ) through an opening in the inguinal ligament known as the inguinal canal. The testicular blood supply also runs through this opening, an anatomical weak point that

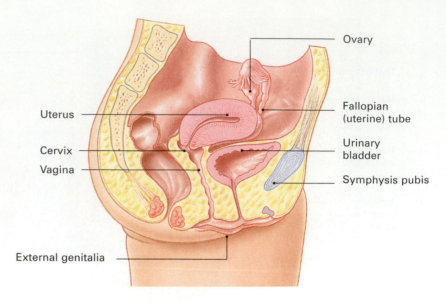

FIGURE 2-43   The female reproductive system.

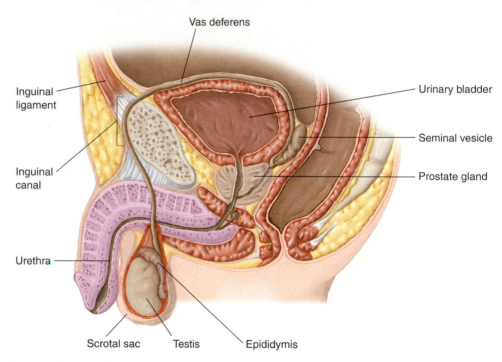

FIGURE 2-44   The male reproductive system.

is the site of male hernias. The vas deferens moves the sperm toward the prostate gland, where it mixes with seminal fluid and is ejected via the penile urethra.

Cardiovascular The large abdominal aorta delivers blood from the heart to all the organs of the abdominal cavity (Figure 2-45). Palpate the aorta just to the left of the umbilicus. The inferior vena cava delivers blood that is deoxygenated and high in carbon dioxide from the abdominal organs and lower extremities to the heart. The mesentery arteries and veins and portal circulation systems deliver blood to and from the intestines and back to the heart for general distribution.

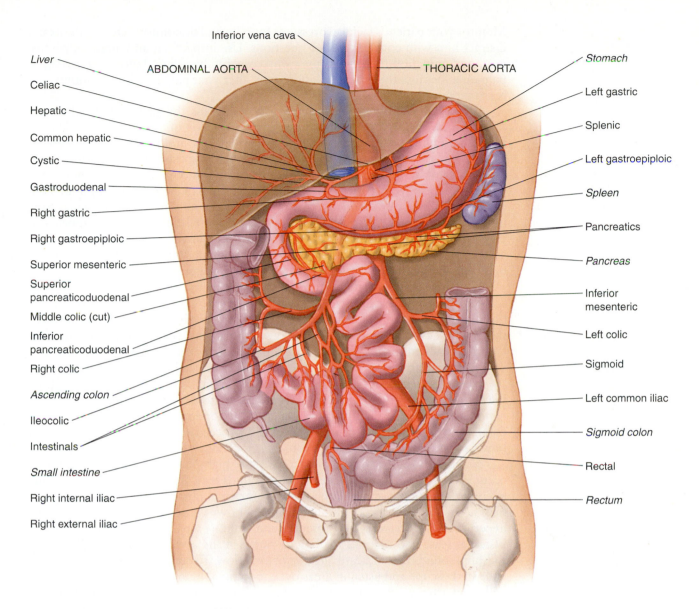

Liver
Celiac
Hepatic
Common hepatic
Cystic
Gastroduodenal
Right gastric
Right gastroepiploic
Superior mesenteric
Superior pancreaticoduodenal
Middle colic (cut)
Inferior pancreaticoduodenal
Right colic
Ascending colon
Ileocolic
Intestinals
Small intestine
Right internal iliac
Right external iliac

Inferior vena cava
ABDOMINAL AORTA
THORACIC AORTA

Stomach
Left gastric
Splenic
Left gastroepiploic
Spleen
Pancreatics
Pancreas
Inferior mesenteric
Left colic
Sigmoid
Left common iliac
Sigmoid colon
Rectal
Rectum

FIGURE 2-45   The abdominal arteries.

Lymphatic   The spleen (LUQ) is the major organ of the lymph system. The vast network of lymph vessels helps drain excessive fluid and return it to the heart and aids the immune and infection control systems.

Abdominal Examination

To examine the abdomen, you need good lighting, a relaxed patient, and exposure from above the xiphoid process to the symphysis pubis. Make sure your patient does not have a full bladder. Make him comfortable in the supine position with one pillow under the head and another under the knees. Have him place his hands at his sides. This helps relax his abdominal muscles, making the examination easier for you and more comfortable for him.

Ask your patient to point out any areas of pain or tenderness. Examine these areas last. Use warm hands and a warm stethoscope and keep your fingernails short. If your hands are cold, palpate your patient through his clothes until your hands warm up. Begin your exam slowly and avoid any quick, unexpected movements.

Monitor your patient's facial expressions for pain and discomfort. During the exam, distract him with conversation or questions. Use inspection, auscultation, percussion, and palpation to perform the exam. Always auscultate before percussing or palpating, because these manipulations may alter your patient's bowel motility and resulting bowel sounds.

When you examine the abdomen you will assess the gastrointestinal organs and other nearby organs and structures. Inspect the skin of the abdomen and flanks for scars, dilated veins, stretch marks, rashes, lesions, and pigmentation changes. Look for discoloration over the umbilicus (**Cullen's sign**) or over the flanks (**Grey-Turner's sign**); these are late signs suggesting intra-abdominal bleeding. Assess the size and shape of your patient's abdomen to determine whether it is scaphoid (concave), flat, round, or distended. Ask the patient if it is its usual size and shape. Note its symmetry. Check for bulges, hernias, or distended flanks. **Ascites** appears as bulges in the flanks and across the abdomen and indicates edema caused by congestive heart failure. A distended bladder or pregnant uterus can cause a suprapubic bulge. Bulges in the inguinal or femoral areas suggest a hernia.

Now look at your patient's umbilicus. Note its location and contour and observe for any signs of herniation or inflammation. Check for any visible pulsation, peristalsis (the wavelike motion of organs moving their contents through the digestive tract), or masses. You may see the normal pulsation of the aorta just lateral to the umbilicus. If you notice a bounding or exaggerated pulsation, suspect an aortic aneurysm. Visible peristalsis may indicate a bowel obstruction.

Next auscultate for bowel sounds and other sounds such as bruits throughout the abdomen. To auscultate for bowel sounds, first warm your diaphragm in your hand, because a cold diaphragm might cause abdominal tension. Gently place the diaphragm on your patient's abdomen and proceed systematically, listening for bowel sounds in each quadrant. Note their location, frequency, and character.

Normal bowel sounds consist of a variety of high-pitched gurgles and clicks that occur every 5–15 seconds. More frequent sounds indicate increased bowel motility in conditions such as diarrhea or an early intestinal obstruction. Occasionally you may hear loud, prolonged, gurgling sounds known as **borborygmi.** These indicate hyperperistalsis. Decreased or absent sounds suggest a paralytic ileus or peritonitis. Listen at least two minutes for bowel sounds if the abdomen is silent. Bruits are swishing sounds that indicate turbulent blood flow. To confirm bruits use the bell of your stethoscope and listen in areas over abdominal blood vessels such as the aorta and renal arteries (Procedure 2-10a on page 96). If you hear a bruit, suspect an arterial disorder such as an abdominal aortic aneurysm or renal artery stenosis.

Percussing the abdomen produces different sounds based on the underlying tissues. These sounds help you detect excessive gas and solid or fluid-filled masses. They also help you determine the size and position of solid organs such as the liver and spleen. Percuss the abdomen in the same sequence you used for auscultation. Note the distribution of tympany and dullness. Expect to hear tympany in most of the abdomen; expect dullness over the solid abdominal organs such as the liver and spleen.

Palpate the abdomen last to detect tenderness, muscular rigidity, and superficial organs and masses. Before you begin palpation, ask your patient if he has any pain or tenderness. If he does, ask him to point to the area with one finger. Palpate that area last, using gentle pressure with a single finger. Ask him to cough and tell you if and where he experiences any pain. If coughing causes pain, suspect peritoneal inflammation.

Now ask your patient to take slow, deep breaths with his mouth open, and have him flex his knees to relax his abdominal muscles. Perform light palpation by moving your hand slowly and just lifting it off the skin (Procedure 2-10b). Palpate all areas in the same sequence you used for auscultation and percussion. Watch your patient's face for signs of discomfort. Identify any masses and note

* **Cullen's sign** discoloration around the umbilicus (occasionally the flanks) suggestive of intra-abdominal hemorrhage.

* **Grey-Turner's sign** discoloration over the flanks suggesting intra-abdominal bleeding.

* **ascites** bulges in the flanks and across the abdomen, indicating edema caused by congestive heart failure.

* **borborygmi** loud, prolonged, gurgling bowel sounds indicating hyperperistalsis.

their size, location, contour, tenderness, pulsations, and mobility. Abdominal pain upon light palpation suggests peritoneal irritation or inflammation. If you feel rigidity or guarding while palpating, determine whether it is voluntary (patient anticipates the pain or is not relaxed) or involuntary (peritoneal inflammation).

Next palpate the abdomen deeply to detect large masses or tenderness. Use one hand on top of another and push down slowly (Procedure 2-10c). Assess for rebound tenderness by pushing down slowly and then releasing your hand quickly off the tender area. If the peritoneum is inflamed, your patient will experience pain when you let go. Alternatively, hold your hand one centimeter above your patient's abdomen at rest. Then ask him to push his abdomen out to touch your hand. Limitation by pain suggests peritoneal irritation.

If you note a protruding abdomen with bulging flanks and dull percussion sounds in dependent areas, you might perform two tests for ascites. First assess for areas of tympany and dullness while your patient is supine. Then ask him to lie on one side. Percuss again, noting once more any areas of tympany and dullness. If your patient has ascites, the area of dullness will shift down to the dependent side and the area of tympany will shift up. To test for fluid wave, ask an assistant to press the edge of his hand firmly down the midline of your patient's abdomen (Procedure 2-10d). With your fingertips, tap one flank and feel for the impulse's transmission to the other flank through excess fluid. If you detect the impulse easily, suspect ascites.

THE FEMALE GENITALIA

The external female genitalia consist of highly-vascular tissues that protect the entrance to the birth canal (Figure 2-46). The mons pubis is the hair-covered fat pad that covers the pubic symphysis. The labia majora and labia minora are

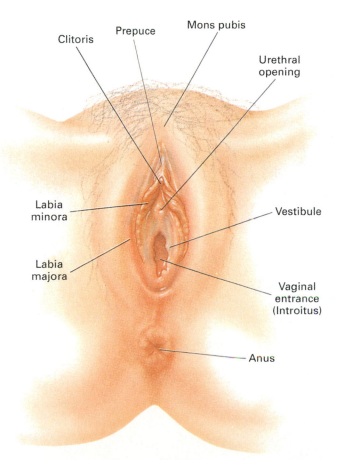

Clitoris
Prepuce
Mons pubis
Urethral opening
Labia minora
Vestibule
Labia majora
Vaginal entrance (Introitus)
Anus

FIGURE 2-46   The external female genitalia.

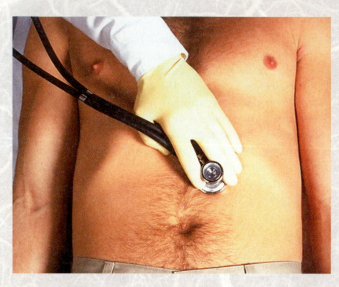

2-10a   Auscultate for renal bruits.

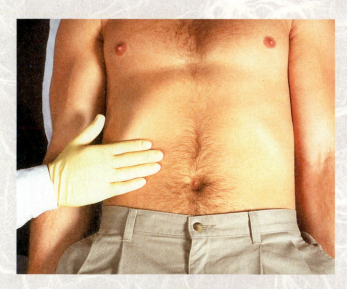

2-10b   Light abdominal palpation.

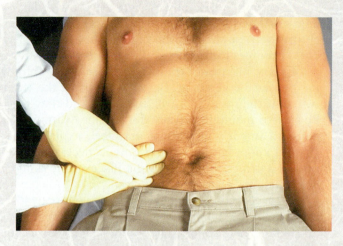

2-10c   Deep abdominal palpation.

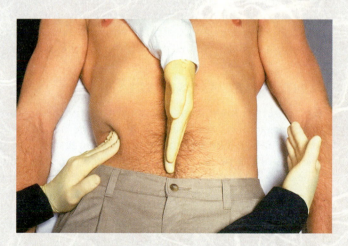

2-10d   Test for ascites.

rounded folds of tissue that protect the opening to the vagina. Extensions of the labia form the prepuce and clitoris. The vagina is the receptacle for the penis during sexual intercourse. The urethral opening lies between the clitoris and the vagina. The perineum refers to the tissue between the vagina and the anus.

The external genital organs begin to mature and take adult proportions during adolescence. Puberty also marks the appearance of breast buds, pubic hair, and the first period (menarche). The age in which sexual development occurs varies among individuals. As women grow older, ovarian function diminishes, menstrual periods cease, and pubic hair becomes gray and sparse. The labia and clitoris become smaller; the vagina narrows and shortens and its lining (the mucosa) becomes thin, pale, and dry. The ovaries and uterus decrease in size.

Except in cases of trauma or abuse, you rarely would be expected to examine the female genitalia. Before examining the external female genitalia, make sure that the room is warm and quiet and that your patient's bladder is empty. Be sure to maintain privacy during this examination. To reduce any anxiety or embarrassment your patient may feel, explain what you are doing during the exam. Expose her body areas only as necessary, be sensitive to her feelings, and project a professional demeanor. Place a pillow under her head and shoulders to help relax her abdominal muscles.

Begin your assessment by inspecting your patient's external genitalia. Look at the mons pubis, labia, and perineum for abnormalities such as inflammation, swelling, or lesions. These abnormalities may signal a sebaceous cyst or a sexually transmitted disease such as syphilis or herpes simplex virus infection. Check the bases of the pubic hair for signs of lice such as excoriation, or small, itchy, red maculopapules.

Now retract the outer labia and inspect the inner labia and urethral meatus (opening). Assess for vaginal discharge. The normal discharge is clear or cloudy and has little or no odor. A white, curd-like discharge with no odor or a yeasty, sweet odor may suggest a fungal infection (candidiasis). A yellow, green, or gray discharge with a foul or fishy odor may suggest a bacterial infection (gonorrhea or Gardnerella). Examining the external female genitalia can be an embarrassing, uncomfortable experience, especially for male clinicians. Remember it is probably twice as awkward for your patient. It is customary for male clinicians to have a female partner present during the examination.

THE MALE GENITALIA

The external male genitalia consist of the penis and scrotum. The penis is the male organ for copulation. It houses the urethra and specialized erectile tissue (Figure 2-47). The scrotum contains the testes. The glans, a conical structure at the end of the penis, is covered by a fold of skin called the foreskin, or prepuce. The foreskin may have been surgically removed by circumcision.

The genital organs begin to mature and take adult proportions during adolescence. Puberty also marks a noticeable increase in the size of the testes. As in the female, the actual age in which sexual development occurs will vary widely. As men grow older, the penis decreases in size and the testes hang lower in the scrotum. The pubic hair becomes gray and sparse.

Except for trauma, you rarely would be expected to inspect the male genitalia. Before examining the male genitalia make sure that the room is warm and quiet and that your patient's bladder is empty. Be sure to maintain privacy during this examination. To reduce any anxiety or embarrassment your patient may feel, explain what you are doing during the exam. Expose his body areas only as necessary, be sensitive to his feelings, and project a professional demeanor.

Begin your assessment by inspecting your patient's penis and scrotum. Note any inflammation, and inspect the skin around the base of the penis for abnormalities such as lesions that may be caused by sexually transmitted diseases. Also

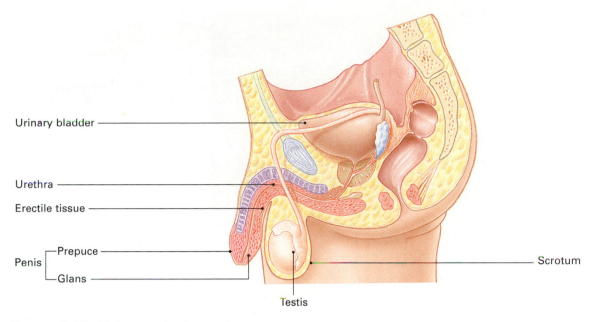

Urinary bladder

Urethra

Erectile tissue

Penis — Prepuce
— Glans

Scrotum

Testis

FIGURE 2-47   Male reproductive anatomy.

check the bases of the pubic hair for signs of lice such as excoriation or small, itchy, red maculopapules. Next inspect the glans for signs of degeneration or other abnormalities. If the foreskin is present, ask your patient to retract it. Note any abnormalities and the location of the urethral meatus. Inspect the anterior surface of the scrotum and note its contour. Then lift the scrotum to inspect its posterior surface and note any swelling or lumps. Expect acute epididymitis or testicular torsion if your patient has scrotal swelling and lower abdominal pain. Testicular torsion requires immediate intervention.

Assess any discharge from the urethral meatus. Normally no discharge is present. A profuse, yellow discharge may be a sign of gonorrhea. A scant, clear or white discharge may suggest a nongonococcal urethritis. Examining the male genitalia can be an embarrassing, uncomfortable experience, especially for female clinicians. Remember it is probably twice as awkward for your patient. It is customary for female clinicians to have a male partner present during the examination.

THE ANUS

The rectum and anus mark the most distal end of the gastrointestinal system (Figure 2-48). The anal canal is approximately 2.5–4.0 cm long and is kept closed by the internal and external anorectal sphincters. The internal ring has smooth muscle that the autonomic nervous system controls. When the rectum fills with feces the internal sphincter relaxes, resulting in the urge to defecate. Because the external sphincter has striated muscle, defecation is under voluntary control. The lower half of the anal canal contains sensory fibers, while the upper half is somewhat insensitive. Hence, many problems of the lower anus cause pain, while those in the upper region do not. The lower anus is also rich in venous circulation, promoting internal and external hemorrhoids.

Examining the anus is normally not a prehospital assessment practice. Unless your patient presents with rectal bleeding, there will be no reason for you to examine this area. Because routine internal rectal and prostate examinations are beyond the scope of this course, this section will focus on the external anal exam. As always, your aim is gentleness, a calm demeanor, and talking to your patient about what you are doing.

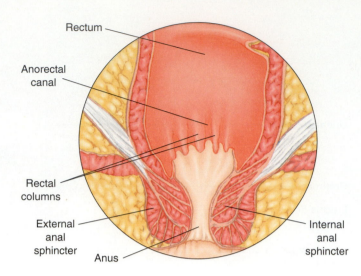

Rectum

Anorectal
canal

Rectal
columns

External
anal
sphincter

Anus

Internal
anal
sphincter

FIGURE 2-48   The anus.

Before examining the anus make sure the room is warm and quiet. Be sure to maintain privacy during this examination. To reduce any anxiety or embarrassment your patient may feel, explain what you are doing during the exam. Drape your patient appropriately and expose his body areas only as necessary; be sensitive to his feelings and project a professional demeanor. Place your patient on his left side with his legs flexed and his buttocks near the edge of the examination table. Glove your hands and spread the buttocks apart. Inspect the sacrococcygeal and perianal areas for lumps, ulcers, inflammations, rashes, or excoriation. Palpate any abnormal areas carefully and note any tenderness or inflammation. If appropriate, obtain a fecal sample and test it for occult blood. Simply smear a small sample onto a special test slide and add a couple drops of developer onto the sample. If it turns blue, there is blood in the stool.

THE MUSCULOSKELETAL SYSTEM

The musculoskeletal system consists of at least 206 bones and their associated muscles, tendons, ligaments, and cartilage. Its main functions are to give form to the body and to allow for movement. Skeletal muscle is attached to bone by a tendon (Figure 2-49). The proximal attachment is the origin, while the distal attachment is the insertion. When a muscle contracts, the distal attachment usually moves toward the origin. Movement of one bone upon another occurs at a joint. In an elaborate system, the muscles and tendons act like ropes, the bones like levers, and the joints like fulcrums to make movement possible.

Each joint's structure, along with the number and size of the surrounding ligaments, determines its range of motion. Hinge joints such as the fingers and elbows allow only flexion and extension (Figure 2-50). Ball-and-socket joints such as the shoulder and hip allow rotation and a wide range of motion. Saddle joints like those in the thumbs permit movement in several planes. Condyloid joints such as the wrist are similar to ball and socket joints but do not allow rotation. Gliding joints such as in the hands and feet permit a movement in which one bone slides across another. Pivot joints, as in the first two cervical vertebra, allow a turning motion.

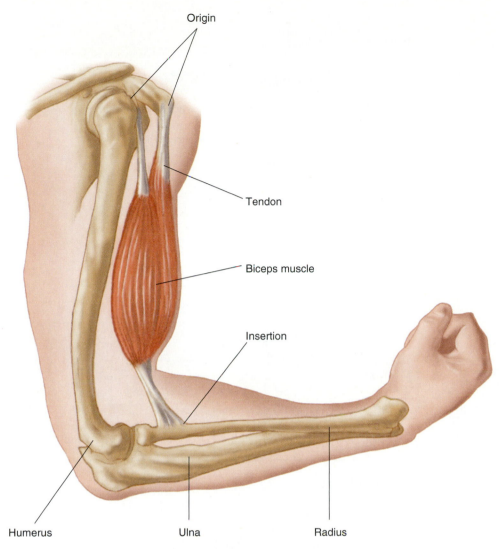

Origin

Tendon

Biceps muscle

Insertion

Humerus

Ulna

Radius

FIGURE 2-49   Interaction of bone, muscle, and tendon.

    The bones within a joint do not touch each other (Figure 2-51). Instead, their articulating surfaces are covered with cartilage. A synovial membrane at the outer margins of the cartilage creates a synovial cavity into which it secretes synovium, a viscous lubricating fluid. A joint capsule surrounds and protects the synovial capsule. In turn, strong ligaments surround the joint capsule and extend to the articulating bones. In some joints such as those in the spinal column, cartilaginous disks instead of synovial cavities separate the bones. These disks cushion the vertebrae and absorb shocks. Bursa—fluid-filled, disk-shaped sacs—lie between the skin and the convex surface of a bone where friction may occur. They appear where tendons or muscles might rub against a bone or ligament or another muscle or tendon, such as in the knee and shoulder.

    The musculoskeletal system's most obvious physical change with age is the gradual shortening in height. This occurs because the intervertebral disks become thinner and even collapse due to osteoporosis. As a result, your patient's limbs may appear longer than they should in proportion to his trunk. The other visible

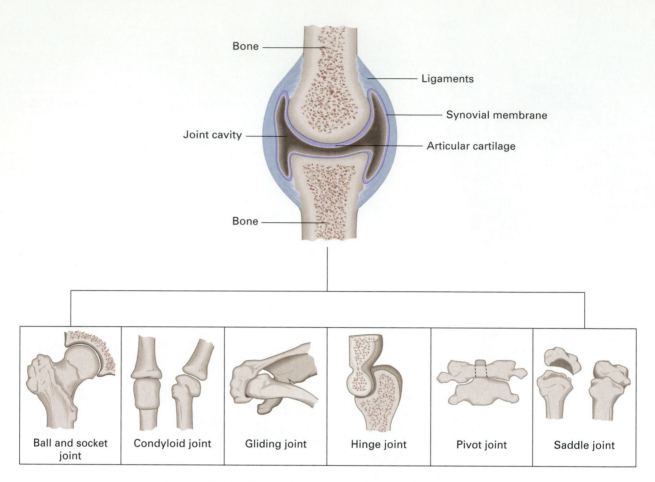

FIGURE 2-50   Types of joints.

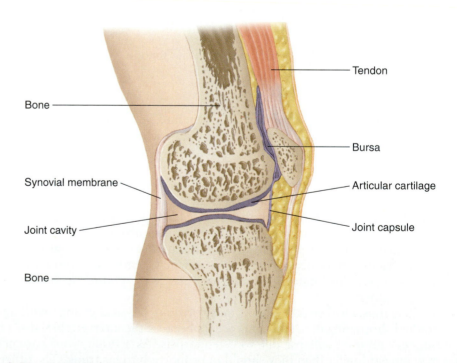

FIGURE 2-51   A synovial joint.

change is in posture. The anteroposterior diameter of the chest increases due to kyphosis (abnormal curvature of the spine), particularly in women. Also, skeletal muscles decrease in size and strength, and the ligaments lose some of their pliability. As a result, the range of motion decreases. Osteoporosis also contributes to this loss of mobility.

An examination of the musculoskeletal system must include a detailed assessment of function and structure. Inspect and palpate your patient's joints, their structure, their range of motion, and the surrounding tissues. Begin your assessment with a general observation of posture, build, and muscular development. Watch how your patient's body parts move, and observe their resting positions. Begin the exam with your patient sitting to evaluate his head, neck, shoulders, and upper extremities. Then have him stand to assess his chest, back, and ilium; ask him to walk so that you can assess his gait. Finally, ask him to lie down to examine his hips, knees, ankles, and feet.

Inspect for swelling in or around joints, changes in the surrounding tissue, redness of the overlying skin, deformities, and symmetry of impairment. Swelling may be caused by trauma to the area or by excess synovial fluid in the joint space or tissues surrounding the joint. Tissue changes may include muscle atrophy, skin changes, and subcutaneous nodules resulting from rheumatoid arthritis or rheumatic fever. Skin redness may suggest inflammation or arthritis. Deformities may be produced by restricted range of motion, misalignment of the articulating bones, dislocation (complete separation of bone ends), or subluxation (partial dislocation). Symmetrical impairment is usually associated with a disorder such as rheumatoid arthritis.

Inspect and palpate each body part, then test its range of motion and muscle strength as explained in the Motor System section later in this chapter. Examine each joint and compare joints on opposite sides for equal size, shape, color, and strength. Swelling in a joint usually involves the synovial membrane or a bursa, which will feel spongy on deep palpation within the joint space. It also may involve the surrounding structures such as ligaments, cartilage, tendons, or the bones themselves. Redness of the overlying skin suggests a nontraumatic joint inflammation such as arthritis, gout, or rheumatic fever. Palpate for tenderness in and around the joint. Try to identify the specific structure that is tender, such as a ligament or tendon. Some common causes of a tender joint include arthritis, tendinitis, bursitis, or osteomyelitis. With the back of your hand, feel over the tender area for increased heat, which suggests arthritis.

After you have inspected and palpated each body part with your patient at rest, assess range of motion. Test each joint for passive range of motion, range of motion against gravity, and range of motion against resistance. First test the joint's passive range of motion by moving it in the directions that it normally allows. For example, test the elbow, a hinge joint, for flexion and extension. Note any resistance and whether the range of motion is within normal limits. Now test range of motion against gravity by asking your patient to perform the same movements by himself. Again, note the range of motion and any difficulties. Finally, test range of motion against resistance. Have your patient perform the same movements while you apply resistance.

Passive and active range should be equal. A discrepancy indicates either a muscle weakness or a joint problem. If your patient has difficulty with passive and active tests, suspect a joint problem. If he has difficulty only with active tests, suspect a weakened muscle or nerve disorder. A decreased range of motion could indicate arthritis or injury, while an increased range of motion suggests a loosening of the structures that support the joint.

Listen for **crepitation** (or **crepitus**), the crunching sounds of unlubricated parts rubbing against each other, while you manipulate the joint. Crepitus may

Content Review

STEPS IN EVALUATING JOINTS

1 Inspection
2 Palpation
3 Passive range of motion
4 Range of motion against gravity
5 Range of motion against resistance

✱ crepitation (or crepitus) crunching sounds of unlubricated parts in joints rubbing against each other.

indicate an inflamed joint or osteoarthritis. An obvious traumatic deformity could indicate a sprained ligament, a bone fracture, or a dislocation. In these cases, modify your manipulation and range of motion exam accordingly. Non-traumatic deformities are caused by arthritis or the misalignment of bones. Avoid manipulating a painful joint.

The Extremities

The extremities are the arms and legs. A complete examination of your patient's extremities will include wrists and hands, elbows, shoulders, ankles and feet, knees, and hips.

Wrists and Hands The radius and ulna articulate with the carpal bones at the wrist, or radiocarpal joint (Figure 2-52). The carpals articulate with the metacarpals. The metacarpals articulate with the proximal phalanges at the metacarpophalangeal (MCP) joint. The proximal phalanges articulate with the middle phalanges at the proximal interphalangeal (PIP) joint. The middle phalanges articulate with the distal phalanges at the distal interphalangeal (DIP) joint. Movement at the wrist includes flexion, extension, radial deviation, and ulnar deviation. Movement at the MCP, PIP, and DIP joints includes flexion and extension. The MCP joints also allow abduction

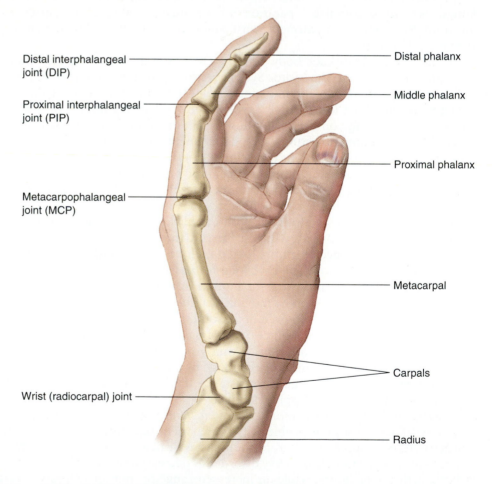

Distal interphalangeal joint (DIP)

Proximal interphalangeal joint (PIP)

Metacarpophalangeal joint (MCP)

Wrist (radiocarpal) joint

Distal phalanx

Middle phalanx

Proximal phalanx

Metacarpal

Carpals

Radius

FIGURE 2-52   Bones and joints of the hand and wrist.

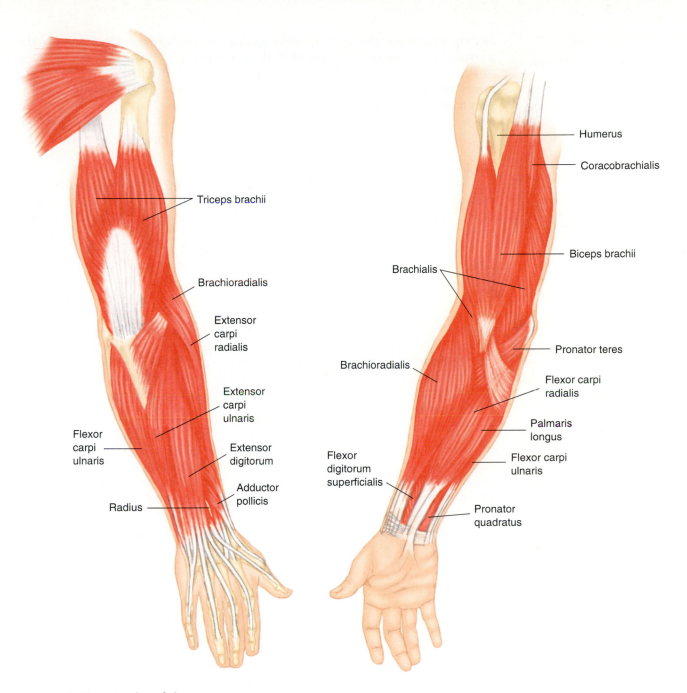

Triceps brachii

Brachioradialis

Extensor
carpi
radialis

Extensor
carpi
ulnaris

Flexor
carpi
ulnaris

Extensor
digitorum

Adductor
pollicis

Radius

Humerus

Coracobrachialis

Biceps brachii

Brachialis

Pronator teres

Flexor carpi
radialis

Palmaris
longus

Flexor carpi
ulnaris

Brachioradialis

Flexor
digitorum
superficialis

Pronator
quadratus

FIGURE 2-53   Muscles of the arm.

(spreading the fingers out) and adduction (bringing them back together). The major flexor muscles are the flexor carpi radialis and flexor carpi ulnaris (Figure 2-53). The major extensor muscles are the extensor carpi radialis longus, extensor carpi radialis brevis, and extensor carpi ulnaris.

Begin by inspecting your patient's hands and wrists. Next palpate them by feeling the medial and lateral aspects of the DIP joints and then the PIP joints with your thumb and forefinger (Procedure 2-11a on page 108). Note any swelling, sponginess, bony enlargement, or tenderness. Then palpate the tops and bottoms of these joints in the same manner. Now ask your patient to flex his hand slightly so you can examine each MCP. Compress the MCP joints by squeezing the hand from side-to-side between your thumbs and fingers and note any swelling, tenderness, or sponginess (Procedure 2-11b). Finally, palpate each wrist joint with your thumbs and note any swelling, sponginess, or tenderness (Procedure 2-11c). If your patient has had swelling of both his wrists or finger joints for several weeks, suspect an inflammatory condition such as rheumatoid arthritis.

To assess range of motion, ask your patient to make a fist with each hand and then open his fist and extend and spread his fingers. He should be able to make a tight fist and spread his fingers smoothly and easily. Next ask him to flex and then extend his wrist. Normal flexion is 90°, extension 70° (Procedure 2-11d). Check for radial and ulnar deviation by asking your patient to flex his wrist and move his hands medially and laterally. Normal radial movement is 20°, ulnar movement 45° (Procedure 2-11e).

If your patient complains of hand pain and numbness, especially at night, suspect carpal tunnel syndrome, the painful inflammation of the median nerve. To detect additional signs of this disorder, hold your patient's wrists in acute flexion for 60 seconds (Procedure 2-11f). In carpal tunnel syndrome, he will develop numbness or tingling in the areas innervated by the median nerve—the palmar surface of his thumb, index, and middle fingers, and part of his ring finger. Throughout these maneuvers watch for deformities, redness, swelling, nodules, or muscular atrophy.

Elbows The lateral and medial epicondyles (large rounded edges) of the distal humerus, the olecranon process of the proximal ulna, and the proximal radius comprise the elbow joint (Figure 2-54). Between the olecranon process and skin lies a bursa. The ulnar nerve (funny bone) extends through the groove between the olecranon process and the medial epicondyle. The elbow is a hinge joint, allowing flexion and extension. The major flexor muscles are the

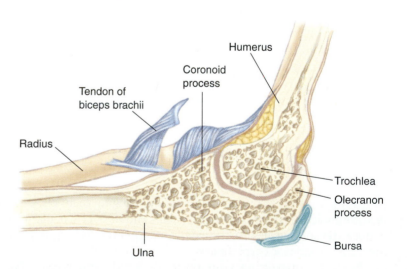

FIGURE 2-54 The elbow.

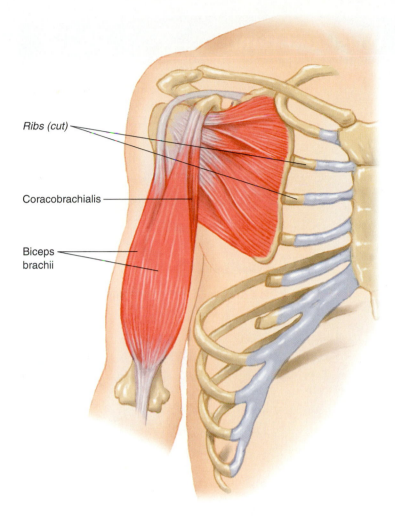

Ribs (cut)

Coracobrachialis

Biceps
brachii

Anterior

FIGURE 2-55   Elbow flexors.

biceps (Figure 2-55). The major extensor muscles are the triceps (Figure 2-56).
Just below the elbow, the relationship of the radius and ulna to the pronator
and supinator muscles allows the forearm to supinate (turn palm up) and
pronate (turn palm down) (Figure 2-57).

To examine the elbow, support your patient's forearm with your hand so that
his elbow is flexed about 70° (Procedure 2-12a on page 109). Inspect the elbow
joint and note any deformities, swelling, or nodules. Palpate the joint structures
for tenderness, swelling, or thickening. Press on the medial and lateral epicondyles (Procedure 2-12b). Inflammation of either the medial epicondyle (ten-
nis elbow) or of the lateral epicondyle (golfer's elbow) suggests tendinitis at those
muscle insertion sites. To assess range of motion, ask your patient to flex and extend his elbow (Procedure 2-12c). Normally he will flex his elbow up to 160° and
return it back to the neutral position. Then ask him to keep his elbows flexed and
his arms at his sides. Now have him turn his palms up and then down. Normally
both supination and pronation are 90° (Procedure 2-12d).

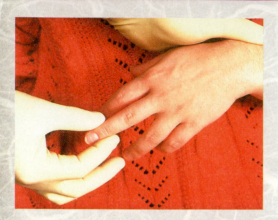

2-11a Palpate the DIP and PIP joints.

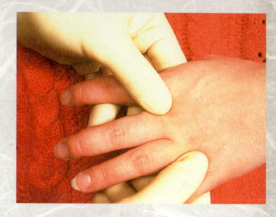

2-11b Palpate the MCP joint.

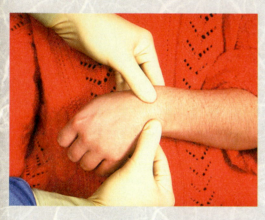

2-11c Palpate the wrist.

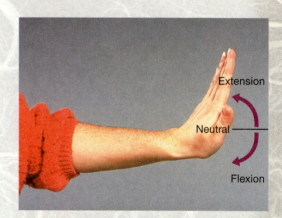

2-11d Assess wrist flexion and extension.

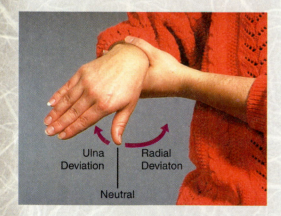

2-11e Assess radial and ulnar deviation.

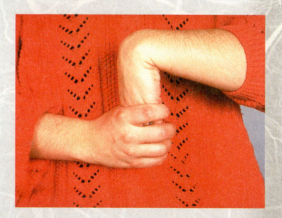

2-11f Test for carpal tunnel syndrome.

Procedure 2-12 Examining the Elbow

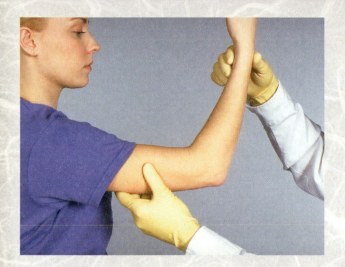

2-12a Inspect the elbow.

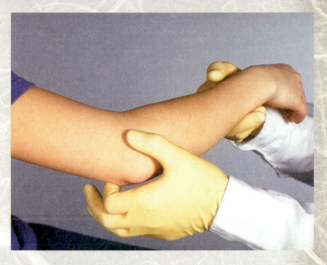

2-12b Palpate the lateral and medial epicondyles.

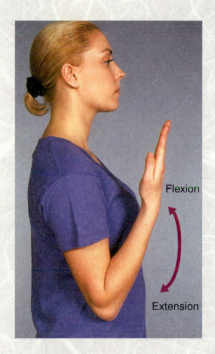

Flexion

Extension

2-12c Assess elbow flexion and extension.

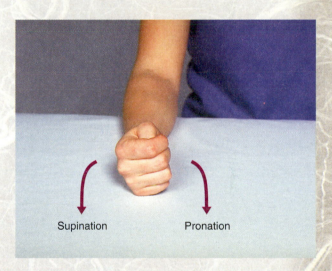

Supination   Pronation

2-12d Assess supination and pronation of the wrist.

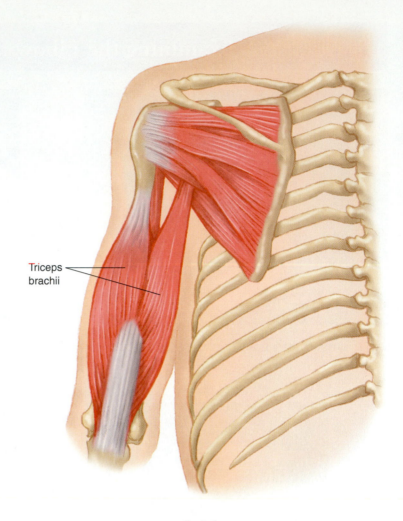

Triceps
brachii

Posterior

FIGURE 2-56   Elbow extensors.

Shoulders The shoulder girdle consists of articulations between the clavicle and the scapula and between the scapula and the head of the humerus (Figure 2-58). The sternoclavicular joint, which joins the clavicle and the manubrium, is the only bony link between the upper extremity and the axial skeleton. Movement at this joint is largely passive and occurs as a result of active movements of the scapula. The distal clavicle articulates with the acromion, or acromion process, of the scapula at the acromioclavicular (AC) joint. The clavicle acts as a strut, keeping the upper limb away from the thorax and permitting a greater range of motion. The AC joint also helps provide stability to the upper limb, reducing the need for muscle energy to keep the shoulder in its proper alignment.

The glenohumeral joint is a ball-and-socket joint that allows flexion, extension, internal and external rotation, abduction, and adduction. It has the greatest range of motion of any joint in the body and as a result is the most frequent site for dislocation. The head of the humerus (ball) fits into the glenoid cavity (socket) of the scapula. The proximal humerus has two rounded protrusions called the greater and lesser tubercles. The biceps tendon runs through the bicipital groove between the greater and lesser tubercles and is easily palpable on the lateral surface of the shoulder. The glenohumeral joint is encapsulated and reinforced by the tendons and four muscles that make up the rotator cuff and by the large deltoid

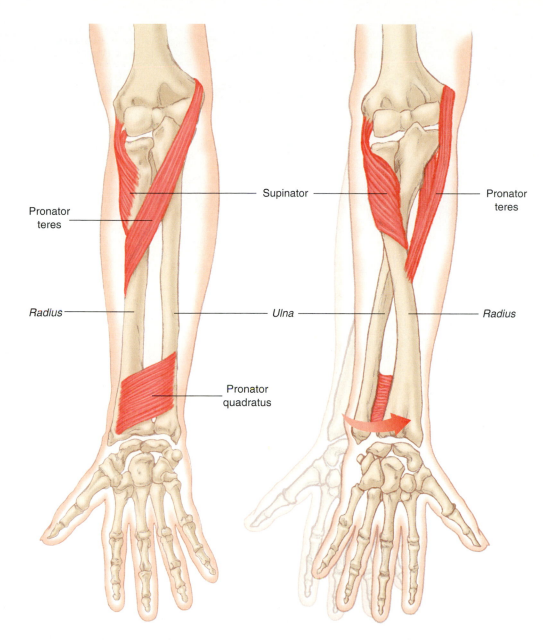

Pronator
teres

Supinator

Pronator
teres

Radius

Ulna

Radius

Pronator
quadratus

FIGURE 2-57   Pronator-supinator muscles.

muscle (Figures 2-59 and 2-60). The muscles of the rotator cuff include the supraspinatus, the infraspinatus, the teres minor, and the subscapularis muscles.

To assess your patient's shoulders look at them from the front and then look at his scapulae from the back. Inspect the entire shoulder girdle for swelling, deformities, or muscular atrophy. Before you palpate, ask your patient if he has any pain in his shoulders. If so, have him point to it with one finger; palpate this area last. Palpate the shoulders with your fingertips, moving along the clavicles out toward the humerus (Procedure 2-13a on page 114). Palpate the sternoclavicular joint, acromioclavicular joint, subacromial region, and the bicipital groove for tenderness (biceps tendinitis) or swelling (bursitis). Now palpate over the greater tubercle of the humerus as you abduct the arm at the shoulder. Then palpate the scapulae.

To assess range of motion ask your patient to raise both arms forward and then straight overhead (flexion) (Procedure 2-13b). Expect to see forward flexion

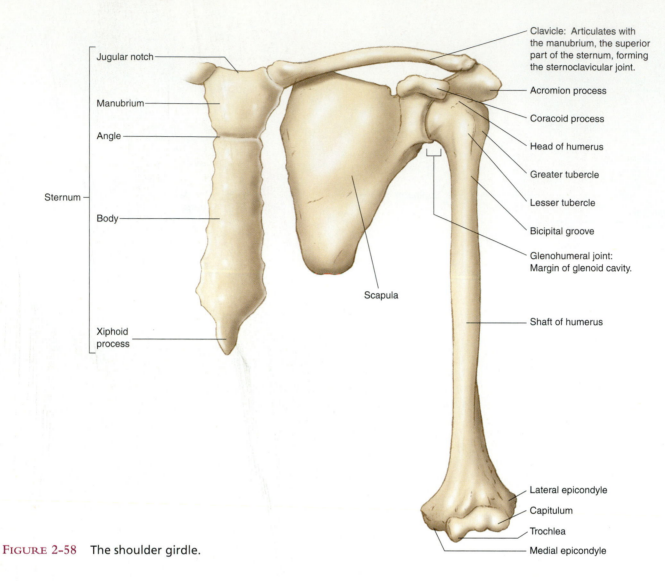

Jugular notch

Manubrium

Angle

Sternum

Body

Xiphoid
process

Clavicle: Articulates with
the manubrium, the superior
part of the sternum, forming
the sternoclavicular joint.

Acromion process

Coracoid process

Head of humerus

Greater tubercle

Lesser tubercle

Bicipital groove

Glenohumeral joint:
Margin of glenoid cavity.

Scapula

Shaft of humerus

Lateral epicondyle

Capitulum

Trochlea

Medial epicondyle

FIGURE 2-58   The shoulder girdle.

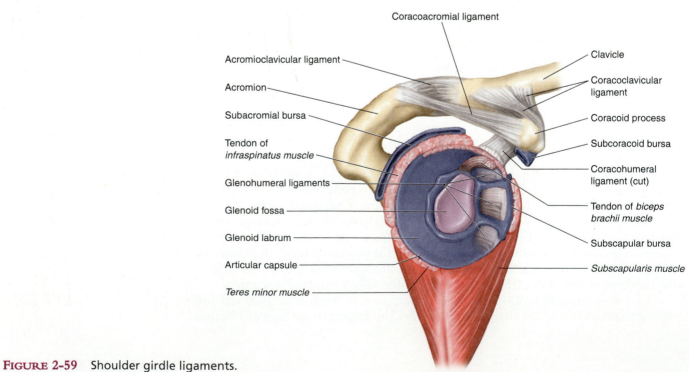

Coracoacromial ligament

Acromioclavicular ligament

Acromion

Subacromial bursa

Tendon of
infraspinatus muscle

Glenohumeral ligaments

Glenoid fossa

Glenoid labrum

Articular capsule

Teres minor muscle

Clavicle

Coracoclavicular
ligament

Coracoid process

Subcoracoid bursa

Coracohumeral
ligament (cut)

Tendon of *biceps
brachii muscle*

Subscapular bursa

Subscapularis muscle

FIGURE 2-59   Shoulder girdle ligaments.

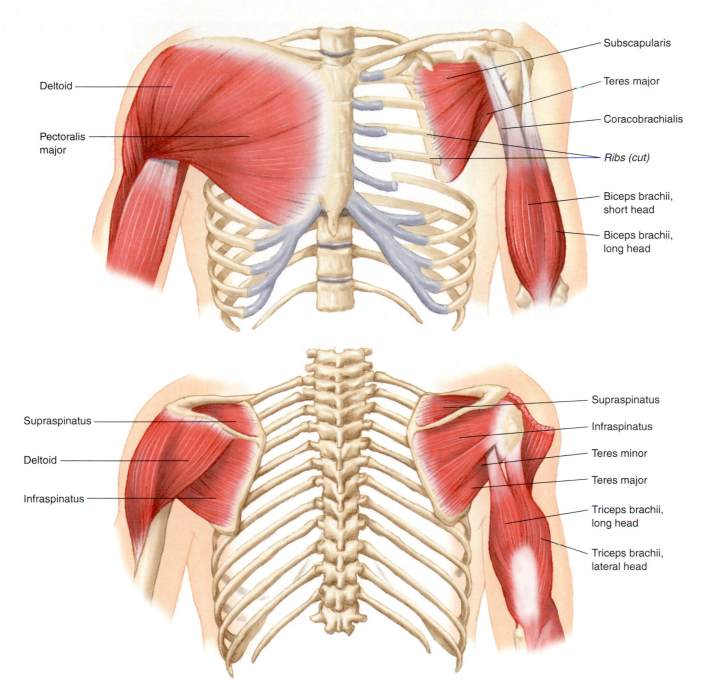

Deltoid

Pectoralis
major

Subscapularis

Teres major

Coracobrachialis

Ribs (cut)

Biceps brachii,
short head

Biceps brachii,
long head

Supraspinatus

Deltoid

Infraspinatus

Supraspinatus

Infraspinatus

Teres minor

Teres major

Triceps brachii,
long head

Triceps brachii,
lateral head

Figure 2-60   Shoulder muscles.

of 180°. Next ask him to extend both arms behind his back (extension). Normal extension is 50°. Now have him raise both arms overhead from the side (abduction) (Procedure 2-13c). Normal abduction is 180°. Then ask him to lower his arms and swing them as far as he can across his body (adduction). Normal shoulder adduction is 75°. Finally have him adduct his shoulders to 90°, pronate, and flex his elbows 90° to the front of his body. Now ask him to rotate his shoulders to the "goal post" position (external rotation) (Procedure 2-13d). Normal external rotation is 90°. Finally, ask him to place both hands behind the small of his back (internal rotation). Normal internal rotation is 90°. During these motions, cup your hands over your patient's shoulders and note any crepitus.

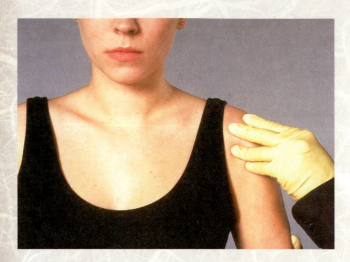

2-13a   Palpate the shoulder with your fingertips.

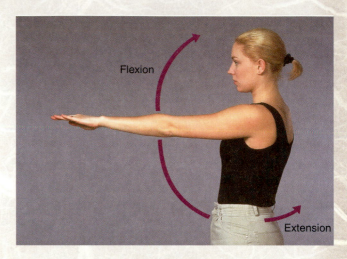

2-13b   Assess shoulder flexion and extension.

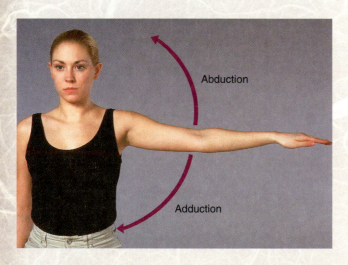

2-13c   Assess shoulder abduction and adduction.

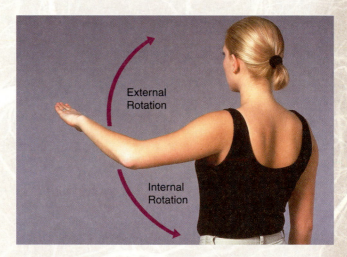

2-13d   Assess internal and external shoulder rotation.

Ankles and Feet The foot comprises seven tarsal bones, five metatarsal bones, and fourteen phalanges (Figure 2-61). The talus, the calcaneus (heel), and the other tarsals articulate in a system of joints that allows inversion (lifting the inside of the foot) and eversion (lifting the outside of the foot). The most distal tarsals articulate with the metatarsals, which articulate with the proximal phalanges at the metatarsophalangeal joints.

At the ankle joint, the distal tibia (medial malleolus) and the distal fibula (lateral malleolus) articulate with the talus (Figure 2-62). Ligaments stretching from each

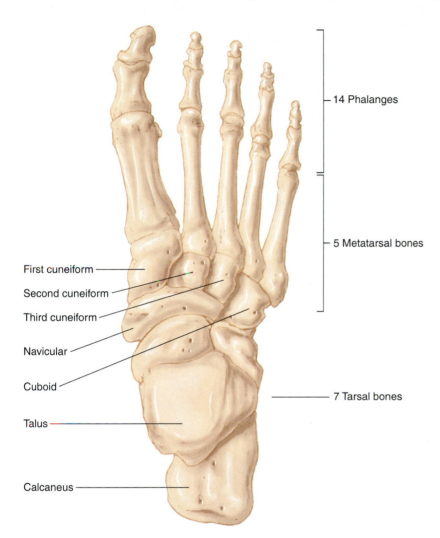

First cuneiform

Second cuneiform

Third cuneiform

Navicular

Cuboid

Talus

Calcaneus

14 Phalanges

5 Metatarsal bones

7 Tarsal bones

FIGURE 2-61   Bones of the foot.

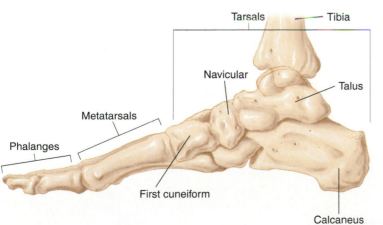

Tarsals   Tibia

Navicular

Talus

Metatarsals

Phalanges

First cuneiform

Calcaneus

FIGURE 2-62   The foot and ankle.

malleolus to the foot itself hold the ankle joint together. The strong Achilles tendon, which inserts on the calcaneus (heel), also helps maintain the ankle's integrity. Movement in the ankle is limited to dorsiflexion (raising the foot) and plantar flexion (lowering the foot). The major dorsiflexor muscle is the tibialis anterior (Figure 2-63). The major plantar flexor is the gastrocnemius (calf muscle) (Figure 2-64).

Inspect the foot and ankle for obvious deformities, nodules, swelling, calluses, or corns. Palpate the anterior aspect of each ankle joint with your thumbs and note any sponginess, swelling, or tenderness (Procedure 2-14a on next page). Feel along the Achilles tendon for tenderness or nodules. Exert pressure between your thumbs and fingers on each metatarsophalangeal joint (Procedure 2-14b). Acute inflammation of these joints suggests gout. Tenderness is an early sign of rheumatoid arthritis.

To test range of motion, ask your patient to bring his foot upward (dorsiflexion) (Procedure 2-14c). Normal dorsiflexion is 20°. Then have him point it downward (plantar flexion). Normal plantar flexion is 45°. Next, while stabilizing the ankle with one hand, grasp the heel with the other hand and invert the foot, then evert it (Procedure 2-14d). Normal inversion is 30°, normal eversion 20°. These four movements test the ankle joint's stability. A sprained ankle will cause your patient pain when the injured ligament is stretched or torn. Since the lateral ligaments are smaller and weaker than the medial ligaments, lateral sprains are more common, causing severe pain upon inversion and plantar flexion. In arthritis, pain and tenderness will accompany movement in any direction. Finally, flex and extend the toes (Procedure 2-14e). Expect a great range of motion in these joints, especially the big toes.

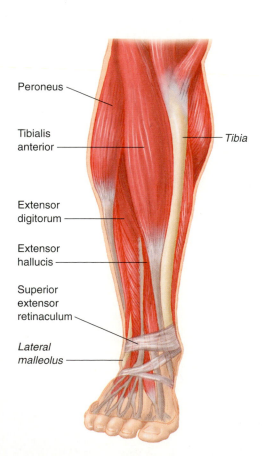

FIGURE 2-63   The dorsiflexors.

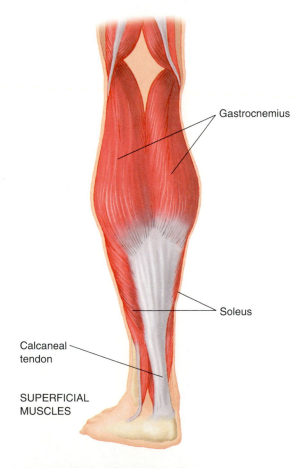

FIGURE 2-64   The plantar flexors.

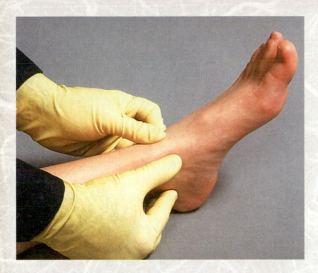

2-14a Palpate the ankle and foot.

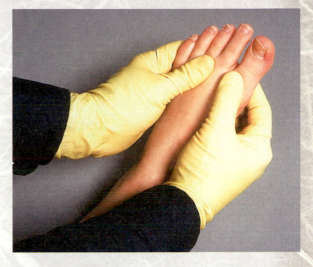

2-14b Palpate the metatarsal-phalangeal joints.

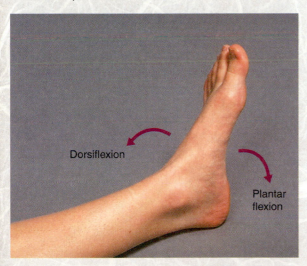

Dorsiflexion

Plantar flexion

2-14c Assess dorsiflexion and plantar flexion.

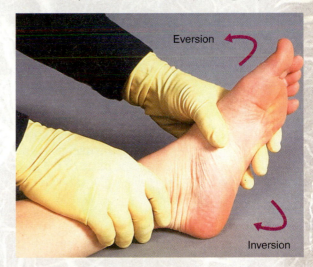

Eversion

Inversion

2-14d Assess inversion and eversion of the foot.

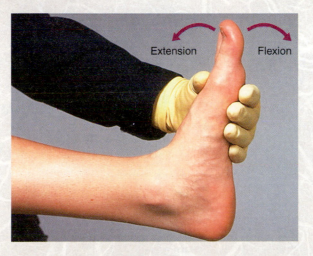

Extension

Flexion

2-14e Test flexion and extension of the toes.

Knee The knee joint involves the distal femur, the proximal tibia, and the patella (Figure 2-65). The distal femur and the proximal tibia meet at this joint and are cushioned by the lateral meniscus and the medial meniscus, which form a cartilaginous surface for painfree movement. The joint capsule contains synovial fluid. Several ligaments surround the knee joint and help maintain its integrity. The medial and lateral collateral ligaments provide side-to-side stability and are easily palpable. The anterior and posterior cruciate ligaments, which give the knee front-to-back stability, lie deep within the joint capsule and are not palpable.

The knee is a modified hinge joint, allowing flexion and extension, with some rotation during flexion. The major flexors are a group of three muscles (biceps femoris, semimembranosus, and semitendinosus) known as the hamstrings (Figure 2-66). The major extensors are a group of four muscles (vastus lateralis, vastus intermedius, vastus medialis, and rectus femoris) known as the quadriceps (Figure 2-67). The femur can rotate on the tibia slightly. The patella lies deep in the middle of the quadriceps tendon, which inserts on the tibial tuberosity below the knee. Concave areas at each side of the patella and below it contain synovial fluid.

Inspect your patient's knees for alignment and deformities. Look for the concave areas that usually appear on each side of the patella and just above it. The absence of these concavities indicates swelling in the knee or the surrounding structures. If swelling is present, milk the medial aspect of the knee firmly upward two or three times to displace the fluid. Then press the knee just behind the lateral margin of the patella and watch for a return of fluid (a positive sign for effusion) (Procedure 2-15a on page 122). Feel for any thickening or swelling around the patella; these suggest synovial thickening or effusion. Compress the patella and move it against the femur (Procedure 2-15b). Note any pain or tenderness.

To test for range of motion, have your patient flex his knee to 90°. Press your thumbs into the joint and palpate along the tibial margins from the patellar tendon laterally. Palpate along the course of each ligament and note any points of tenderness. If your patient has tenderness, expect damage to the meniscus or to lateral ligaments. If you feel irregular bony ridges, suspect osteoarthritis. Now test for stability of the medial and collateral ligaments by moving the knee joint from side to

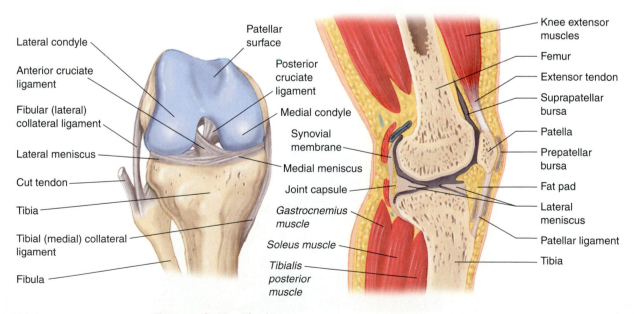

FIGURE 2-65 The knee.

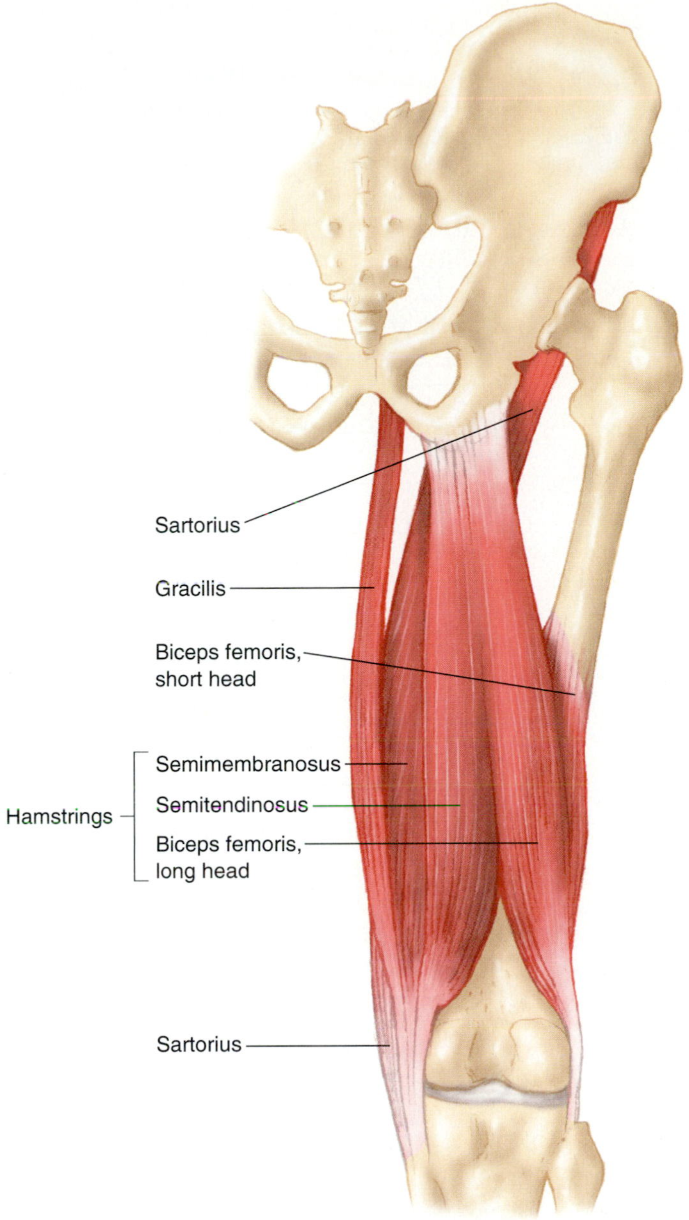

FIGURE 2-66   The knee flexors.

Sartorius

Gracilis

Biceps femoris, short head

Semimembranosus

Hamstrings — Semitendinosus

Biceps femoris, long head

Sartorius

side with the knee flexed to 30° (Procedure 2-15c). There should be little movement if the joint is stable. Evaluate the anterior and posterior cruciate ligaments by using the "drawer" test. Try to move the knee joint anterior and posterior, much like opening and closing a drawer (Procedure 2-15d). Again, if the ligaments are strong, there should be little movement.

Now have your patient sit at the edge of the exam table with his lower legs dangling. Ask him to extend his leg. Normal extension is 90° (Procedure 2-15e). Ask him to roll over and try to touch his foot to his back. Normal flexion is 135°. With your patient standing, inspect the posterior surface of his legs, especially the popliteal region behind his knees. Note any deformity or abnormalities such as bowlegs, knock-knee, or flexion contracture, the inability to fully extend the knee.

Hips The hip joint involves the head of the proximal femur (ball) and the acetabulum (socket) of the ischium (Figure 2-68). Although the hip is a ball-and-socket joint like the shoulder, the two are very different. While the shoulder has

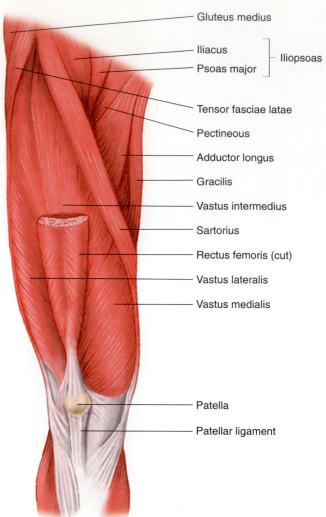

FIGURE 2-67   The knee extensors.
(The vastus intermedius is behind
the rectus femoris.)

Gluteus medius

Iliacus ⎤
Psoas major ⎦ Iliopsoas

Tensor fasciae latae

Pectineous

Adductor longus

Gracilis

Vastus intermedius

Sartorius

Rectus femoris (cut)

Vastus lateralis

Vastus medialis

Patella

Patellar ligament

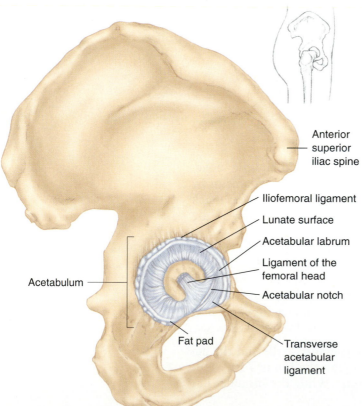

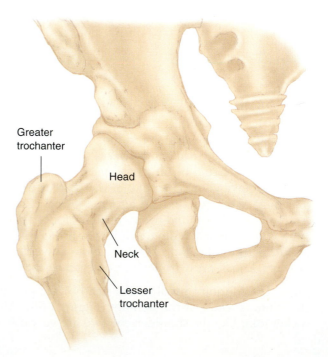

Anterior
superior
iliac spine

Iliofemoral ligament

Lunate surface

Acetabular labrum

Ligament of the
femoral head

Acetabular notch

Transverse
acetabular
ligament

Acetabulum

Fat pad

Greater
trochanter

Head

Neck

Lesser
trochanter

FIGURE 2-68   The hip joint.

a wide range of motion, the hip joint is restricted by many large ligaments, a bony ridge in the pelvis, and capsular fibers. Hip flexion, the most important movement, occurs via the iliopsoas muscle group (Figure 2-69). Other movements, though much more limited in range than the shoulder, include extension, abduction, adduction, and internal and external rotation. A number of muscle groups control these movements. One of these is the gluteus, a series of adductor muscles and lateral rotators (Figure 2-70). Three bursa in the hip play an important role in painfree movement. The iliopectineal bursa sits just anterior to the hip joint. The trochanteric bursa lies just to the side and behind the greater trochanter. The ischiogluteal bursa resides under the ischial tuberosity.

Inspect the hips for deformities, symmetry, and swelling. Palpate for tenderness all around the joint, including the three bursa and greater trochanter of the femur (Procedure 2-16a on page 123). Test the hip's range of motion with your patient supine. Ask him to raise his knee to his chest and pull it firmly against his abdomen. Observe the degree of flexion at the knee and hip (normally 120°) (Procedure 2-16b). Now flex the hip at 90° and stabilize the thigh

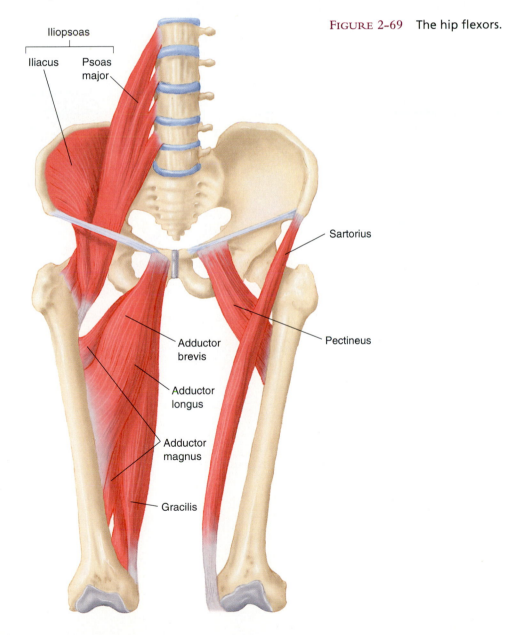

Iliopsoas
Iliacus   Psoas major

FIGURE 2-69   The hip flexors.

Sartorius

Adductor brevis

Pectineus

Adductor longus

Adductor magnus

Gracilis

Procedure 2-15   Examining the Knee

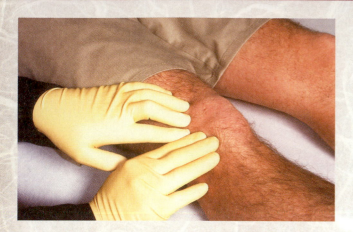

2-15a   Palpate the knee.

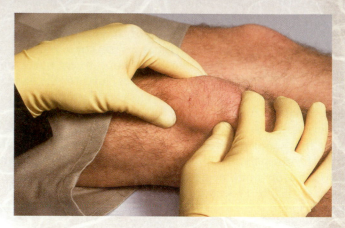

2-15b   Palpate the patella.

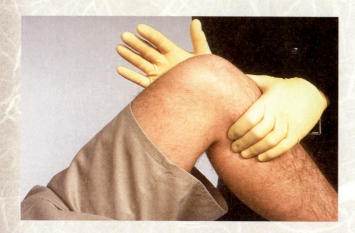

2-15c   Test the collateral ligaments of the knee.

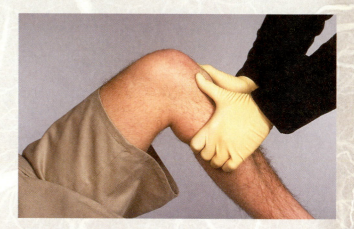

2-15d   Test the cruciate ligaments of the knee.

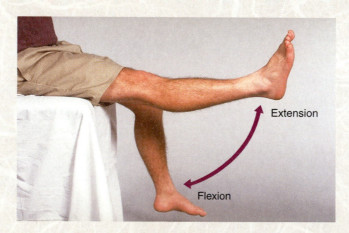

2-15e   Assess knee flexion and extension.

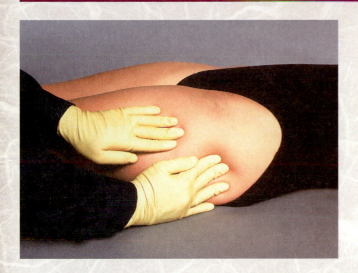

2-16a   Palpate the hip.

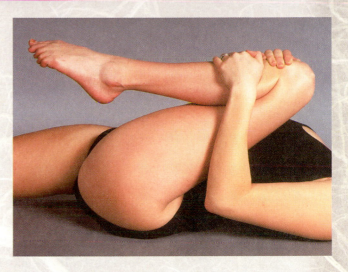

2-16b   Assess hip flexion with the knee flexed.

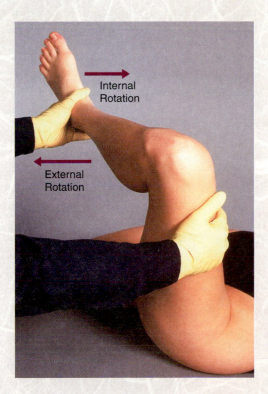

Internal
Rotation

External
Rotation

2-16c   Assess external and internal rotation of the hip.

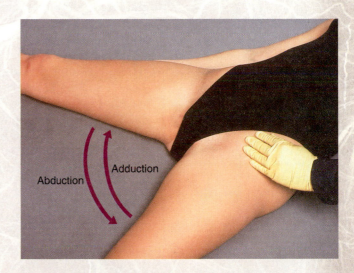

Abduction

Adduction

2-16d   Assess hip abduction and adduction.

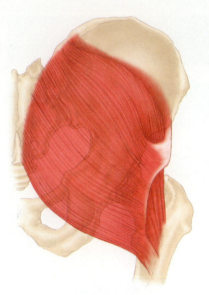
Gluteus maximus

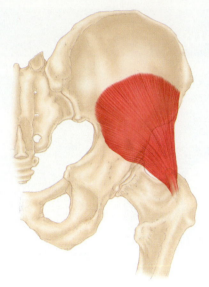
Gluteus minimus

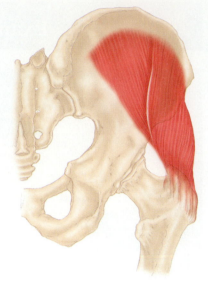
Gluteus medius

FIGURE 2-70   The gluteus muscles.

with one hand while you grasp the ankle with the other. Swing the lower leg medially to evaluate external rotation and laterally to evaluate internal rotation (Procedure 2-16c). Normal external rotation is 40°, normal internal rotation 45°. Arthritis restricts internal rotation. To test for hip abduction, have your patient extend his legs. Then while you stabilize the anterior superior iliac spine with one hand, abduct the other leg until you feel the iliac spine move. This marks the degree of hip abduction, which is normally 90° (Procedure 2-16d). If your patient complains of hip pain or if range of motion is limited, palpate the three bursa for swelling (bursitis) and tenderness.

The Spine

The spine comprises the cervical, thoracic, lumbar, sacral, and coccygeal vertebrae (Figure 2-71). Cartilaginous disks separate the vertebrae from one another, except for those in the sacrum and coccyx, which fuse in adulthood. The vertebrae form a series of gliding joints that permit a variety of movements.

The cervical vertebrae are the most mobile. C1 and C2 share a special structural relationship. C1, also known as the atlas because it supports the head much as the mythical Atlas supported the world, allows flexion and extension between itself and the skull. This enables us to look up and down. C2, also known as the axis, has a finger-like projection called the odontoid process. The atlas sits atop the odontoid process and rotates around it. The cervical spine (C2 through C7) permits flexion, extension, lateral bending, and rotation in a fairly wide range of motion in all directions. The thoracic vertebrae (T1 through T12) articulate with the 12 sets of ribs that protect the vital organs of the chest. The lumbar vertebrae (L1 through L5) are the most massive because they bear most of the body's weight when it is standing erect. Like the cervical vertebrae, they are not well protected and are the site of frequent back problems. They, too, allow flexion, extension, lateral bending, and rotation.

The spinal cord runs through a foramen (opening) in the center of each vertebra. Nerve roots for both sensory and motor nerves leave the spinal cord bilaterally at each level and innervate the various body regions (Figure 2-72).

When the vertebrae's supporting structures are injured, the risk of damage to the spinal column, and ultimately to the spinal cord, becomes a priority concern.

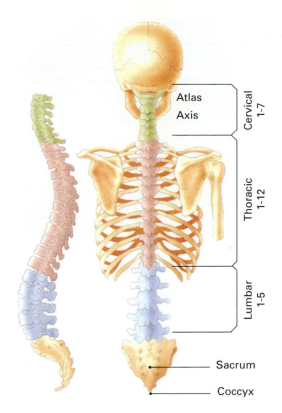

Atlas

Axis

Cervical 1-7

Thoracic 1-12

Lumbar 1-5

Sacrum

Coccyx

FIGURE 2-71   The spinal column.

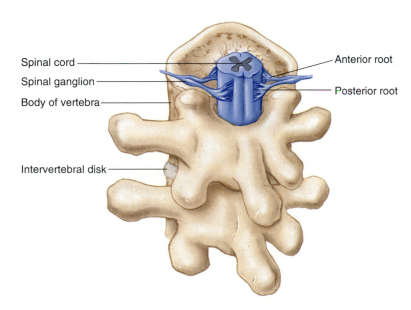

Spinal cord

Spinal ganglion

Body of vertebra

Intervertebral disk

Anterior root

Posterior root

FIGURE 2-72   The vertebrae.

Damage to the cord or nerve roots can render those regions numb and immobile. Ligaments, tendons, muscles, and various other connective tissues hold the vertebrae in place. When these supporting structures are injured, the risk of damage to the spinal column, and ultimately to the spinal cord, becomes a priority concern.

Table 2-7	SPINAL CURVATURES
Condition	**Description**
Normal	Concave in cervical and lumbar regions, convex in thorax
Lordosis	Exaggerated lumbar concavity (swayback)
Kyphosis	Exaggerated thoracic concavity (hunchback)
Scoliosis	Lateral curvature

To assess your patient's spine, first inspect his head and neck for deformities, abnormal posture, and asymmetrical skin folds. The head should be erect and the spine straight. Ask your patient to bend forward slightly while you visually identify the spinous processes, the paravertebral muscles, the scapulae, the iliac crests, and the posterior iliac spines (usually marked by dimples). Draw imaginary horizontal lines across the shoulders and iliac crests. Now draw an imaginary vertical line from T1 to the space between the buttocks (gluteal cleft). Any deviations suggest a variety of pathologies.

Next observe your patient from the side. Evaluate the curves of the cervical, thoracic, and lumbar spine and note any irregularities. Common abnormalities of the spine include lordosis, scoliosis, and kyphosis (Table 2-7). Using the pads of your fingers, palpate the spinous processes for tenderness (Procedure 2-17a on next page). Feel the supporting structures for muscle tone, symmetry, size, and tenderness or spasms. If your patient exhibits tenderness of the spinous processes and paravertebral muscles, suspect a herniated intervertebral disk, most commonly found between L4 and S1.

Now test range of motion. First test for flexion by asking your patient to touch his chin to his chest (Procedure 2-17b). Flexion is normally 45°. Next, ask him to bend his head backward. This tests extension, which normally is up to 55°. Now test for rotation by asking your patient to touch his chin to each shoulder (Procedure 2-17c). Normal rotation is 70° on each side. Finally ask him to touch his ears to his shoulders without raising his shoulders. This assesses lateral bending, which normally is 40° on each side (Procedure 2-17d). Now test for flexion of the lower spine with your patient standing. Ask him to bend and touch his toes (Procedure 2-17e). Note the smoothness and symmetry of movement, the range of motion, and the curves in the lumbar region. Normal flexion ranges from 75° to 90°. If the lumbar area remains concave or appears asymmetrical during this exam, your patient may have a muscle spasm. Next stabilize your patient's pelvis with your hands and have him bend sideways; normal lateral bending is 35° on each side (Procedure 2-17f). To assess hyperextension, ask him to bend backwards toward you; normal hyperextension is 30° (Procedure 2-17g). Finally test spinal rotation by asking your patient to twist his shoulders one way, then the other. Normally they will rotate 30° to each side (Procedure 2-17h).

If your patient complains of lower back pain radiating down the back of one leg, assess it by having him lie supine on the table. Ask him to raise his straightened leg until he feels pain. Note the angle of elevation at which the pain occurs, as well as the quality and distribution of the pain. Now dorsiflex your patient's foot. If this causes a sharp pain that radiates from your patient's back down his leg, suspect compression of the nerve roots of the lower lumbar region. Repeat this test with the other leg. Increased pain in the affected leg when the opposite leg is raised confirms the finding.

Procedure 2-17 Assessing the Spine

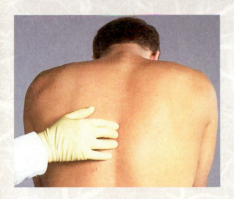

2-17a   Palpate the spine.

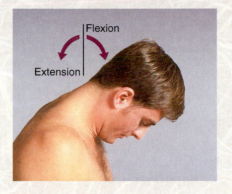

2-17b   Test flexion and extension of the head and neck.

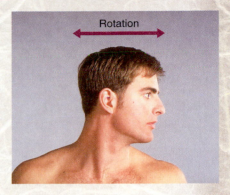

2-17c   Test rotation of the head and neck.

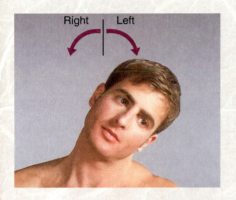

2-17d   Assess lateral bending of the head and neck.

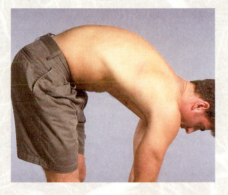

2-17e   Assess flexion of the lower spine.

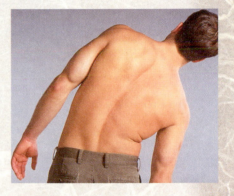

2-17f   Assess lateral bending of the lower spine.

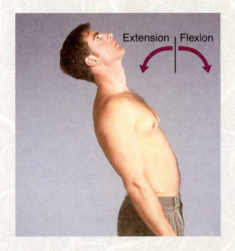

2-17g   Assess spinal extension.

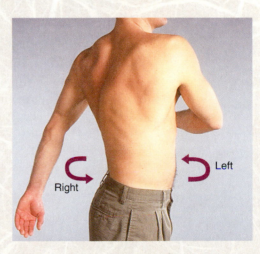

2-17h   Assess spinal rotation.

THE PERIPHERAL VASCULAR SYSTEM

The peripheral arterial system delivers oxygenated blood to the tissues of the extremities (Figure 2-73). Where the arteries lie close to the skin, the pulse is palpable. The brachial artery runs along the medial humerus and delivers blood to the arm and hands. Palpate the brachial pulse just above the elbow and medial to the biceps tendon and muscle. The brachial artery splits into the radial and ulnar arteries that deliver blood to the forearm and hands. Palpate the radial artery just above the wrist on the thumb side; palpate the ulnar artery just above the wrist on the other side.

In the lower extremities, the femoral artery delivers blood to the legs and feet. Palpate the femoral artery just below the inguinal ligament midway between the anterior superior iliac spine and the symphysis pubis. The femoral artery then branches into the popliteal artery, which passes behind the knee and is easily palpated there. Below the knee the popliteal artery branches into the posterior tibial artery, which travels behind the tibia and can be felt just below the medial malleolus. The anterior branch can be felt as the dorsalis pedis pulse on top of the foot just lateral to the extensor tendon of the big toe.

The venous system comprises deep, superficial, and communicating veins that return blood to the heart. In the upper extremities, superficial veins are visible in the back of the hand, the inside of the arms, and in the antecubital fossa (crook of the elbow). These veins are used for venous access in the emergency setting. They eventually deliver their blood into the superior vena cava en route to the right atrium. In the legs, the vast majority of venous return happens via deep veins. The superficial veins, however, also play an important role. The great saphenous vein originates in the foot and joins the deep vein system near the inguinal ligament. The small saphenous vein, which also begins in the foot, joins the deep system in the popliteal space behind the knee. The two saphenous systems and the deep system are connected in other places by communicating veins and anastomotic vessels. The veins of the lower extremities deliver their blood into the inferior vena cava en route to the heart. Venous flow occurs via muscular contractions that push the blood against gravity toward the heart and one-way valves that prohibit backflow.

The lymphatic system is a network of valveless vessels that drains fluid, called lymph, from the body tissues and delivers it to the subclavian vein (Figure 2-74). Lymph nodes in the neck, the axilla, and the groin help filter impurities en route to the heart. They are palpable when congested with infectious products.

The lymph system plays an important role in the body's immune system. It also plays an important role in our circulatory system. When arterial blood flows into a capillary bed, hydrostatic pressure pushes fluid across the capillary membrane into the tissues. As the blood flows through the capillary bed, this pressure diminishes. Plasma proteins in the capillaries create an oncotic pressure gradient that draws fluid back into the blood stream. On the venous side of the capillary bed, the oncotic pressure drawing fluid in is greater than the hydrostatic pressure pushing fluid out. The net effect is that fluid returns to the capillary for its return to the heart. In a perfect system, whatever fluid enters the tissues should exit at the other end. In reality, some fluid usually remains. The lymph system acts as an auxiliary drainage system, collecting the remaining fluid from the tissues and returning it to the heart. Tissue edema can occur because of an increase in hydrostatic pressure, a decrease in plasma proteins, or a lymph system blockage.

As we age, the arteries lengthen, stiffen, and develop atherosclerosis. A complete evaluation of your patient's circulatory system is an essential component of any physical exam. Many diseases result from poor circulation, either localized (specific artery occlusion) or generalized (cardiovascular collapse). Carefully assess your elderly patient's end-organ perfusion.

A complete evaluation of your patient's circulatory system is an essential component of any physical exam.

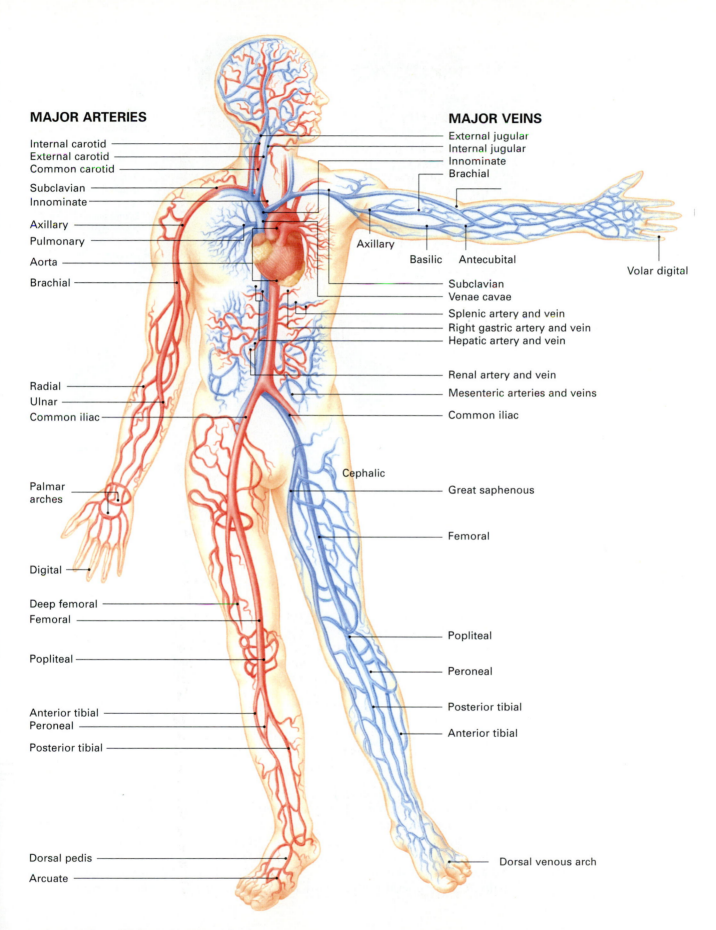

MAJOR ARTERIES

Internal carotid
External carotid
Common carotid

Subclavian
Innominate

Axillary
Pulmonary

Aorta

Brachial

Radial
Ulnar
Common iliac

Palmar arches

Digital

Deep femoral
Femoral

Popliteal

Anterior tibial
Peroneal

Posterior tibial

Dorsal pedis

Arcuate

MAJOR VEINS

External jugular
Internal jugular
Innominate
Brachial

Axillary

Basilic   Antecubital

Volar digital

Subclavian
Venae cavae

Splenic artery and vein
Right gastric artery and vein
Hepatic artery and vein

Renal artery and vein
Mesenteric arteries and veins

Common iliac

Cephalic

Great saphenous

Femoral

Popliteal

Peroneal

Posterior tibial

Anterior tibial

Dorsal venous arch

FIGURE 2-73   The circulatory system.

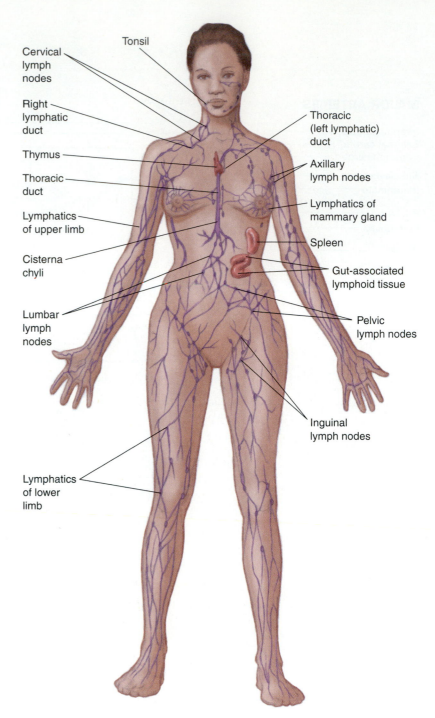

Cervical
lymph
nodes

Tonsil

Right
lymphatic
duct

Thoracic
(left lymphatic)
duct

Thymus

Axillary
lymph nodes

Thoracic
duct

Lymphatics of
mammary gland

Lymphatics
of upper limb

Spleen

Cisterna
chyli

Gut-associated
lymphoid tissue

Lumbar
lymph
nodes

Pelvic
lymph nodes

Inguinal
lymph nodes

Lymphatics
of lower
limb

FIGURE 2-74   The lymphatic system.

To assess your patient's peripheral vascular system, inspect both arms from the fingertips to the shoulders. Note their size and symmetry. Observe swelling, venous congestion, the color of the skin and nail beds, and the skin texture. Yellow or brittle nails or poor color in the fingertips indicates chronic arterial insufficiency. Palpate the peripheral arteries to evaluate pulsation and capillary refill and to assess skin temperature (Procedure 2-18a and 2-18b on page 132). To palpate a peripheral pulse, lightly place your fingerpads over the artery's pulse

Table 2-8	ASSESSING A PERIPHERAL PULSE
Score	**Description**
0	Absent pulse
1+	Weak or thready
2+	Normal
3+	Bounding

point. Slowly increase the pressure until you feel a maximum pulsation. Note the rate, regularity, equality, and quality of the pulses. Count the number of beats in one minute. Then determine whether the pulse is regular, regularly irregular, or irregularly irregular. Finally, assess the quality of the pulse by noting its amplitude and contour; rate its quality from 0 to 3+ as shown in Table 2-8. Determine if it is absent, normal, weak, or bounding, and note any thrills, humming vibrations that feel similar to the throat of a purring cat. Thrills suggest a cardiac murmur or vascular narrowing. Expect the pulse of a normal adult to range between 60 and 100 beats per minute with a regular rhythm and normal amplitude.

Compare peripheral pulses bilaterally. If you detect a weak or absent pulse in one extremity, suspect an arterial occlusion proximal to the pulse point. Also compare distal and proximal pulses for equality. If you cannot palpate a distal artery move proximally to another artery. For example, if you cannot palpate the radial artery, move to the the brachial artery in the antecubital area. While you are at the elbow, you can also assess the epitrochlear lymph nodes; they will be palpable only if inflamed.

Next assess the feet and legs. Have your patient lie down and ask him to remove his socks. Inspect the legs from the feet to the groin. Note their size and symmetry. Evaluate the presence of swelling, venous congestion, the color of the skin and nail beds, and the skin texture. Note any venous enlargement. Evaluate scars, pigmentation, rashes, and ulcers. Palpate and compare the femoral pulses (Procedure 2-18c). Note the rate, regularity, equality, and quality of the pulses. Palpate the popliteal pulse behind the knee, the dorsalis pedis pulse on top of the foot, and the posterior tibial pulse just behind the medial malleolus (Procedure 2-18d through 2-18f). Feel the temperature of the legs, feet, and toes with the back of your fingers and compare both sides. Unilateral coldness indicates an arterial occlusion. Bilateral coldness is due to an environmental problem, bilateral occlusion (saddle embolus) or to a general circulatory problem (shock). Palpate the superficial inguinal lymph nodes for enlargement and tenderness.

Observe the legs for edema, the presence of an abnormal amount of fluid in the tissues. Compare one leg and foot with the other. Note their relative size and symmetry. Are veins, tendons, and bones easily visible under the skin? Edema will usually obscure these structures. Palpate for pitting edema by pressing firmly with your thumb for five seconds over the top of the foot, behind each medial ankle, and over the shins (Procedure 2-18g). **Pitting** is a depression left by the pressure of your thumb. Normally there should be no depression. If edema is present evaluate the degree of pitting that can range from slight to marked (Figure 2-75). You can grade the depth of the pitting according to the appropriate scale in Table 2-9. Expect the pit to disappear within ten seconds after you release the pressure. Bilateral edema suggests a central circulatory problem such as congestive heart failure or renal failure; unilateral edema suggests a lower extremity circulation abnormality such as deep vein thrombosis or venous occlusion. Note the extent of the edema. How far up the leg does it spread? The higher the edema, the more severe the problem.

✱ **pitting** depression that results from pressure against skin when pitting edema is present.

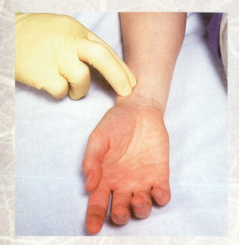

2-18a   Palpate the radial artery.

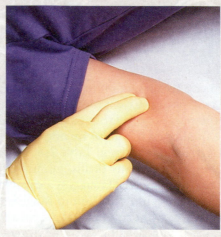

2-18b   Palpate the brachial artery.

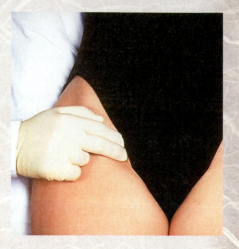

2-18c   Palpate and compare the femoral arteries.

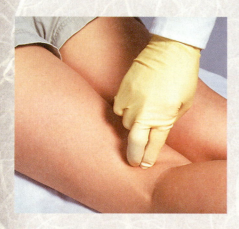

2-18d   Palpate the popliteal pulse.

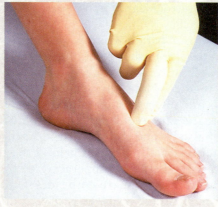

2-18e   Palpate the dorsalis pedis pulse.

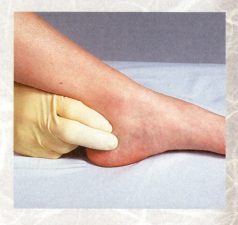

2-18f   Palpate the posterior tibial pulse.

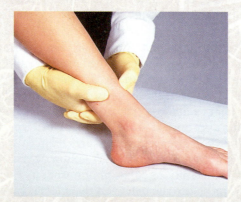

2-18g   Palpate for edema.

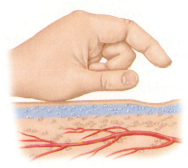
+1 Slight pitting edema

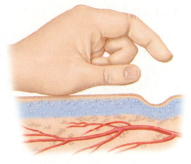
+4 Deep pitting edema

FIGURE 2-75   Assessing for edema.

Table 2-9	PITTING EDEMA SCALE
Score	**Description**
1+	One quarter inch or less
2+	One quarter to one half inch
3+	One half to one inch
4+	One inch or more

During your assessment, look for visible venous distention. An associated swollen, painful leg suggests a deep vein thrombosis (DVT). Palpate the femoral vein just medial to the femoral artery. If you detect a tender femoral vein, flex the knee and palpate the calf for tenderness, another classic sign of DVT. Is there a local redness or warmth? Feel for a cordlike vessel. Evaluate the skin for discoloration, ulcers, and unusual thickness. Finally, ask your patient to stand. Evaluate his legs for varicose veins and, if present, palpate them for signs of thrombophlebitis (redness, swelling, pain, and tenderness).

THE NERVOUS SYSTEM

A comprehensive physical exam includes a thorough evaluation of your patient's mental status and thought processes. On the scene of an emergency, you would limit your mental exam to level of consciousness and basic orientation questions such as "What is your name?" "Where are you right now?" "What day is it today?" If you are conducting a full physical exam or evaluating someone with altered mentation, some or all of the following techniques will be useful.

When you conduct a neurological exam, you are attempting to answer two vital questions. First, are the findings symmetrical or unilateral? Second, if the signs are unilateral, is the site of origin in the central nervous system (brain and spinal cord) or in the peripheral nervous system (everything else). You will conduct many parts of the neuro exam while you assess other anatomical areas and systems. For example, you can examine the cranial nerves while evaluating the head and face. You can note any weaknesses or abnormal neurological findings while evaluating the arms and legs during the musculoskeletal exam.

A nervous system exam covers five areas: mental status and speech, the cranial nerves, the motor system, the reflexes, and the sensory system. This section presents the complete neuro exam. The chief complaint, clinical condition of your patient, and time constraints will determine which parts you actually use.

A neurological exam attempts to answer two vital questions: are the findings symmetrical or unilateral, and if unilateral, where do they originate?

Content Review

FIVE AREAS OF NEUROLOGICAL EXAM

- Mental status and speech
- Cranial nerves
- Motor system
- Sensory system
- Reflexes

Mental Status and Speech

The central nervous system consists of the brain and spinal cord. The brain is the nerve center for the human body. It has three major regions, the brainstem; the cerebrum, or cerebral cortex; and the cerebellum (Figure 2-76). The brain stem consists of the midbrain, pons, and medulla. The cerebrum and the cerebellum are each divided into left and right hemispheres. Each cerebral hemisphere comprises four lobes, frontal, parietal, temporal, and occipital, which serve diverse functions (Figure 2-77). Myelin-coated axons (white matter) allow areas of the brain to communicate with one another and transmit their messages to the rest of the body via the spinal cord and peripheral nerves.

The cerebral cortex (gray matter) is the center for conscious thought, sensory awareness, movement, emotions, rational thought and behavior, foresight and planning, memory, speech, and language and interpretation. The frontal lobe contains a special speech area and the motor strip that controls voluntary skeletal muscle movement. It is also the area associated with personality and behavior. The parietal lobe is responsible for processing sensory data from the peripheral nerves. The occipital lobe houses the primary vision center and interprets visual data. The temporal lobe perceives and interprets sounds and integrates the senses of taste, smell, and balance.

Generally you will evaluate your patient's mental status and speech when you begin your interview. During this time you will assess his level of response, general appearance and behavior, and speech. If you detect abnormalities, continue your assessment with more specific questioning or testing as presented here.

Appearance and Behavior First, assess your patient's level of response. Is he alert and awake? Does he understand your questions? Are his responses appropriate and timely, or does he drift off the topic easily or lose interest? If you detect an abnormality, continue with more specific questions. Is he lethargic (drowsy, but answers questions appropriately before falling asleep again)? Is he obtunded (opens his eyes and looks at you but gives slow, confused responses)? Sometimes you must arouse your patient repeatedly by gently shaking him or

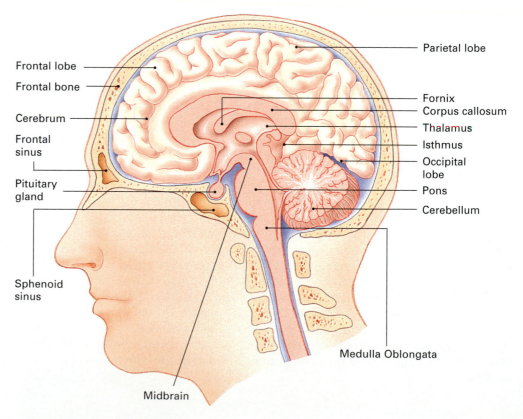

FIGURE 2-76   The brain.

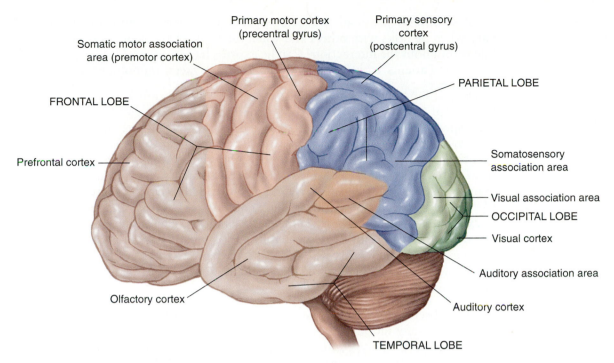

FIGURE 2-77 The cerebrum.

shouting his name. If he does not respond to your verbal cues, assess him with painful stimuli for coma or stupor. The stuporous patient is arousable for short periods but is not aware of his surroundings. The comatose patient is in a state of profound unconsciousness and is totally unarousable.

If your patient is awake and alert, observe his posture and motor behavior. Does he lie in bed or prefer to walk around? His posture should be erect and he should look at you. A slumped posture and a lack of facial expression may indicate depression. Excessive energetic movements or constantly watchful eyes suggest tension, anxiety, or a metabolic disorder. Watch the pace, range, and character of his movements. Are they voluntary? Are any parts immobile? Do his posture and motor activity change with the environment? Some possible findings are listed in Table 2-10.

Observe your patient's grooming and personal hygiene. How is he dressed? Are his clothes clean, pressed, and properly fastened? Is his appearance appropriate for the season, climate, and occasion? A deterioration in grooming and personal hygiene in the previously well-groomed person may suggest an emotional problem, a psychiatric disorder, or an organic brain disease. Patients with obsessive-compulsive behavior may exhibit excessive attention to their appearance. Note your patient's hair, teeth, nails, skin, and beard. Are they well groomed? Compare one side to another. One-sided neglect may suggest a brain lesion.

Table 2-10	POSTURE AND BEHAVIOR
Motor Activity	**Meaning**
Tense posture, restlessness, fidgeting	Anxiety
Crying, hand wringing, pacing	Agitated, depression
Hopeless, slumped posture, slowed movements	Depression
Singing, dancing, expansive movements	Manic

Also observe your patient's facial expressions. Are they appropriate? Do they vary when he talks with others and when the topic changes or is his face immobile throughout the interaction? Can he express happiness, sadness, anger, or depression? Patients with Parkinson's disease have facial immobility, a mask-like appearance.

Speech and Language Note your patient's speech pattern. Normally a person's speech is inflected, clear and strong, fluent and articulate, and varies in volume. It should express thoughts clearly. Is your patient excessively talkative or silent? Does he speak spontaneously or only when you ask him a direct question? Is his speech slow and quiet, as in depression? Is it fast and loud, as in a manic episode? Does he speak clearly and distinctly? Does he have dysarthria (defective speech caused by motor deficits), dysphonia (voice changes caused by vocal cord problems), or aphasia (defective language caused by neurologic damage to the brain)? With expressive aphasia his words will be garbled; with receptive aphasia, his words will be clear but unrelated to your questions. Your patient with aphasia may have such difficulty talking that you mistakenly suspect a psychotic disorder.

Mood Observe your patient's verbal and nonverbal behavior for clues to his mood. Note any mood swings or behaviors that suggest anxiety or depression. Is he sad, elated, angry, enraged, anxious, worried, detached, or indifferent? Assess the intensity of your patient's mood. How long has he been this way? Is his behavior normal for the circumstances? For example, anxiety is normal for someone having a heart attack; if your heart attack patient did not act frightened and concerned, that would be abnormal. If your patient is depressed, is he suicidal? If you suspect the possibility of suicide, ask him directly, "Have you ever thought of committing suicide? Are you currently thinking of committing suicide?"

Thought and Perceptions Assess how well your patient organizes his thoughts when he speaks. Is he logical and coherent? Does he shift from one topic to an unrelated topic without realizing that the thoughts are not connected? These "loose associations" are typical in schizophrenia, manic episodes, and other psychiatric disorders. Does he speak constantly in related areas with no real conclusion or end-point? Such "flight of ideas" is most often associated with mania. Does he ramble with unrelated, illogical thoughts and disordered grammar? You may see this "incoherence" in severe psychosis. Does he make up facts or events in response to questions? You may see this "confabulation" in amnesia. Does he suddenly lose his train of thought and stop in mid-sentence before completing an idea? Such blocking occurs in normal people but is pronounced in schizophrenia.

Assess the thought content of your patient's responses as they occur during the interview. For example, "You said you thought you were allergic to your mother. Can you tell me why you think that way?" In this way you can ask about your patient's unpleasant or unusual comments. Allow him the freedom to explore these thoughts with you. Is your patient driven to try to prevent some unrealistic future result (compulsion)? Does he have a recurrent, uncontrollable feeling of dread and doom (obsession)? Does he sense that things in the environment are strange or unreal (feelings of unreality)? Does he have false personal beliefs that other members of his group don't share (delusions)? Compulsions and obsessions are neurotic disorders, while delusions and feelings of unreality are psychotic disorders.

Determine whether your patient perceives imaginary things. Does he see visions, hear voices, smell odors, or feel things that aren't there? Ask him about these false perceptions just as you would ask about anything else. For example, "When you see the pink elephants, what are they doing?" Decide whether your patient is misinterpreting what is real (illusions) or seeing things that are not real (hallucinations). Both illusions and hallucinations may occur in schizophrenia, post traumatic stress disorders, and organic brain syndrome. Auditory and visual hallucinations are common in psychedelic drug ingestion, while tactile hallucinations suggest alcohol withdrawal.

Insight and Judgment During the interview you will most likely evaluate your patient's insight and judgment. Does he understand what is happening to him? Does he realize that what he thinks and how he feels is part of the illness? Patients with psychotic disorders may not have insight into their illness. Judgment refers to your patient's ability to reason appropriately. Does your mature patient respond appropriately to questions concerning his family and personal life? Ask him what he would do if he cut himself shaving. Proper judgment means that your patient can evaluate the data and provide an adequate response. Impaired judgment is common in emotional problems, mental retardation, and organic brain syndrome.

Memory and Attention Assess your patient's orientation. Does he know his name? Person disorientation suggests trauma, seizures, or amnesia. Does he know the time of day, day of the week, month, season, and year? Time disorientation may suggest anxiety, depression, or organic brain syndrome. Does he know where he is, where he lives, the name of the city and state? Place disorientation suggests a psychiatric disorder or organic brain syndrome. Your patient should be oriented to person, time, and place and respond appropriately to your questions.

Your patient should be oriented to person, time, and place and respond appropriately to your questions.

To assess your patient's ability to concentrate, use the following three exercises. First, have him repeat a series of numbers back to you (digit span). Normally, a person can repeat at least five numbers forward and backward. Then, ask him to start from 100 and subtract seven each time (serial sevens). A normal person can complete this in ninety seconds with fewer than four errors. Finally, ask your patient to spell a common five-letter word backward (spelling backward). Poor performance in these tests may suggest delirium, dementia, mental retardation, loss of calculating ability, anxiety, or depression.

Memory can be divided into three grades, immediate, recent, and remote. First, test your patient's immediate memory. Ask him to repeat three or four words that have no correlation such as "desk," "toothbrush," "six," and "blue." This tests immediate recall and is similar to digit span. Next, test your patient's recent memory by asking him what he had for lunch or to repeat something he told you earlier in the interview. Make sure the information you ask for is verifiable. Finally, test for remote memory by asking about facts such as his wife's name, son's birthday, or his social security number. Ask him to describe the house in which he grew up or the schools he attended. Long-term and short-term memory problems may be due to amnesia, anxiety, or organic causes. Finally, test your patient's ability to learn new things. Give him the names of three or four items such as "man, chair, grass, and hot dog." Ask him to repeat them. This tests registration and immediate recall. About five minutes later ask him to repeat them again. Normally, he will be able to name all four. Note his accuracy, his awareness of whether he is correct, or if he tries to confabulate by making up new words.

The Cranial Nerves

The 12 pairs of cranial nerves originate from the base of the brain and provide sensory and motor innervation, mostly to the head and face (Figure 2-78). Each pair bears the name of its function and carries either sensory fibers, motor fibers, or both (Figures 2-79 through 2-87). Table 2-11 lists the cranial nerves' names, their specific functions, and the areas they innervate.

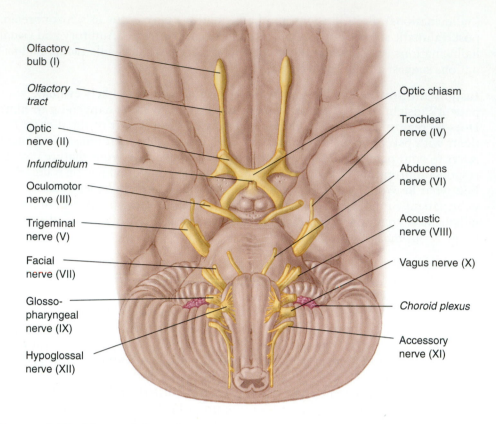

Olfactory bulb (I)

Olfactory tract

Optic nerve (II)

Infundibulum

Oculomotor nerve (III)

Trigeminal nerve (V)

Facial nerve (VII)

Glosso-pharyngeal nerve (IX)

Hypoglossal nerve (XII)

Optic chiasm

Trochlear nerve (IV)

Abducens nerve (VI)

Acoustic nerve (VIII)

Vagus nerve (X)

Choroid plexus

Accessory nerve (XI)

FIGURE 2-78   The cranial nerves.

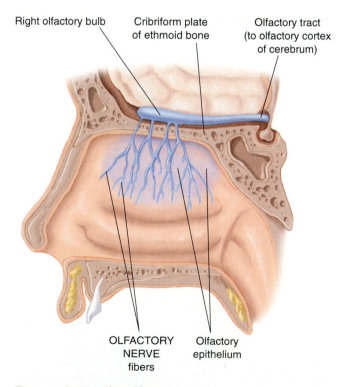

Right olfactory bulb

Cribriform plate of ethmoid bone

Olfactory tract (to olfactory cortex of cerebrum)

OLFACTORY NERVE fibers

Olfactory epithelium

FIGURE 2-79   The olfactory nerve.

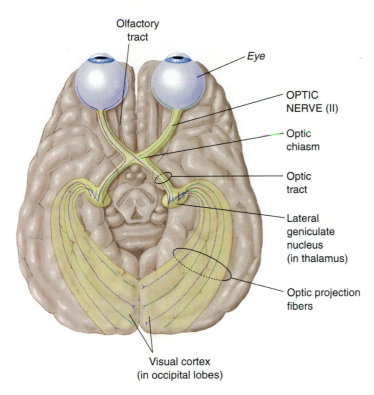

Olfactory
tract

Eye

OPTIC
NERVE (II)

Optic
chiasm

Optic
tract

Lateral
geniculate
nucleus
(in thalamus)

Optic projection
fibers

Visual cortex
(in occipital lobes)

FIGURE 2-80   The optic nerve.

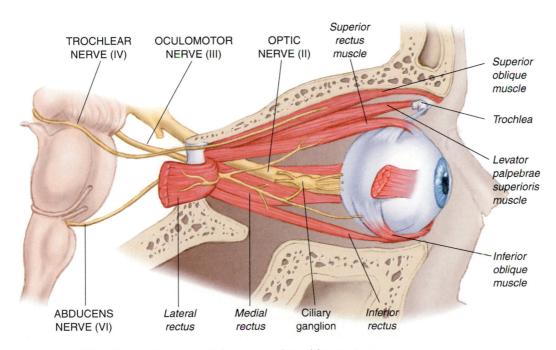

TROCHLEAR
NERVE (IV)

OCULOMOTOR
NERVE (III)

OPTIC
NERVE (II)

Superior
rectus
muscle

Superior
oblique
muscle

Trochlea

Levator
palpebrae
superioris
muscle

Inferior
oblique
muscle

ABDUCENS
NERVE (VI)

Lateral
rectus

Medial
rectus

Ciliary
ganglion

Inferior
rectus

FIGURE 2-81   The oculomotor, abducens, and trochlear nerves.

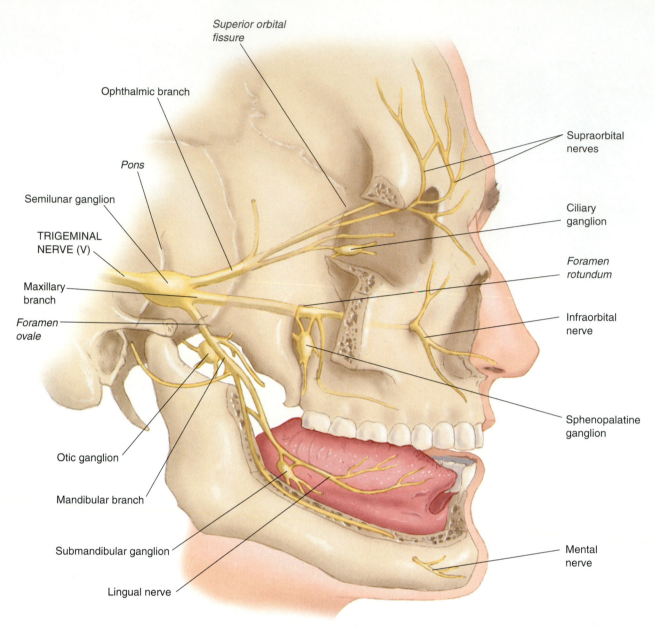

Superior orbital fissure

Ophthalmic branch

Pons

Semilunar ganglion

TRIGEMINAL NERVE (V)

Maxillary branch

Foramen ovale

Otic ganglion

Mandibular branch

Submandibular ganglion

Lingual nerve

Supraorbital nerves

Ciliary ganglion

Foramen rotundum

Infraorbital nerve

Sphenopalatine ganglion

Mental nerve

FIGURE 2-82　The trigeminal nerve.

Most likely you will conduct parts of the cranial nerve exam when you assess other areas such as the eyes, ears, throat, and musculoskeletal system. The following is the cranial nerve exam in its entirety.

CN-I Test your patient's olfactory nerve by having him close his eyes and compress one nostril while you present him with a variety of common, nonirritating odors (Procedure 2-19a on page 146). Repeat the test with each nostril. Ask him to identify the odor. Most people will do so easily. If your patient cannot, several causes are possible. Bilateral loss of smell suggests head trauma, nasal stuffiness, smoking, cocaine use, or a congenital defect. A unilateral loss of smell without nasal disease suggests a frontal lobe lesion.

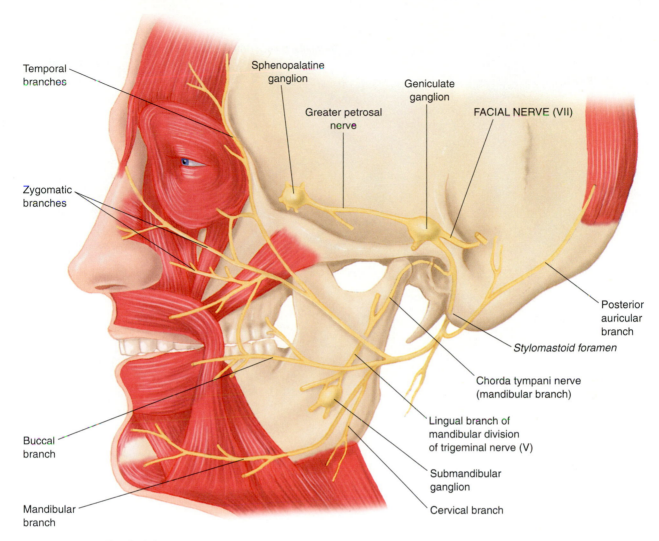

Temporal
branches

Sphenopalatine
ganglion

Greater petrosal
nerve

Geniculate
ganglion

FACIAL NERVE (VII)

Zygomatic
branches

Posterior
auricular
branch

Stylomastoid foramen

Chorda tympani nerve
(mandibular branch)

Lingual branch of
mandibular division
of trigeminal nerve (V)

Buccal
branch

Submandibular
ganglion

Mandibular
branch

Cervical branch

FIGURE 2-83   The facial nerve.

CN-II Test the optic nerve with the visual acuity and visual field tests described earlier in this chapter in the anatomical regions section on the eyes.

CN-III Test the oculomotor nerve with the optic nerve when you perform pupil reaction tests. Inspect the size and shape of your patient's pupils and compare one side to the other. A slight inequality may be normal. Usually the pupil is mid-point. Constricted or dilated pupils may result from medications, drug abuse, glaucoma, and neurologic disease. Darken the room, if possible, to test for pupillary reaction. Ask your patient to look straight ahead. Shine a bright light obliquely into one of his pupils. Watch for direct reaction (pupillary constriction in the same eye) and for consensual reaction (pupillary constriction in the opposite eye). Repeat this test on the other side. Now assess for the near response, asking your patient to follow your finger as you move it in toward the bridge of his nose. Watch for his pupils to constrict and his eyes to converge.

CN-III, IV, VI Test the oculomotor, trochlear, and abducens nerves by evaluating your patient's extraocular movements (EOM). Ask him to follow your finger

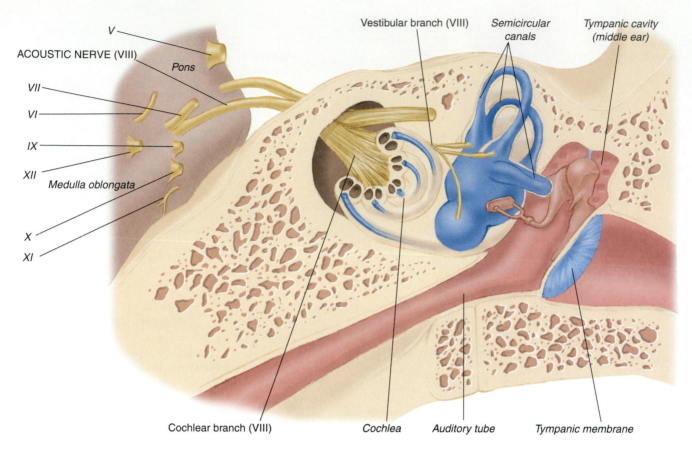

Figure 2-84   The acoustic nerve.

Labels in Figure 2-84:

- V
- ACOUSTIC NERVE (VIII)
- *Pons*
- VII
- VI
- IX
- XII
- *Medulla oblongata*
- X
- XI
- Vestibular branch (VIII)
- *Semicircular canals*
- *Tympanic cavity (middle ear)*
- Cochlear branch (VIII)
- *Cochlea*
- Auditory tube
- *Tympanic membrane*

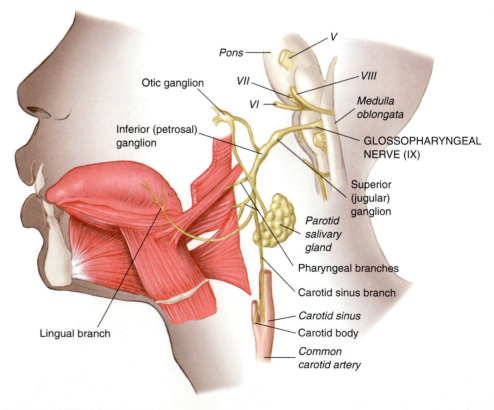

Figure 2-85   The glossopharyngeal nerve.

Labels in Figure 2-85:

- Otic ganglion
- Inferior (petrosal) ganglion
- Lingual branch
- *Pons*
- V
- VII
- VI
- VIII
- *Medulla oblongata*
- GLOSSOPHARYNGEAL NERVE (IX)
- Superior (jugular) ganglion
- *Parotid salivary gland*
- Pharyngeal branches
- Carotid sinus branch
- *Carotid sinus*
- Carotid body
- *Common carotid artery*

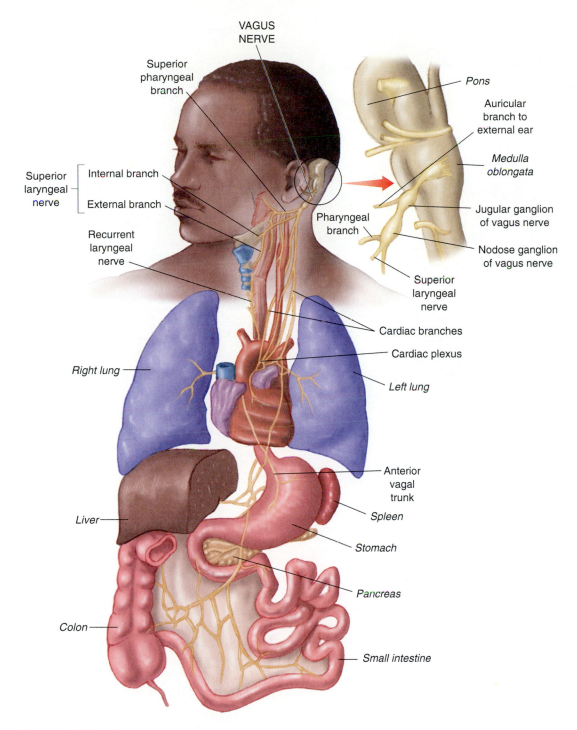

VAGUS
NERVE

Superior
pharyngeal
branch

Pons

Auricular
branch to
external ear

Superior
laryngeal
nerve

Internal branch

External branch

Medulla
oblongata

Recurrent
laryngeal
nerve

Pharyngeal
branch

Jugular ganglion
of vagus nerve

Nodose ganglion
of vagus nerve

Superior
laryngeal
nerve

Cardiac branches

Cardiac plexus

Right lung

Left lung

Anterior
vagal
trunk

Liver

Spleen

Stomach

Pancreas

Colon

Small intestine

FIGURE 2-86   The vagus nerve.

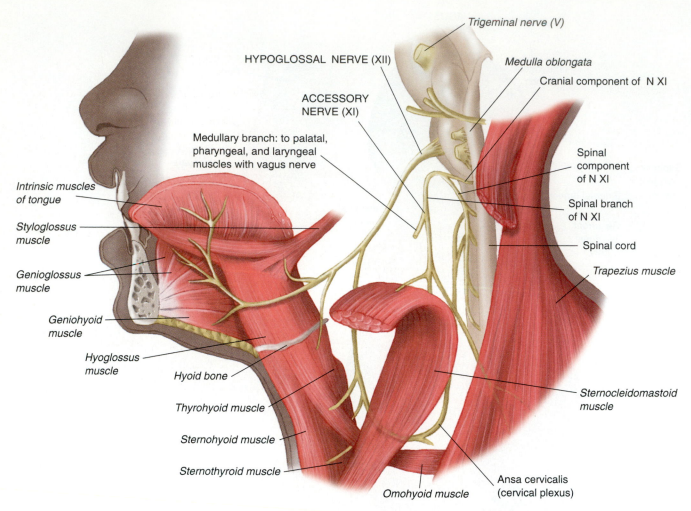

Trigeminal nerve (V)

HYPOGLOSSAL NERVE (XII)

Medulla oblongata

Cranial component of N XI

ACCESSORY
NERVE (XI)

Medullary branch: to palatal,
pharyngeal, and laryngeal
muscles with vagus nerve

*Intrinsic muscles
of tongue*

*Styloglossus
muscle*

*Genioglossus
muscle*

*Geniohyoid
muscle*

*Hyoglossus
muscle*

Hyoid bone

Thyrohyoid muscle

Sternohyoid muscle

Sternothyroid muscle

Spinal
component
of N XI

Spinal branch
of N XI

Spinal cord

Trapezius muscle

*Sternocleidomastoid
muscle*

Ansa cervicalis
(cervical plexus)

Omohyoid muscle

FIGURE 2-87   The accessory and hypoglossal nerves.

with only his eyes as you move it through the six cardinal positions of gaze (Procedure 2-19b). Make a wide "H" in the air with your finger. Observe for conjugate (together) movements of your patient's eyes in each direction. Normally your patient can follow your finger with no strabismus (deviation) or nystagmus (involuntary movements). Inability to move in any direction can be the result of a problem with a cranial nerve, an ocular muscle, or an eye orbit that may be fractured and impinging on the muscle or nerve. Finally, look for ptosis (a droopy eyelid) that may be the result of CN-III palsy or myasthenia gravis.

CN-V   Test motor function by asking your patient to clench his teeth while you palpate the temporal and masseter muscles (Procedure 2-19c). Note the strength of the muscle contraction. Unilateral weakness or the inability to contract suggests a trigeminal nerve lesion. Bilateral dysfunction suggests motor neuron involvement.

To test for sensory function in the three main divisions of the trigeminal nerve, first ask your patient to close his eyes. Using something sharp and something dull, lightly scrape the objects across the forehead, cheek, and chin on both sides and ask your patient to distinguish the sensations (Procedure 2-19d). The two ends of a paper clip work well for this procedure; straighten one end and use its tip as the sharp object. Unilateral loss of sensation suggests a trigeminal nerve lesion. Finally, test the corneal reflex. Ask your patient to look up and away as you touch his cornea lightly with some fine cotton fibers. He should blink. Repeat this test on the other eye.

Table 2-11 CRANIAL NERVES

CN	Name	Function	Innervation
I	Olfactory	Sensory	Smell
II	Optic	Sensory	Sight
III	Oculomotor	Motor	Pupil constriction; superior rectus, inferior rectus, inferior oblique muscles
IV	Trochlear	Motor	Superior oblique muscles
V	Trigeminal	Sensory	Opthalmic (forehead), maxillary (cheek), and mandibular (chin) regions
		Motor	Chewing muscles
VI	Abducens	Motor	Lateral rectus muscle
VII	Facial	Sensory	Tongue
		Motor	Face muscles
VIII	Acoustic	Sensory	Hearing balance
IX	Glossopharyngeal	Sensory	Posterior pharynx, taste to anterior tongue
		Motor	Posterior pharynx
X	Vagus	Sensory	Taste to posterior tongue
		Motor	Posterior palate and pharynx
XI	Accessory	Motor	Trapezius muscles Sternocleidomastoid muscles
XII	Hypoglossal	Motor	Tongue

CN-VII First assess your patient's face at rest and during conversation. Note any asymmetry, eyelid drooping, or abnormal movements such as tics. Test the facial nerve by having your patient assume a variety of facial expressions. Ask him to raise his eyebrows, frown, show his upper and lower teeth or smile, and puff out his cheeks. Also ask him to close his eyes tightly so that you cannot open them; then to test muscle strength, try to open them. Bell's palsy is an inflammation of CN-VII. Your patient will present with unilateral facial drooping from paralysis of this nerve.

CN-VIII Ask your patient to occlude one ear with a finger. Then whisper something softly into the other ear. Ask him to repeat what you said. Any loss of hearing warrants further testing to detect air and bone conduction problems. Test the acoustic nerve for the senses of hearing and balance. Ask your patient to stand erect and close his eyes. Now evaluate his balance and then ask him to open his eyes. If he doesn't become dizzy and opens his eyes to your command, the eighth nerve is functioning appropriately.

CN-IX, X Test the glossopharyngeal and vagus nerves together. Listen to your patient's voice. Hoarseness suggests a vocal cord problem; a nasal quality suggests a palate problem. Ask your patient to swallow; note any difficulties. Ask him to open his mouth and say "aaahhh"; watch for the soft palate and uvula to rise symmetrically. The posterior pharynx should move medially. If the vagus nerve is paralyzed, the soft palate and uvula will deviate toward the side of the lesion. Test the gag reflex with a tongue blade on the posterior tongue (Procedure 2-19e). Absence of a gag reflex suggests a lesion in one of these nerves.

CN-XI Inspect the upper portions of your patient's trapezius muscles and sternocleidomastoid muscles for symmetry at rest. To test his trapezius muscles,

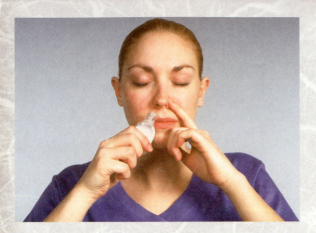

2-19a   Test the olfactory nerve by having your patient identify common odors.

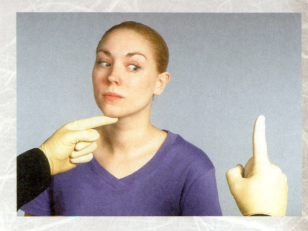

2-19b   Test the oculomotor, trochlear, and abducens nerves by evaluating your patient's extraocular movements.

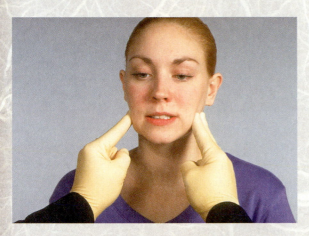

2-19c   Test motor function of the trigeminal nerve by palpating the temporal and masseter muscles.

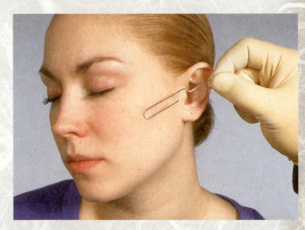

2-19d   Test sensory function of the trigeminal nerve with sharp and dull objects.

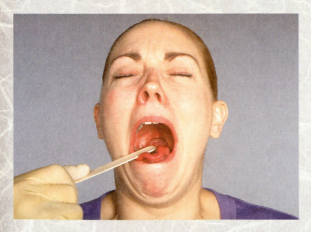

2-19e   Test the glossopharyngeal and vagus nerves with a tongue blade.

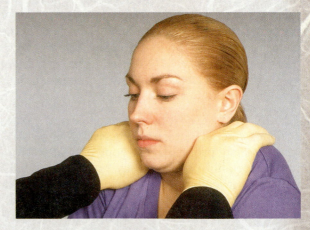

2-19f   Test the spinal accessory nerve by having your patient shrug her shoulders against resistance.

place your hands on his shoulders and ask him to raise his shoulders against resistance (Procedure 2-19f). Now test his sternocleidomastoid muscles. Place your hands along his face and ask him to turn his head to each side as you apply resistance. Note any bilateral or unilateral weaknesses. A supine patient with bilateral weakness of the sternocleidomastoids will have trouble lifting his head.

CN-XII First evaluate your patient's speech articulation. Then ask him to stick out his tongue; watch for a midline projection. A CN-XII lesion will make the tongue deviate away from the affected side. Have your patient move his tongue from side to side as you watch for symmetry.

You may conduct a cranial nerve exam according to this sequence. More likely, you will develop your own efficient system of testing these nerves.

The Motor System

Thirty-one pairs of nerves arise from the spinal foramina on both sides of the spinal column (Figure 2-88). The anterior root of the peripheral nerves carries the motor, or efferent, nerve fibers from the brain and spinal cord through three pathways:

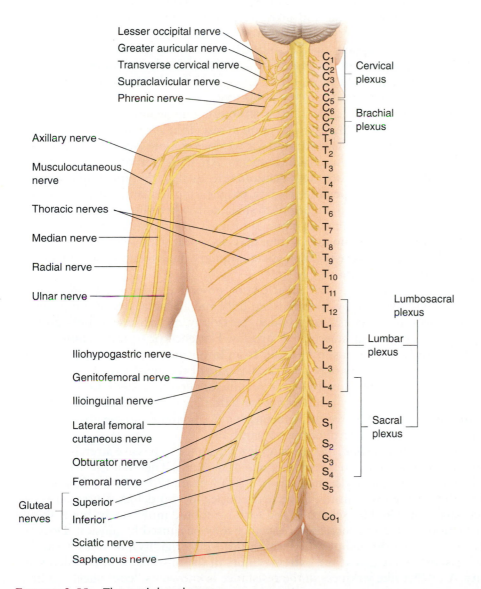

FIGURE 2-88   The peripheral nerves.

the pyramidal, extrapyramidal, and cerebellar systems. The pyramidal tract, which begins in the motor cortex of the brain, mediates voluntary movements. Its fibers travel down the brainstem, where they crisscross to innervate the opposite sides of the body. These tracts guide voluntary skeletal muscle movement and allow for fine motor movements by stimulating some muscles and inhibiting others. The motor system's net effect is coordinated, skilled movements.

When this system is damaged, function is lost below the level of the injury, and movements become weak or paralyzed. Inhibition is lost, so muscle tone is increased and deep tendon reflexes are exaggerated. If the damage occurs above the crossover point in the brainstem, then the effects will be seen on the opposite (contralateral) side of the body. If the damage is below the crossover point, the damage will be on the same (ipsilateral) side. For example, if your patient suffers a stroke on the left motor strip controlling the hands, then the motor deficiencies will appear in the right hand. If your patient has swelling of the spinal cord from an injury that impinges on the left motor nucleus, the motor deficiencies will appear on the left side of his body.

The extrapyramidal tract controls body movements and maintains muscle tone through motor fibers and pathways outside the pyramidal system. Since the extrapyramidal tract is mostly inhibitory, damage to this system causes increased muscle tone, abnormal gait and posture, and involuntary movements. This is commonly seen in patients who have adverse reactions to drugs in the phenothiazine class. They appear flushed and stiff, with motor control problems. The cerebellar system coordinates muscular activity, and helps to maintain equilibrium and posture through its motor fibers. Cerebellar damage causes abnormal changes in gait, coordination, and equilibrium.

Inspect your patient's general body structure, muscle development, positioning, and coordination. What is his position at rest? Is he erect or does he slump to one side, suggesting unilateral paralysis or weakness? Note any obvious asymmetries, deformities, or involuntary movements. Are there tremors, tics, or fasciculations (twitches)? If so, note their location, rate, quality, rhythm, amplitude, and relation to your patient's posture, activity, fatigue, emotion, and other factors. For example, if your patient's hand begins to shake only when you ask him to perform a task with it such as writing his name or lifting a spoon, this suggests a postural tremor. Conversely, a tremor at rest that may disappear with voluntary movement suggests Parkinson's disease. To assess involuntary movement, observe your patient throughout the exam.

To determine your patient's muscle bulk, observe the size and contour of his muscles. Look for atrophy, a decrease in bulk and strength; hypertrophy, an increase in bulk and strength; or pseudohypertrophy, an increase in bulk and decrease in strength, as in muscular dystrophy. Flattened or concave contours, especially with fasciculations, may result from lower motor neuron disease. Some degree of muscle atrophy may be a normal part of the aging process or may result from the effects of diabetes on the peripheral nervous system. Look for signs of general muscle atrophy by checking for flattening of the thenar (thumb) muscle and for furrowing between the metacarpals. Unilateral muscle atrophy in the hands suggests median or ulnar nerve paralysis.

To assess muscle tone, feel the muscle's resistance to passive stretching in the extremities. Ask your patient to relax one of his arms. Then put the arm, wrists, and hands through a moderate range-of-motion exam (Procedure 2-20a on page 150). Repeat the exam in the lower extremities. If you detect decreased resistance, shake the hand loosely back and forth. It should move freely, but it should not be floppy (flaccid). Increased resistance may be caused by tension. Does the resistance persist throughout the motion (lead-pipe rigidity), or does it vary? If the resistance increases at the extreme limits of the movement, it is called spasticity. A ratchet-like jerkiness in the resistance is known as "cog-wheel rigidity," a common finding in a patient faking his symptoms or trying to resist your examination. Table 2-12 describes some common muscle tone findings.

Table 2-12	MUSCLE TONE
Finding	**Description**
Spasticity	Increased tone when passive movement applied, especially at the end of range. Common in stroke.
Rigidity	Increased rigidity throughout movement (lead-pipe). Common in Parkinson's disease and extra pyramidal reactions. Cog-wheel motion is a patient-applied resistance.
Flaccidity	Loss of muscle tone causing limb to be loose. Common in stroke, spinal cord lesion, and Guillain-Barré syndrome.
Paratonia	Sudden changes in tone with passive movement. Can be increased or decreased resistance. Common in dementia.

Table 2-13	MUSCLE STRENGTH TESTS	
Muscles	**Nerves**	**Test**
Biceps	C5, C6	Flexion of the elbow
Triceps	C6, C7, C8	Extension of the elbow
Wrist extensors	C6, C7, C8, radial nerve	Extension of the wrist
Fingers	C8, T1, ulnar nerve	Finger abduction
Thumb	C8, T1, median nerve	Thumb opposition
Iliopsoas	L2, L3, L4	Hip flexion
Hip extensor	S1	Hip extension
Hip abductors	L4, L5, S1	Hip abduction
Hip adductors	L2, L3, L4	Hip adduction
Quadriceps	L2, L3, L4	Knee extension
Hamstrings	L4, L5, S1, S2	Knee flexion
Feet	L4, L5	Dorsiflexion
Calf muscles	S1	Plantar flexion

Now focus on your patient's muscle strength. First, assess the strength of his grip. Test both grips simultaneously and compare them. Cross your middle finger over the top of your index finger to prevent your fingers from being hurt; then ask your patient to squeeze them as hard as possible (Procedure 2-20b). Normally you will have difficulty removing your fingers from your patient's grip. Continue testing all of the muscle groups listed in Table 2-13. While assessing muscle strength remember that each patient's age, gender, size, and muscular training will affect your exam results. When comparing sides, your patient's dominant side will be stronger. Test for muscle strength by having your patient move actively against your resistance (Procedure 2-20c). If the muscle is too weak to perform against resistance, have him try the movement against gravity or with gravity eliminated (you support the limb). Grade muscle strength on a scale from 1 to 5 (Table 2-14).

To assess your patient's position sense and coordination, first observe his gait. Ask him to walk across the room, turn, and come back. Normally he will be able to maintain his balance, swing his arms at his side, and turn easily. If his gait is ataxic—uncoordinated, reeling, or unstable—suspect cerebellar disease, loss of position sense, or intoxication. Next ask him to walk heel-to-toe in a straight line. This "tandem walking" may reveal an ataxia not previously seen. Now ask your patient to walk first on his toes, then on his heels. This will assess plantar flexion and dorsiflexion of the ankle as well as balance. Next, ask him to hop in place on

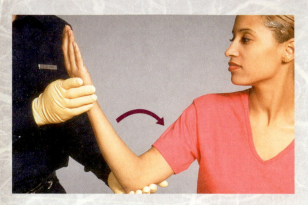

2-20a   Assess the elbow's range of motion.

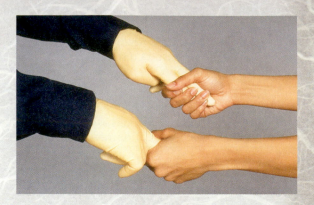

2-20b   Test your patient's grip.

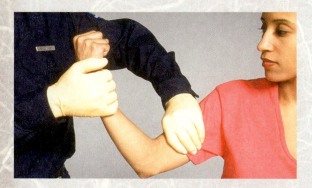

2-20c   Test arm strength.

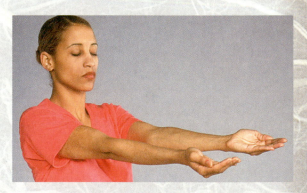

2-20d   Test for pronator drift.

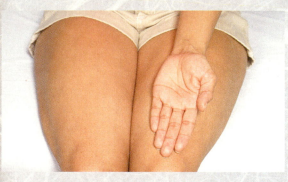

2-20e   Test for coordination with rapid alternating movements.

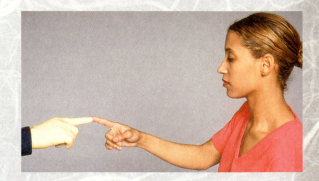

2-20f   Test coordination with point-to-point testing.

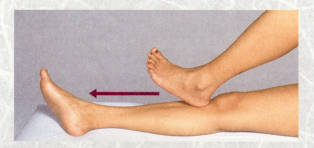

2-20g   Assess coordination with heel-to-shin testing.

Table 2-14	MUSCLE STRENGTH SCALE
Score	**Description**
5	Active movement against full resistance with no fatigue
4	Active movement against some resistance and gravity
3	Active movement against gravity
2	Active movement with gravity eliminated
1	Barely palpable muscle contraction with no movement
0	No visible or palpable muscle contraction

each foot in turn. Difficulty hopping may result from leg muscle weakness, lack of position sense, or cerebellar dysfunction. Now ask him to do a shallow knee bend on each leg in turn. Difficulty doing this suggests muscle weakness in the pelvic girdle and legs. If your patient is old and unable to hop or do knee bends, have him rise from a sitting position without arm support, or step up onto a stool.

Next perform the Romberg test. Ask him to stand with his feet together and his eyes open. Now have him close his eyes for 20 to 30 seconds. Observe his ability to remain upright with minimal swaying and no support. Losing his balance indicates a positive Romberg test caused by ataxia from a loss of position sense. An inability to maintain his balance with his eyes open and feet together represents a cerebellar ataxia. Now check your patient for pronator drift. Ask him to stand with his arms straight out in front of him with his palms up and his eyes closed (Procedure 2-20d). Ask him to maintain this position for 20 to 30 seconds. Normally your patient can do this easily. If one forearm pronates, suspect a mild hemiparesis. If it drifts sideways or upward, suspect a loss of position sense.

To assess your patient's coordination, test for rapid alternating movements. These maneuvers can be difficult to describe, so you should always demonstrate them to your patient. Ask him to repeat them as rapidly as possible while you observe for speed, rhythm, and smoothness. He should repeat all movements with both sides of the body. Keep in mind that his dominant hand usually will perform better than his nondominant hand. If his movements are slow, irregular and clumsy, suspect cerebellar or extrapyramidal tract disease or upper motor neuron weakness.

First, have your patient tap the distal joint of his thumb with the tip of his index finger as rapidly as possible. Then ask him to place his hand, palm up, on his thigh, quickly turn it over palm down, and return it palm up (Procedure 2-20e). Have him repeat this movement as quickly as possible for 15 seconds; evaluate both hands. Next have him perform point-to-point testing. Ask him to alternate touching your index finger and his nose several times while you observe for accuracy and smoothness (Procedure 2-20f). Note any tremors or difficulty performing this task, indicating cerebellar disease; evaluate both hands. Now assess for point-to-point testing in his legs. Ask him to touch his heel to the opposite knee, then run it down his shin to his big toe (Procedure 2-20g). Note the smoothness and accuracy of his actions. Repeat the test with the other leg. To test your patient's position sense, have him close his eyes and repeat this test for both legs. Abnormalities suggest cerebellar disease.

The Sensory System

The posterior root of the peripheral nerves carries the sensory, or afferent, nerve fibers to the spinal cord and brain along two pathways. The spinothalamic tracts conduct the sensations of pain, temperature, and crude touch. The posterior column

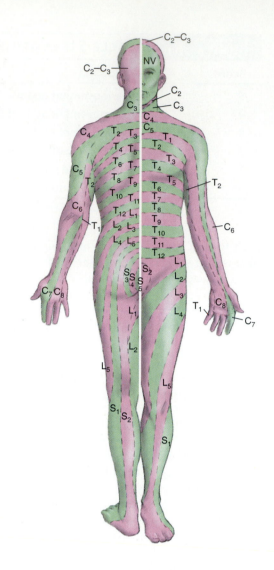

FIGURE 2-89 Dermatome chart. Knowing basic landmarks enables you to locate spinal cord lesions.

of the spinal cord conducts the sensations of position, vibration, and fine touch. Areas of the skin innervated by these afferent fibers are known as dermatomes. A dermatome chart is a road map depicting bands of skin innervated by sensory nerve fibers at each particular spinal level (Figure 2-89). By learning some basic landmarks, you can begin to identify approximate areas of spinal cord lesions according to the absence of skin sensation.

To assess the sensory system, test for pain, light touch, temperature, position, vibration, and discriminative sensations. Remember to compare distal areas to proximal areas, to compare symmetrical areas bilaterally, and to scatter the stimuli to assess most of the dermatomes. Ask your patient to close his eyes for each of these tests. To test for pain sensation, touch your patient's skin with a sharp object and ask him to tell you whether it is sharp or dull. Compare areas as you move along the different regions, intermittently substituting a dull object for the sharp one. To test for light touch, softly touch him with a fine piece of cotton. Ask him to tell you whenever he feels the cotton. An abnormality suggests a peripheral neuropathy. Test for temperature sensation by touching his skin with a vial filled with either hot or cold liquid. Then test for

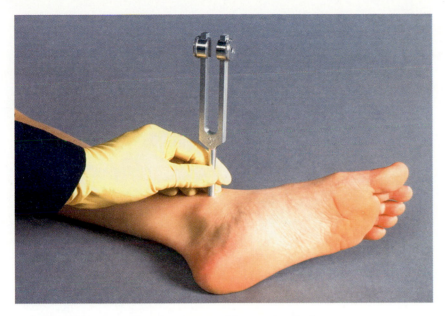

FIGURE 2-90   Test vibration sense with a tuning fork.

position sense by pulling one of his toe's upward and asking him to tell you whether it is up or down. Test for vibration sense by placing the stem of a vibrating tuning fork against a bony prominence (Figure 2-90). Finally, test for discriminative sensation by putting a familiar object such as a key in your patient's hand and asking him to identify it.

Reflexes

The sensory pathways manage conscious sensation and participate in the reflex arc. The reflex arc connects some sensory impulses directly to motor neurons, triggering immediate responses to noxious stimuli such as touching your hand to a flame. Deep tendon reflexes are a similar involuntary response to direct muscular stretch. Striking a slightly flexed tendon with a reflex hammer sends an impulse to the spinal cord, where a reflex arc occurs (Figure 2-91). This immediately sends a motor response back to the tendon, which begins the muscle contraction.

When you perform a nervous system exam, also test your patient's superficial and deep tendon reflexes. Always compare one side to the other. Grade the reflexes on a scale of 0 to 4+ (Table 2-15) and record your findings on a stick figure (Figure 2-92). A hyperactive response suggests upper motor neuron disease. A diminished response or no response suggests damage to the lower motor neurons or spinal cord.

Deep tendon reflexes can be tested at several places on the body. Use the pointed end of a reflex hammer for striking small areas, the flat end for striking larger areas. First ask your patient to relax. Then properly position the limb you are testing. Quickly strike the tendon using wrist motion only.

Biceps Support your patient's arm in the slightly flexed position with your thumb directly over the distal biceps tendon in the antecubital space (Procedure 2-21a on page 156). Strike your thumbnail with the point of the reflex hammer

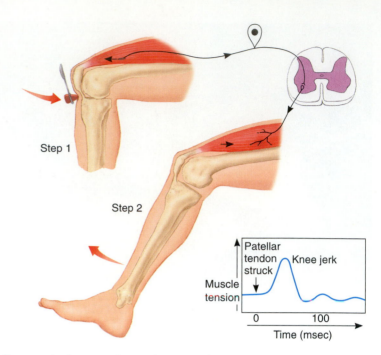

FIGURE 2-91   A reflex arc depicts muscle tension over time.

Table 2-15	REFLEX SCALE
Grade	**Description**
0	No response
+	Diminished, below normal
++	Average, normal
+++	Brisker than normal
++++	Hyperactive, associated with clonus

and watch for contraction of the biceps muscle and the resulting flexion of the elbow. This tests for spinal nerves C5 and C6.

Triceps Flex your patient's arm at a right angle. With the point of your reflex hammer, strike the triceps tendon along the posterior aspect of the distal humerus (Procedure 2-21b). Watch for triceps contraction and the resulting elbow extension. This tests spinal nerves C6, C7, and C8.

Brachioradialis Support your patient's arm with the forearm slightly pronated (Procedure 2-21c). Now strike his radius about two inches above his wrist. Watch for contraction of the brachioradialis and the resulting flexion and supination of the forearm. This tests cervical nerves C5 and C6.

Quadriceps Have your patient sit with his leg hanging off the end of the exam table. Tap the tendon just below the patella and watch for the quadriceps to contract and extend the knee (Procedure 2-21d). This tests lumbar nerves L2, L3, and L4.

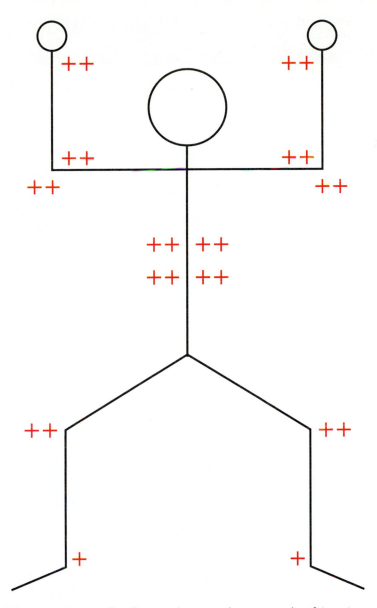

FIGURE 2-92   Reflex figures show grades on a scale of 0 to 4+.

Achilles With your patient sitting, dorsiflex the foot at the ankle and strike the Achilles tendon (Procedure 2-21e). Watch for the calf muscles to contract and cause plantar flexion of the foot. This tests sacral nerves S1 and S2.

Abdominal/Plantar Now test the superficial abdominal reflexes and plantar response. These are initiated by stimulating the skin instead of muscle. Assess the plantar reflex by stroking the lateral aspect of the sole from the heel to the ball of your patient's foot, curving medially across the ball (Procedure 2-21f). Begin with the lightest stimulus that will elicit a response. If you detect no response, be more firm. Watch for plantar flexion of the toes. Note if the big toe dorsiflexes while the other toes fan out. Known as a positive **Babinski response**, this indicates a central nervous system lesion.

✱ **Babinski response** big toe dorsiflexes and the other toes fan out when sole is stimulated.

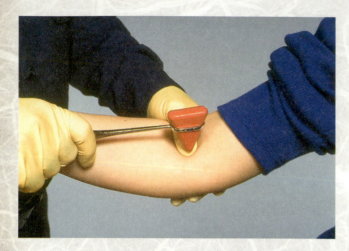

2-21a   Test the biceps reflex (cervical nerves C5 and C6).

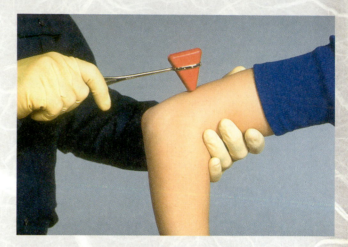

2-21b   Test the triceps reflex (cervical nerves C6, C7, and C8).

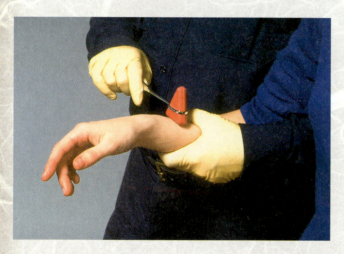

2-21c   Test the brachioradialis reflex (cervical nerves C5 and C6).

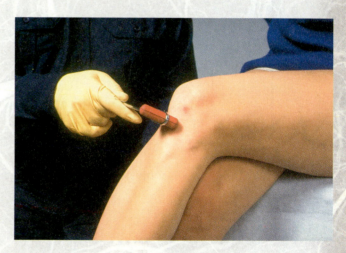

2-21d   Test the quadriceps reflex (lumbar nerves L2, L3, and L4).

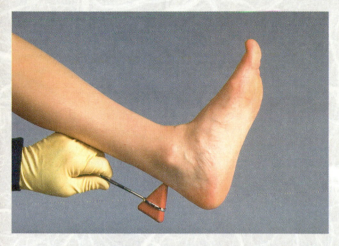

2-21e   Test the Achilles reflex (sacral nerves S1 and S2).

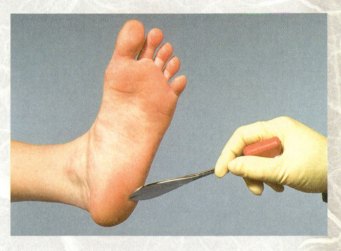

2-21f   Test the plantar reflex (central nervous system).

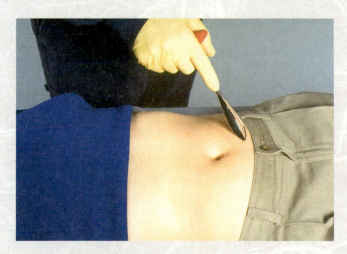

2-21g   Test abdominal reflexes (thoracic nerves T8, T9, T10, T11, and T12).

Test the abdominal reflex by lightly stroking each side of the abdomen above and below the umbilicus with an irregular object such as a reflex hammer, a broken cotton swab or a split tongue blade (Procedure 2-21g). Note the contraction of the abdominal muscles and how the umbilicus deviates to the stimulus. The area above the umbilicus is innervated by thoracic nerves T8, T9, and T10. The area below the umbilicus is innervated by thoracic nerves T10, T11, and T12. The absence of abdominal reflexes can suggest either a central or peripheral nervous system disorder.

PHYSICAL EXAMINATION OF INFANTS AND CHILDREN

Conducting a physical examination of a sick or injured child can challenge any clinician. Your success will depend on several factors. First, you must be familiar with the anatomical differences between children and adults. Second, you must understand the physical and psychological developmental stages of the different age groups. Most importantly, you must practice these skills daily.

BUILDING PATIENT AND FAMILY RAPPORT

Children are not just small adults, and you cannot treat them as if they were.

Children are not just small adults, and you cannot treat them as if they were. Children are naturally apprehensive of strangers and new things. A sick or injured child is a frightened child. He fears pain, separation from his family, and unfamiliar surroundings. Dealing with these fears paves the way for a successful encounter with the child and his parents. You are a stranger. In uniform, you become even more ominous. Gaining your pediatric patient's trust becomes a vital part of your assessment. Unless he requires emergency critical care, take time to establish a rapport with him. This will help to ensure continuous cooperation.

The more invasive the procedure, the later in the exam you should perform it.

While different age groups have specific fears and characteristics, the following general rules apply to pediatrics as a whole. Remain calm and confident. Be direct and honest about what you are doing, especially if you are performing a painful procedure. If possible, do not separate the child from his parents. Instead, elicit their help in obtaining the history and allow them to help hold the child while you conduct your exam. The more invasive the procedure, the later in the exam you should perform it—unless, of course, your patient is critically ill or injured. (Never delay important procedures or techniques on the critically ill or injured child.) Once your patient begins crying and carrying on, the more difficult the rest of your exam will be, if not impossible. Finally, provide continuous reassurance and feedback to your patient and his family members. This helps reduce everyone's anxiety over what is wrong, what you are doing, and what comes next.

Position yourself at the child's eye level, use a soft voice, and smile a lot. Often a small toy, such as a teddy bear, can distract your patient while you examine him. If you are using diagnostic equipment, allow the child to handle it while you explain how it works. Make sure your movements are slow and deliberate, and explain everything you are doing.

GENERAL APPEARANCE AND BEHAVIOR

Evaluate the child's general appearance and behavior. Ask the parents if his behavior seems normal. Observe his body position and muscle tone, keeping in mind the normal physical and psychological developmental stages of children.

Ask yourself two questions. Does your patient look and act like a normal child in the same age group? Do his actions appear normal to you and to his parents?

Infants (Newborn–1 Year) In the newborn or young infant, the arms and legs will flex slightly and move equally (Figure 2-93). Infants recognize their parents' faces and voices at about two months. They are normally alert and like to look around. They also like to be held and kept warm. They are frightened by loud noises and bright lights and may be soothed by having something to suck on. They are somewhat easy to assess because they are not very strong. At four to six months, they begin to sit up, and they can do so without assistance by eight months. They are easily distracted by a toy or shiny object. They are very distressed by separation from their parents. Since they will not understand what you are doing or why you are there, they probably will resist being examined. It is best to leave children in a parent's arms while you examine them (Figure 2-94). It is best to examine any child under the age of one from toe to head.

Toddlers (1–3 Years) Toddlers should be able to walk by their 18th month (Figure 2-95). They love to disagree with everyone and everything, and they trust no one but their parents. They are the most difficult age group to examine, even when they are not sick or hurt. They do not want you to touch them, so be prepared to take opportunities to assess areas as they become available. You may want to limit your assessment of the very ill or injured child to the most important areas. For example, focus on the chest and lungs of any child in respiratory distress. Do the vital areas first, before the child becomes agitated and makes the rest of your exam nearly impossible. Toddlers do like to be distracted with toys; if possible, make a game of the examination. In addition, because toddlers are beginning to sense their dignity, always respect their modesty.

Preschoolers (3–6 Years) Preschoolers (Figure 2-96) are particularly distrusting of strangers. Talk with them, gain their trust, and answer their questions honestly. Always prepare them if something you are going to do may hurt. Tell them it may hurt and that it's all right to cry. They have a great fear of being hurt and of the sight of

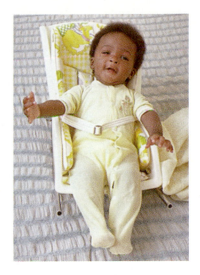

FIGURE 2-93 Infant (newborn–1 year).

Always cover a preschooler's wounds quickly, so he won't have to look at them.

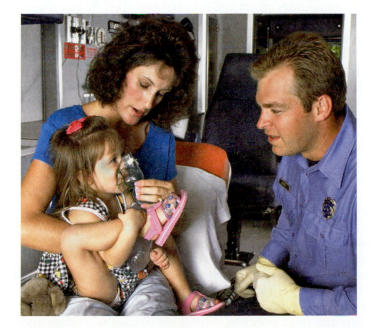

FIGURE 2-94 Have parents hold young children while you examine them.

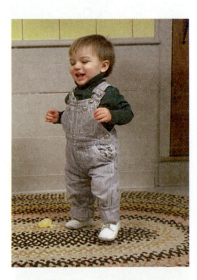

FIGURE 2-95 Toddler (1–3 years).

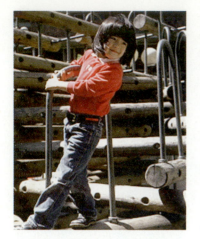

FIGURE 2-96 Preschooler
(3–6 years).

Allow school-age children to participate in the exam and to make treatment choices whenever possible.

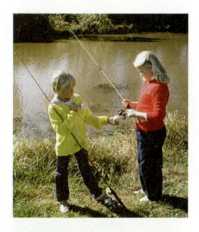

FIGURE 2-97 School-age
(6–12 years).

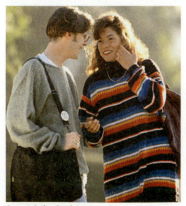

Source: Index Stock Imagery, Inc.

FIGURE 2-98 Adolescent
(13–18 years).

their own blood. They fear mutilation of their bodies, and the slightest injury may result in a temporarily hysterical child. Always cover a preschooler's wounds quickly, so he won't have to look at them. Often, injured or sick children in this age group feel guilty about their problem, as if it is their fault, regardless of the circumstances. Approach them slowly and offer a calming reassurance that they will be all right.

School-age (6–12 Years) School-age children (Figure 2-97) will cooperate with you if you gain their trust. They want to participate and to remain somewhat in control. Allow them to participate in the exam and to make treatment choices whenever possible. They have a basic understanding of their bodies, but they still fear separation, pain, and punishment. Modesty becomes more important, and they will not like being examined. Talk honestly with them about what you are doing and prepare them for what will come next as you proceed.

Adolescents (13–18 Years) Adolescents (Figure 2-98) can be treated much the same as adults. Since a teenager's modesty is extremely important, have a person of the same sex examine this patient if possible. Otherwise, conduct the physical exam just as you would for an adult patient.

ANATOMY AND THE PHYSICAL EXAM

To assess a child properly, you must understand his unique anatomy (Figure 2-99). The anatomical differences among age groups will alter your interpretation of physical findings. For example, since an infant's skin is thinner and contains less subcutaneous fat, you can expect environmental temperature extremes to affect him more severely.

This section deals with examining infants and children in the clinical situation. The pediatric chapter in Volume 5, *Special Considerations/Operations*, discusses a more detailed pediatric assessment.

General Appearance

Especially in the emergency setting, note whether your patient looks toxic, or sick. A toxic child appears not to recognize or respond to his parents. He may look tired and have a decreased respiratory effort and may have mottled skin or a generalized rash. He may be gray or cyanotic and just look very sick, usually from some type of bacterial process. These children, who present with the signs and symptoms of respiratory failure or shock, usually require rapid transport while you provide aggressive resuscitation procedures (advanced airway management, oxygenation and ventilation, intravenous access, and rapid fluid administration).

Head and Neck

The bones of the skull are soft and the fontanelles ("soft spots," spaces between a child's cranial bones) stay opened until about 18 months (Figure 2-100). From this time until about age five, cartilage connects the sutures. This allows the skull to expand as the brain grows. Check the sutures for bulging (increased intracranial pressure) or sunkenness (dehydration). In infants, a soft bulging spot following a history of trauma suggests a head injury with increasing intracranial pressure. The same finding associated with a fever suggests meningitis.

Because a child's airways are so much smaller than an adult's, a minor obstruction can create an acute respiratory problem. Watch the child's face for signs of distress and increased respiratory effort, such as nasal flaring. Children in acute respiratory distress will appear anxious and not interested in their surroundings. Also watch for retractions and head bobbing. Listen for stridor, wheezing, and grunting as further signs of severe breathing problems. As the child speaks, listen for hoarseness (upper airway obstruction) or moaning (decreasing level of consciousness). These findings always require appropriate intervention and rapid transport. Remember, a crying or screaming child has a patent airway.

Observe the child's face for signs of pain and discomfort as you continue your examination. Inspect his eyes as you would an adult's. Assess the outer ear for position. The top of the ear should be on a horizontal line with the outer corner of the eye. As a child grows, the anatomy of the external ear canal changes. In infancy the canal curves downward, so you should pull down the auricle to see the tympanic membrane at the distal end of the canal. As the child grows, the canal starts to move up and backward, and the ear is relatively higher and farther back on the head. Remember to pull the auricle upward and backward to afford the best view with the otoscope. Brace your hand against the child's skull to prevent injury from sudden movement.

Choose the largest speculum that will fit comfortably into the child's ear. Tilt the child's head away from you. Hold the otoscope firmly in one hand and, with your free hand, pull the ear appropriately to straighten the ear canal. Slowly insert the speculum one-fourth to one-half inch into the canal. Observe the amount, texture, and color of wax and the presence of foreign bodies. Inspect the tympanic membrane for color, light reflex, and bony landmarks. Repeat the same steps for the other ear.

Inspect the child's mouth much the same as you would for the adult. A young child's mouth is small, while the tongue is relatively large, so examining his oral cavity will be a challenge. Examine the nose using the nasal speculum and penlight or the appropriate attachment to the otoscope. To examine the mucous membrane, tip the child's head back and use the otoscope to inspect for color or swelling.

Evaluate the child's neck for stiffness, which—when associated with a fever—suggests meningitis. Evaluate for lymphadenopathy (enlarged lymph

Hoarseness, suggesting an upper airway obstruction, or moaning, suggesting decreased consciousness, requires intervention and rapid transport.

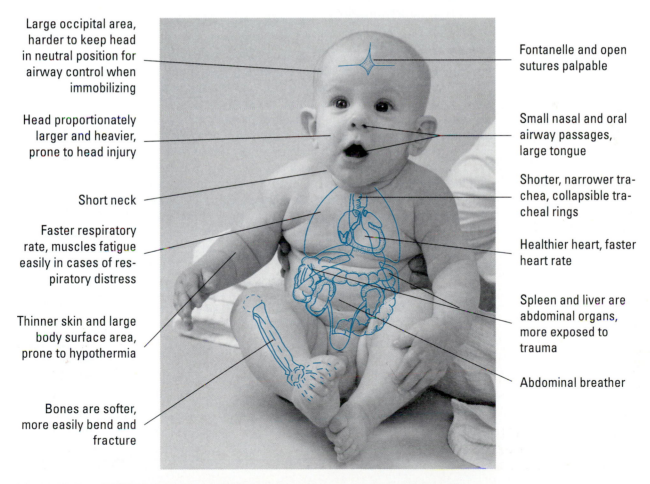

Large occipital area, harder to keep head in neutral position for airway control when immobilizing

Head proportionately larger and heavier, prone to head injury

Short neck

Faster respiratory rate, muscles fatigue easily in cases of respiratory distress

Thinner skin and large body surface area, prone to hypothermia

Bones are softer, more easily bend and fracture

Fontanelle and open sutures palpable

Small nasal and oral airway passages, large tongue

Shorter, narrower trachea, collapsible tracheal rings

Healthier heart, faster heart rate

Spleen and liver are abdominal organs, more exposed to trauma

Abdominal breather

FIGURE 2-99 Pediatric anatomy and physiology. You must understand a child's unique anatomy to assess him properly.

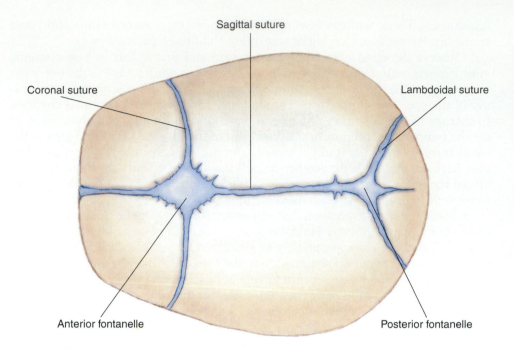

Sagittal suture

Coronal suture

Lambdoidal suture

Anterior fontanelle

Posterior fontanelle

FIGURE 2-100   Fontanelle of the infant skull.

nodes) in the neck by assessing the nodes' size, warmth, tenderness, and mobility. Certain infectious diseases like mononucleosis, rubella, and mumps are associated with lymphadenopathy. Nodes commonly feel enlarged due to recurrent upper respiratory infection.

Chest and Lungs

The rib cage in infants and small children is elastic and flexible. Because it comprises more cartilage than bone at this age, rib fractures are rare. On the other hand, lung contusions are common, because the lung tissue is very fragile. Small children also have a mobile mediastinum with a greater tendency to develop a tension pneumothorax. The chest muscles are not well developed, so children are mostly diaphragm breathers until about age seven.

The chest muscles are considered accessory muscles in the young child; to evaluate his breathing, observe both the chest and abdomen for movement. A child in severe respiratory distress may exhibit a "see-saw" pattern in which his sternum and abdomen rise and fall in opposition to each other. Count the respiratory rate without touching your patient, if possible. Assess the rate, quality, and depth of his respirations. Normal respiratory rates vary with age, but generally they decrease as the child grows older. Table 2-16 gives normal vital signs

Table 2-16	NORMAL PEDIATRIC VITAL SIGNS		
Age Group	Respiratory Rate	Heart Rate	Systolic BP
Newborn	30–60	100–180	60–90
Infant	30–60	100–160	87–105
Toddler	24–40	80–110	95–105
Preschooler	22–34	70–110	95–110
School Age	18–30	65–110	97–112
Adolescent	12–26	60–90	112–128

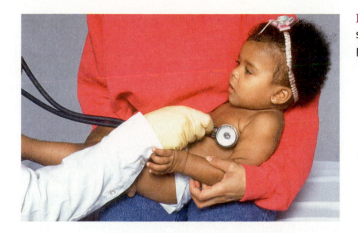

FIGURE 2-101   Place your stethoscope along your young patient's mid-axillary line.

for the various pediatric age groups. Auscultate for breath sounds with the bell of your stethoscope at the mid-axillary lines (Figure 2-101). Use this location to avoid hearing transmitted breath sounds from the opposite lung fields.

Cardiovascular

Unless the child has a congenital defect, his heart will be strong and healthy. His heart rate will vary with age, but generally it will decrease as he gets older. If the child is alert and uncooperative, measure his pulse rate by listening to the heart. Place your stethoscope between the sternum and nipple on your patient's left side. Children have thin chest walls, so you will usually be able to observe the apical impulse of the heart. Remember that tachycardia or bradycardia can both be a response to hypoxia in infants and young children. Bradycardia is the initial response to this condition in the newborn; without aggressive intervention, cardiopulmonary arrest will soon follow. Blood pressure will vary in children, but generally it will rise as they grow older. Children respond to hypovolemia by increasing cardiac function.

Tachycardia or bradycardia can both be a response to hypoxia in infants and young children; without aggressive intervention, cardiopulmonary arrest will soon follow.

Abdomen

A child's liver and spleen are proportionally larger and more vascular than an adult's. Thus they extend beyond the rib cage and are more exposed. Likewise, the child's immature abdominal muscles provide less protection than an adult's. Inspect the abdomen first for movement. Normally only respiratory movements should be visible; peristalsis is not normally observable. Next, assess contour. The abdomen normally bulges by the end of inspiration. Note any asymmetry. Inspect the groin area for inguinal hernias, common in male children. Finally, look at the umbilicus for any hernias, common in children under three years. Percuss and auscultate the abdomen as in the adult.

Before you begin palpating the abdomen, make sure the child is comfortable. Bend his knees to relax the abdominal muscles and make palpation easier.

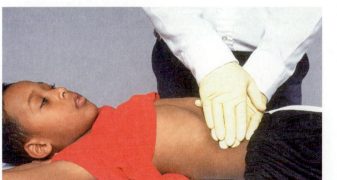

FIGURE 2-102   Gradually increase the pressure when palpating a young patient's abdomen.

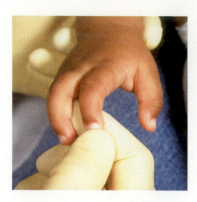

FIGURE 2-103 Pressing a child's fingernail is one of several ways to assess capillary refill. The child's capillary refill time is a good indicator of the child's peripheral perfusion status.

Your hands should be warm. If the child is ticklish, cover his hands with yours as you palpate. Begin with light palpation and gradually increase the pressure (Figure 2-102). Palpate all four quadrants. Deep palpation is performed next. You are feeling for masses and tenderness. The child's facial expression is a better guide to pain than his words, since he may interpret your pressure as pain.

Musculoskeletal

Evaluate pulses, sensation, movement, and warmth in all four extremities. Check for capillary refill and feel for peripheral pulses (Figure 2-103). Evaluate the skin, which reveals important clues in children. Its color, turgor, moisture, and temperature are key indicators of his cardiovascular system's condition. Unlike the adult's, the child's capillary refill time accurately reflects his peripheral perfusion status. When examining the musculoskeletal system, remember the growth and posture at different stages of the child's development. For example, a toddler walks with a broad base for support and is likely to appear bowlegged. A teenager with poor posture may suffer from a skeletal problem such as scoliosis.

Palpate the upper and lower extremities for swelling, tenderness, and contractions. Next have the child demonstrate the range of motion of his joints while you feel for smoothness of movement. Examine all joints. Check muscle strength in all muscle groups by asking the child to prevent you from moving a part of his body. A child's bones are more likely to break at the ends, where growth takes place. Until the child reaches adolescence, when these areas become as strong as the rest of the bone, injuries that occur near the joints are more likely to damage the bone than the ligaments or tendons. Assess the child's muscle coordination by having him stand and then hop on one foot. Repeat this for the other foot. Children usually enjoy this aspect of the physical examination. You can also have the child skip or jump.

Nervous System

The child's general behavior, level of consciousness, and orientation are signs of cerebral function. You have asked the parents to comment on their child's behavior during the history taking. You have observed the child's behavior throughout the examination and already have learned much about his cerebral function by interacting with him. Now test specific functions such as language and recall. You will have checked most of the 12 cranial nerves during your head and neck exam.

You can test for cerebellar function with several games that children usually enjoy. First, as you move your finger, ask the child to touch his nose and then your finger. Consistent past-pointing should arouse your suspicion. An alternate test is to have the child pat his knees alternately with the palms and backs of his hands. Check for sensation over the child's face, trunk, arms, and leg. Check for hot and cold sensation by alternately touching the skin with warm and cold test tubes. Ask the child to close his eyes and tell you which he feels. Be sure to test for reflexes on both sides of the body, just as with an adult. If the child has difficulty relaxing, test the parent's reflexes to show that it does not hurt.

The most important characteristic of a physical assessment is thoroughness.

Remember, the most important characteristic of a physical assessment is thoroughness. Be systematic in your approach and, with practice, you will be able to do a complete and accurate physical assessment.

RECORDING EXAMINATION FINDINGS

The patient record is only as good as the accuracy, depth, and detail you provide.

After you perform the history and physical examination, it is time to record the findings on your patient's chart, or permanent medical record. The information you enter enables you and other members of the health care team to identify health problems, make a diagnosis, plan the appropriate care, and monitor your patient's response to treatment. The patient record is only as good as the accuracy, depth, and detail you provide.

All health care clinicians follow a standard format when charting patient information. Using it and appropriate medical terminology will allow everyone to easily read and understand your assessment findings. While your first attempts at writing a complete history and physical exam will be lengthy and possibly disorganized, clinical experience will eventually lead to a more efficient and organized record.

Your patient's chart is a legal document, and any information you enter may be used in court. Proper documentation is vital to your protection. Present the data legibly, accurately, and truthfully. They should represent the findings of your history and physical examination—no more, no less. State your assessment, your analysis of the problem, and your management plan clearly and exactly. No question should ever arise about your assessment or care of your patient if you document it properly.

Be sure to include all data about your assessment. You cannot formulate an impression unless you have clearly spelled out the positive and negative details upon which it was made. Remember that the absence of a sign or symptom (pertinent negative) may be just as important as its presence. Record everything in writing. If you do not document a neuro exam, you will never convince anyone that you performed it, especially not a plaintiff's lawyer or a jury. Be complete but avoid unnecessary words. For example, say "pale," not "pale in color." Also avoid lengthy repetitive phrases such as "patient states." Use accepted abbreviations and symbols whenever possible. Avoid using vague adjectives such as *good, normal,* and *poor,* because they are open to interpretation by other providers. Document what your patient tells you, not what you infer or interpret. Use direct quotes whenever possible.

The universally accepted organization for patient charts follows the SOAP format. SOAP stands for Subjective, Objective, Assessment, and Plan. Use this format when writing your patient's chart. Subjective information is what your patient tells you. It comprises the chief complaint, the history of present illness, the past history, the current health status, and the review of systems. Objective information includes the data collected from the general survey, vital signs, head-to-toe anatomical exam, systems-oriented exam, and neurological exam, including the mental status. These are the data you gathered by inspection, palpation, percussion, auscultation, and other techniques of physical examination. Objective information also includes the results of any laboratory tests. The assessment summarizes the relevant data for each problem identified in the history and physical exam. The plan outlines your management strategy in three categories: diagnostic (how you will assess progress), therapeutic (any treatments), and educational (what you need to teach your patient). Figure 2-104 offers an example of documentation for a comprehensive physical examination. Chapter 5, "Documentation," deals with prehospital documentation in detail.

> *Record* everything *in writing.*

Content Review

SOAP

- Subjective
- Objective
- Assessment
- Plan

SUMMARY

This chapter has presented both a regional and a systems approach to physical examination. The setting, chief complaint, and clinical status of your patient will dictate how much of the physical exam you actually use. For example, if you are hired to conduct preemployment physicals, you may decide to conduct a complete examination. If you are at the scene of a critically ill or injured patient, you will assess only those areas relevant to the situation. If your patient presents with a minor, isolated musculoskeletal injury, you may focus your exam on that area and system. As you become more experienced, making these decisions will become easier.

Screening Exam Report

Patient: Jane Doe
Location: University Hospital
Date: 11/11/1998
Examiner: David Cywinski, MD
Jane Doe is a healthy appearing 24 yo white female who has come into the office for a physical for entrance into medical school.

Past History
    General Health Good
    Childhood illnesses   Measles and chicken pox
    Adult illnesses   2 year history of PUD
        Appendectomy 1992 without sequelae
        Last physical exam 1995 for college athletics
    Psychiatric illnesses   None
    Injuries   None
    Operations   None

Current Health Status
    Medications   Zantac
    Allergies   Sulfa drugs
        Bee stings
    Tobacco   5 pack year smoker (no desire to quit, will follow up)
    Alcohol/drugs   2-3 drinks/week, CAGE negative
    Tests   PAP smear 05/1997 normal, no mammograms
    Exercise/leisure   No time

Family History   Single female living with female partner
    Mother   54 yo — healthy
    Father   57 yo — MI 1993
    Brother   20 yo — healthy
    Grandparents both deceased prior to patient's birth, no information available
    Patient denies history of genetic diseases

Psychosocial History   Born in Syracuse, NY. Grew up here.
    Graduated from University of Rochester (Biology)

Review of Systems

General: Patient reports to be in good health.

HEENT: Denies headaches, diplopia, blurred vision, eye pain or redness, decreased visual acuity. Also denies hearing loss, tinnitus, vertigo. No report of sinusitis, PND, epistaxis, bleeding from gums, oral ulceration or growths, sore throats.

Pulmonary: Denies cough, hemoptysis, dyspnea, pleuritic chest pain, wheezing, asthma, or recurrent infections. No history of occupational exposures. Last TB test done 3 weeks ago by school. Results — negative.

Cardiac: Denies chest pain or pressure, palpitations, orthopnea, PND, SOB, pedal edema, heart murmur, HTN, or MVP.

GU: Denies dysuria, hematuria, polyuria. No history of UTIs or renal calculi. Onset of menses at 13 yoa. States she has a regular 28 day cycle with 4 days of bleeding. No history of abnormal vaginal discharge, STDs. No history of pregnancy. SBE done monthly, instructed by her OB/GYN physician.

GI: Denies weight gain or loss, nausea, vomiting, diarrhea, melena, hemorrhoids. History of PUD that started 2 years ago when she decided to go to medical school and had to "buckle down" and do well in school. Pain becomes worse when her workload increases and when she eats spicy food. She describes the pain as burning and sometimes ascending into esophagus. Medication and relaxation alleviate the symptoms.

Neuro: Denies dizziness, syncope, seizures, paresthesia, weakness, or tremors.

Rheum: Denies arthritic pain, joint stiffness or swelling. No history of Lyme disease, back pain.

Vascular: Denies phlebitis, varicose veins, cramping or Raynauds.

Endocrine: Denies polyuria, polydipsia, polyphagia, cold-heat intolerance, tachycardia, fatigue.

FIGURE 2-104   Patient documentation for a comprehensive physical examination.

Heme: Denies easy bruising, bleeding, or anemia. No prior history of transfusion. Patient reports A+ blood group, does donate blood with Red Cross. Denies lymph node enlargement.

Derm: Denies rashes, nevi, dryness, pruritis, or pigmentation change.

Psych: Denies depression, panic-anxiety attacks, memory disturbances, personality changes, or hallucinations.

Physical Exam

General appearance: Jane Doe is an alert, oriented, well developed 24 yo white female in no apparent distress.

VS: BP — 124/78, Pulse — 64 regular both radials, Resp — 16, Temp — not taken, appears afebrile.

HEENT: Head — Normocephalic with scar above OS, pt had sutures above OS from falling off coffee table when she was 2 yoa. Eyes — Visual acuity 20/20 with pocket chart, does not wear glasses. PERLA, EOM intact, sclera white, visual fields intact. Retinal vessels visualized and appeared normal. Ears — Pinnae nontender as well as external ear canal. Gross hearing intact to whispers. Weber test lateralizes to left ear with a normal Rhinne test. Tympanic membrane grey without erythema. Nose — mucosa pink with exudate, no polyps noted. Throat — mucosa, buccal and gingival, pink without exudate, no ulcers or growths noted. Uvula midline.

Neck: Trachea midline, no JVD noted at 45 degrees, thyroid not palpable. Good cartoid pulses. ROM intact. No carotid bruits heard.

Pulmonary: Chest symmetrical, normal respiratory expansion, breath sounds clear bilaterally, no egophony or whispered pectoriloquy. Diaphragmatic excursion equal at 6 cm. Normal resonance to percussion.

Cardiac: PMI not palpated, S1, S2 heard at aortic and pulmonic locations. Tricuspid and mitral valves not auscultated. S1, S2 at above noted sites sounded clear without murmurs, clicks or snaps.

Abdomen: Small scar 3 cm noted in right lower quadrant, appears to have healed well. Otherwise, abdomen is symmetrical. Bowel sounds heard in all four quadrants. No bruits heard over renals, iliacs, or aorta. Liver not palpable, span 8 cm with percussion and scratch test. Spleen not palpable. No CVA tenderness. No masses noted on palpation. Aorta 2 cm in width.

GU/Rectal: Not done.

Musculoskeletal: General muscle tone appears good, no atrophy noted, gross symmetry apparent. No joint swelling or deformity noted. Range of motion intact for all four extremities. Spinal contour appropriate without scoliosis noted.

Nodes: Submental, submandibular, preauricular, postauricular, occipital, cervical chain, supraclavicular, axillary, epitrochlear, inguinal nodes not palpable.

Breast: Not done.

Vascular/Pulses:

	Left	Right
Carotid	2+	2+
Radial	2+	2+
Aorta		2+
Femoral	2+	2+
Popliteal		1+ (equal bilateral)
Dorsalis	1+	1+

No varicose veins noted, bruits were not heard in carotid, aorta, renal, femoral regions.

Extremities: No clubbing, cyanosis, edema, pigmentation change noted. Capillary refill < 2 seconds, nails nonpitted.

Neuro: Patient is alert and responsive.
Cranial Nerves I — XII
  I — not tested
  II — PERLA
  III — PERLA EOM, intact
  IV — EOM intact
  V — Facial sensation intact, muscles of mastication intact/operable
  VI — EOM intact
  VII — Muscles of facial expression intact, symmetrical
  VIII — Hearing grossly intact to whispers, balance intact

FIGURE 2-104 (CONTINUED)   Patient documentation for a comprehensive physical examination.

IX — Gag reflex intact
X — Gag reflex intact, uvula midline
XI — Sternocleidomastoid, trapezius functioning symmetrically
XII — Tongue protrudes midline

Sensory intact to both sharp and dull stimuli. Rhomberg negative. Joint position and sense intact. Two-point discrimination intact and appropriate. Reflexes as follows:

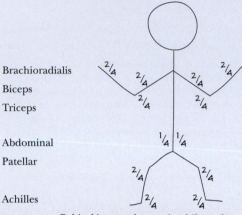

Brachioradialis

Biceps

Triceps

Abdominal

Patellar

Achilles

Babinskis were downgoing bilateral.

Problem list: 1. PUD
2. Abnormal Weber test
3. Smoker

Plan: 1. Continue medications for PUD and instruct patient on stress reduction techniques. If PUD continues, consider biopsy for *H. Pylori*.
2. Refer patient for audiogram
3. At next visit, discuss perils of smoking and advantages of cessation program

David Cywinski, MD
SUNY HSC @ Syracuse

FIGURE 2-104 (CONTINUED) Patient documentation for a comprehensive physical examination.

YOU MAKE THE CALL

Your crew from the Barnes Ambulance Service is at a standby at the annual 10K fun run to benefit the St. Joseph's Hospital pediatric clinic. Several hundred runners began the race on this very warm and muggy day. Thirty minutes into the race, when the serious runners begin crossing the finish line, you receive a call to the turnaround point three miles away. Approaching the scene, you find a woman in her 30s on the side of the road. She is in moderate distress, clutching her right ankle. You ask the runner what happened. The runner says that she stepped into a small pothole and twisted her ankle. You instruct your partner, EMT-basic Darlene Harris, to remove the victim's shoes and socks.

1. How would you begin the exam?
2. What is your differential field diagnosis?
3. What elements of the history are appropriate to ask this patient?
4. Outline your physical exam.

See Suggested Responses at the back of this book.

FURTHER READING

Bates, Barbara, Lynn S. Bickley, and Robert A. Hoekelman. *A Guide to Physical Examination and History Taking*. 6th ed. Philadelphia: J.B. Lippincott, 1995.

Chameides, Leon, and Mary Fran Hazinski, eds. *Textbook of Pediatric Advanced Life Support*. Dallas: American Heart Association, 1994.

DeLorenzo, Robert. "Sneezes, Wheezes, and Breezes—Listening to the Chest." *JEMS* 20 (October 1995): 58–69.

Eichelberger, Martin R., et al. *Pediatric Emergencies: A Manual for Prehospital Care Providers*. 2nd ed. Upper Saddle River, N.J.: Brady, 1998.

Epstein, Owen, et al. *Clinical Examination*. St. Louis: Mosby, 1997.

Foltin, George, et al. *Teaching Resource for Instructors in Prehospital Pediatrics*. New York: Center for Pediatric Medicine, 1998.

Martini, Frederick. *Fundamentals of Anatomy and Physiology*. 4th ed. Upper Saddle River, N.J.: Prentice Hall, 1998.

Martini, Frederick, and Edwin F. Bartholomew. *Fundamentals of Anatomy and Physiology*. Upper Saddle River, N.J.: Prentice Hall, 1989.

Seidel, Henry M., et al. *Mosby's Guide to Physical Examination*. St. Louis: Mosby, 1987.

Spaite, David W., et al. "A Prospective Evaluation of Prehospital Patient Assessment by Direct In-field Observation: Failure of ALS Personnel to Measure Vital Signs." *Prehospital and Disaster Medicine* 5 (October–December 1990): 325–333.

Willms, Janice L., Henry Schniederman, and Paula S. Algranati. *Physical Diagnosis: Bedside Evaluation of Diagnosis and Function*. Baltimore: Williams & Wilkins, 1994.

ON THE WEB

Visit Brady's Paramedic Website at www.bradybooks.com/paramedic.

CHAPTER 3

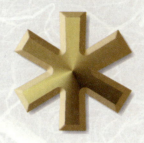

Patient Assessment in the Field

Objectives

After reading this chapter, you should be able to:

1. Recognize hazards/potential hazards associated with the medical and trauma scene. (pp. 174–182)
2. Identify unsafe scenes and describe methods for making them safe. (pp. 174–182)
3. Discuss common mechanisms of injury/nature of illness. (pp. 184–185)
4. Predict patterns of injury based on mechanism of injury. (pp. 184–185, 200–201)
5. Discuss the reason for identifying the total number of patients at the scene. (pp. 182–183)
6. Organize the management of a scene following size-up. (pp. 185–200)
7. Explain the reasons for identifying the need for additional help or assistance during the scene size-up. (pp. 176–183)
8. Summarize the reasons for forming a general impression of the patient. (pp. 186–187)
9. Discuss methods of assessing mental status/levels of consciousness in the adult, infant, and child patient. (pp. 187–189)

Continued

Objectives Continued

10. Discuss methods of assessing and securing the airway in the adult, child, and infant patient. (pp. 189–195)
11. State reasons for cervical spine management for the trauma patient. (p. 187)
12. Analyze a scene to determine if spinal precautions are required. (pp. 184–185, 200–202)
13. Describe methods for assessing respiration in the adult, child, and infant patient. (pp. 194–195)
14. Describe the methods used to locate and assess a pulse in an adult, child, and infant patient. (pp. 195–196)
15. Discuss the need for assessing the patient for external bleeding. (pp. 195–198)
16. Describe normal and abnormal findings when assessing skin color, temperature, and condition. (p. 198)
17. Explain the reason and process for prioritizing a patient for care and transport. (pp. 198–200)
18. Use the findings of the initial assessment to determine the patient's perfusion status. (p. 199)
19. Describe orthostatic vital signs and evaluate their usefulness in assessing a patient in shock. (p. 218)
20. Describe the medical patient physical examination. (pp. 214–218)
21. Differentiate between the assessment for an unresponsive, altered mental status, and alert medical patients. (pp. 213–220)
22. Discuss the reasons for reconsidering the mechanism of injury. (pp. 202–203)
23. Recite examples and explain why patients should receive a rapid trauma assessment. (p. 202)
24. Describe the trauma patient physical examination. (pp. 203–212)

25. Describe the elements of the rapid trauma assessment and discuss their evaluation. (pp. 202–211)
26. Identify cases when the rapid assessment is suspended to provide patient care. (pp. 202–203)
27. Discuss the reason for performing a focused history and physical exam. (pp. 213–215)
28. Describe when and why a detailed physical examination is necessary. (p. 222)
29. Discuss the components of the detailed physical examination. (pp. 222–228)
30. Explain what additional care is provided while performing the detailed physical exam. (pp. 222–228)
31. Distinguish between the detailed physical exam that is performed on a trauma patient and that of the medical patient. (pp. 222–228)
32. Differentiate between patients requiring a detailed physical exam and those who do not. (p. 222)
33. Discuss the rationale for repeating the initial assessment as part of the ongoing assessment. (pp. 229–232)
34. Describe the components of the ongoing assessment. (pp. 229–232)
35. Describe trending of assessment components. (pp. 229–232)
36. Discuss medical identification devices/systems. (p. 208)
37. Given several preprogrammed and moulaged medical and trauma patients, provide the appropriate scene survey, initial assessment, focused assessment, detailed assessment, and ongoing assessments. (pp. 173–232)

CASE STUDY

En route to the scene, paramedic Chris Johnson and EMT-Basic Nick Farina prepare for the worst. The initial report from bystanders at the scene says that a woman jumped from a fourth-floor balcony at the downtown shopping mall. She reportedly landed four stories below on the marble floor and lies bleeding with multiple injuries. If this is true, Chris thinks, she and Nick will find a significant mechanism of injury and probable serious injuries.

Upon arrival, Chris's worst fears come true. A woman in her mid-thirties lies on the floor in a pool of blood with signs of obvious multiple trauma. Immediately, Chris directs her partner to stabilize the woman's head and neck and manually open her airway with a jaw thrust. Nick, also a part-time respiratory therapist, is well-suited for the job.

Chris begins the initial assessment by evaluating their patient's level of response. She quickly notes that their patient is unresponsive to all stimuli. She then assesses the airway, which is noisy with gurgling blood. She immediately suctions the oropharynx and listens for air movement. Their patient has shallow respirations at a rate of 38 per minute. Chris instructs Nick to insert an oropharyngeal airway and begin ventilation with a bag-valve mask and supplemental oxygen at a rate of 12 per minute while she continues her assessment.

Because the patient exhibits signs of severe respiratory distress, Chris decides to assess her neck and chest before proceeding with the initial assessment. Chris quickly exposes their patient's chest and notices deformity to the right side with probable multiple rib fractures. She auscultates the chest and, noticing decreased breath sounds on the right side, suspects a pneumothorax or pulmonary contusion. Chris feels for radial and carotid pulses. She notes the absence of a radial pulse and the cool, pale look of their patient's skin. The carotid pulse is weak at a rate of approximately 130 beats per minute. Nick comments that their patient is in shock. Chris designates her as a priority 1, indicating rapid transport to the appropriate medical facility.

While Nick continues to maintain manual stabilization of their patient's neck, Chris begins a rapid trauma assessment. She starts at the head and quickly palpates a depressed skull fracture. Chris notes that her patient's trachea is midline and jugular veins are flat, temporarily ruling out a tension pneumothorax. She notices a rigid, distended abdomen and suspects an intra-abdominal bleed, which is most likely causing the profound shock. Next Chris palpates the pelvis and notes an unstable pelvic ring, indicating fracture. She also notes severe deformity and angulation to both femurs, suggesting bilateral fractures. As additional help from the fire department arrives, Chris instructs them to immobilize her patient with the pneumatic antishock garment while she prepares the back of the ambulance for transport.

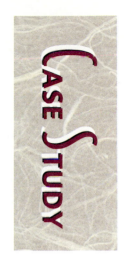

Once in the ambulance, Chris reassesses her patient's mental status and ABCs during the four-minute ride to Duethorn Memorial Hospital. At this time, she takes a full set of vital signs and notes the following: heart rate—130 and weak; blood pressure—76/40; respirations—38 and shallow. Chris decides to start two large-bore IV lines to begin fluid resuscitation. Firefighter EMT-Intermediate Joe Armstrong performs the procedure and runs both lines "wide-open." Chris contacts the hospital and gives a quick report to Dr. Prasad, the attending physician. Upon arrival, they transfer their patient to the emergency department staff and watch as an experienced team of trauma specialists prepares their patient for a quick ride to surgery.

INTRODUCTION

Patient assessment means conducting a problem-oriented evaluation of your patient and establishing priorities of care based on existing and potential threats to human life. In the previous two chapters you studied the techniques of performing a comprehensive history and physical exam. Such all-inclusive evaluations are best suited for patients without a chief complaint. They also establish a baseline health evaluation for patients admitted to the hospital. As a paramedic, however, you will certainly never perform a comprehensive exam in the acute setting. It is too time consuming and yields too much irrelevant information. Instead you will use your foundation of knowledge, skills, and tools to assess the acutely ill or injured patient. With time and clinical experience you will learn which components of the comprehensive exam apply to your particular patient.

Now you can use the pertinent components of the comprehensive history and physical exam to perform patient assessments—problem-oriented assessments based on your patient's chief complaint. The basic components of patient assessment include the initial assessment; the focused history and physical exam, including vital signs; an ongoing assessment; and in some cases, a detailed physical exam.

Your patient's condition will determine which components you use and how you use them. For example, for trauma patients with a significant mechanism of injury, you will perform an initial assessment followed by a rapid trauma assessment (a head-to-toe exam aimed at traumatic signs and symptoms) and, if time allows, a detailed physical exam en route to the hospital. For patients with minor, isolated trauma, an initial assessment followed by a focused physical exam is warranted. For the responsive medical patient, you will conduct an initial assessment followed by a focused history and physical exam. Finally, for the unresponsive medical patient, you will perform an initial assessment followed by a rapid medical assessment (a head-to-toe exam aimed at medical signs and symptoms). In all cases, you will perform an ongoing assessment en route to the hospital to detect changes in patient condition.

The initial assessment's goal is to identify and correct immediately life-threatening conditions. These include airway compromise, inadequate ventilation, and major hemorrhage. During this rapid evaluation you use a variety of maneuvers and special equipment to manage any life threats as you find them. Immediately following the initial assessment you will establish the priorities of

* **patient assessment** problem-oriented evaluation of patient and establishment of priorities based on existing and potential threats to human life.

> **Content Review**
>
> **COMPONENTS OF PATIENT ASSESSMENT**
> Initial assessment
> Focused history and physical exam
> Ongoing assessment
> Detailed physical exam

care. People such as the trauma patient with unstable vital signs and the unresponsive medical patient require a rapid head-to-toe exam and immediate transport to the hospital. Patients with minor, isolated trauma and most medical emergencies allow time to perform further assessments and provide care before transport.

Your proficiency in performing a systematic patient assessment will determine your ability to deliver the highest quality of prehospital advanced life support (**ALS**) to sick and injured people. Paramedic patient assessment is a straightforward skill, similar to the assessment you might have performed as an EMT-Basic. It differs, however, in depth and in the kind of care you will provide as a result. Your assessment must be thorough, because many advanced life support procedures are potentially dangerous. Safely and appropriately performing advanced procedures such as administration of drugs, defibrillation, synchronized cardioversion, needle decompression of the chest, or endotracheal intubation will depend upon your assessment and correct field diagnosis. If your assessment does not reveal your patient's true problem, the consequences can be devastating.

As always, common sense dictates how you proceed in the field. When you assess the responsive medical patient, the history reveals the most important diagnostic information and takes priority over the physical exam. For the trauma patient and the unresponsive medical patient, the reverse is true. Yet trauma may cause a medical emergency, and conversely, a medical emergency may cause trauma. Only by performing a thorough patient assessment can you discover the true cause of your patient's problems. This chapter provides problem-oriented patient assessment templates based on the information and techniques presented in the previous two chapters. You will need to refer to those chapters for the details of taking a history and conducting a physical exam.

SCENE SIZE-UP

Scene size-up is the essential first step at any emergency. Before you enter a scene, take the necessary time to judge the situation. Fire officers drive just past a burning house so they can see three of its sides before they make strategic decisions. Follow their lead. Never rush into any situation; first stop and look around (Figure 3-1).

Upon arrival, determine whether the scene is safe. Does the situation require special body substance isolation precautions? Is the mechanism of injury or the nature of illness obvious? Are there multiple patients? Do you need immediate additional resources? After an initial scene assessment, if necessary, report to your dispatcher what you have, what you need, and what you are doing. This way, you keep everyone informed and your dispatcher can send any necessary additional support.

While size-up is your initial responsibility, remember that it is also an ongoing process. Emergency scenes are dynamic and can change suddenly. An injury to a child call can erupt into a violent domestic dispute if one parent blames the other. A hazardous material spill can ignite. An improperly stabilized car can shift. Always be alert for subtle signs of danger, and avoid becoming a patient yourself.

Sizing up the scene gives you important information that will guide your actions. In trauma, a brief size-up of the accident scene reveals the mechanism of injury. From this, you can estimate the degree of energy transfer and possible seriousness of injuries. In a medical emergency, you can sometimes determine the nature of your patient's illness from clues at the scene. The smell of a lower gastrointestinal bleed, the sound of a hissing oxygen tank, or the sight of drug para-

---

* ALS advanced life support.

If your assessment does not reveal your patient's true problem, the consequences can be devastating.

Only by performing a thorough patient assessment can you discover the true cause of your patient's problems.

Never rush into any situation; first stop and look around.

Always be alert for subtle signs of danger.

Sizing up the scene gives you important information that will guide your actions.

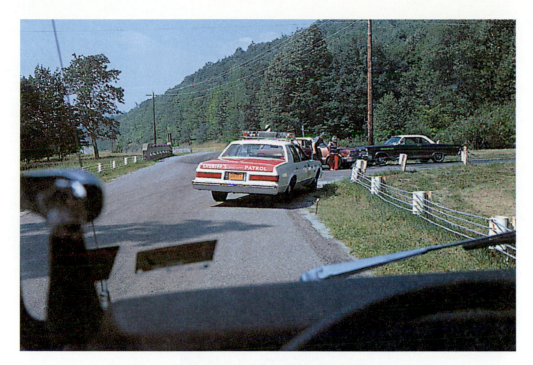

FIGURE 3-1   Always stop to size up the scene before going in.

phernalia provides clues and an initial insight into your patient's situation. Learn to use all your senses when sizing up the scene.

The components of a scene size-up include:

- Body substance isolation
- Scene safety
- Location of all patients
- Mechanism of injury
- Nature of the illness

BODY SUBSTANCE ISOLATION

Body fluids frequently contain health-threatening pathogens. The best defense against bloodborne, body-fluid-borne, and airborne agents is to take appropriate body substance isolation precautions. Your goal is to prevent infectious disease from spreading to yourself or to others. Make sure that personal protective equipment such as gloves, masks, gowns, and eye protection is available on every emergency vehicle, and take the appropriate precautions on every emergency call (Figure 3-2). Your patient's clinical condition and the procedures you perform will determine the required precautions.

Most body isolation procedures are simply common sense. Wash your hands thoroughly before and after treating each patient whenever possible (Figure 3-3). This simple technique is the most effective method of preventing disease transmission between patients and their health care workers. Wear latex or vinyl gloves anytime you expect to contact blood or other body fluids. This includes the mucous membranes, any areas with broken skin, or items soiled with blood or body fluids. Since you often cannot wash your hands before examining your

The best defense against bloodborne, body-fluid-borne, and airborne pathogens is to take body substance isolation precautions.

Washing your hands is the most effective method of preventing disease transmission between you and your patients.

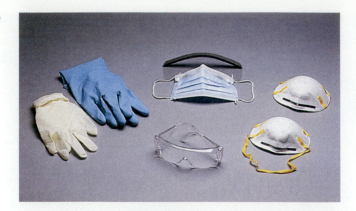

FIGURE 3-2 Always wear the appropriate personal protective equipment (PPE) to prevent exposure to contagious diseases.

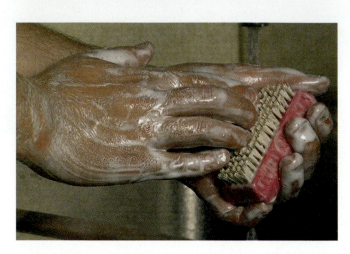

FIGURE 3-3 Careful, methodical hand washing helps reduce exposure to contagious disease.

Always use all the equipment recommended for a particular procedure or patient to maximize your protection against communicable diseases.

★ **scene safety** doing everything possible to ensure a safe environment.

patient, you should wear gloves also to avoid exposing your patient to your germs. If you are managing multiple patients, you should attempt to change gloves between patients in order to prevent cross-contamination. Discard all contaminated gloves in the appropriate biohazard bag (Figure 3-4).

Always use all the equipment recommended for a particular procedure or patient to maximize your protection against communicable diseases. If blood, vomit, or secretions might splash near your eyes, nose, or mouth, wear a face mask and protective eyewear. Such situations may include arterial bleeding, childbirth, invasive procedures such as endotracheal intubation, and oral suctioning, as well as during clean-up when heavy scrubbing is necessary. If you expect large blood splashes, such as in emergency childbirth, wear a gown to protect your clothing.

Consider masking both yourself and your patient whenever the potential for airborne transmission of disease exists (Figure 3-5). The National Institute of Occupational Safety and Health has designed high-efficiency particulate air (**HEPA**) respirators to filter out the tuberculosis bacillus (**TB**). Always wear a properly fitted HEPA mask if you are managing a patient with suspected TB, especially when performing procedures like endotracheal intubation, oral suctioning, and administering nebulized medications. These procedures present a high risk for the transmission of airborne particles.

SCENE SAFETY

Scene safety simply means doing everything possible to ensure a safe environment for yourself, your crew, other responding personnel, your patient, and any bystanders—in that order. Your personal safety is the top priority at any emer-

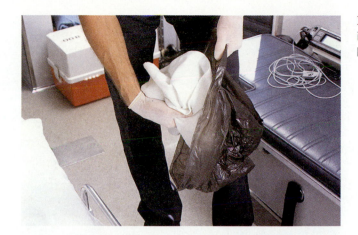

FIGURE 3-4 Place all contaminated items in the appropriate biohazard bag.

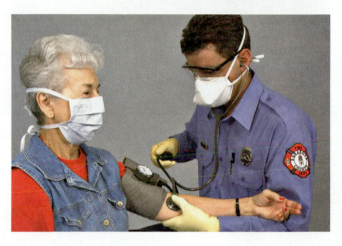

FIGURE 3-5 With a suspected tuberculosis patient, you may place a surgical-type mask on the patient while you wear a NIOSH-approved respirator. Monitor the patient's airway and breathing carefully.

gency scene. Make sure you are not injured while providing care. If you become a patient yourself, you will do your own patient little good. You must determine that no hazards may endanger the lives of people on the scene. If your scene is unsafe, either make it safe or wait until someone else does (Figure 3-6).

As the first unit on the scene, you may overestimate your capability to manage a rescue situation. Do not attempt a hazardous rescue unless you are properly clothed, equipped, and trained. Individual acts of courage are sometimes necessary, but modern rescue operations emphasize safety first, not heroics. Foolish heroics often end in tragedy. If in doubt, it is better to err on the side of caution than to risk personal harm.

Many factors can make an emergency scene unsafe. Through experience you will learn to identify them quickly. Do not become complacent. Sometimes even the most nonthreatening, harmless-looking scene can turn into a disaster (Figure 3-7). If you are not sure the scene is safe, do not enter. As you approach a scene, immediately evaluate the surrounding area. Is it as your dispatcher's information has led you to expect, or does something just not look right? What do the bystanders' faces tell you? Are they angry, scared, or panicked? Be alert for situations that look or feel suspicious. If necessary, wait until law enforcement personnel secure the scene. Use all your senses to evaluate a scene and learn to trust your intuition. If your instincts tell you not to enter or to get out, follow them. They are the subconscious sum of your experiences. Listen to them; they are probably correct.

Carefully look for and identify on-scene hazards before even attempting to reach your patient. To do otherwise places you, other rescuers, and your patient at risk. Remember that you may find such dangers at either medical or trauma

Your personal safety is the top priority at any emergency scene.

Listen to your instincts; they are probably correct.

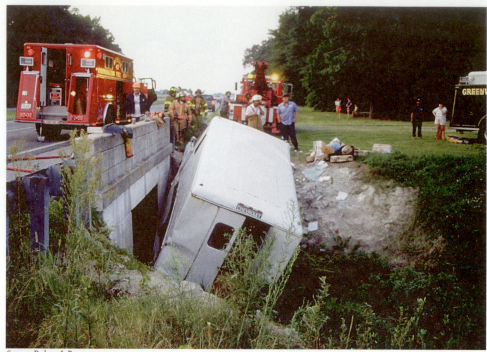

Source: Robert J. Bennett

FIGURE 3-6 Look for potential hazards during scene size-up.

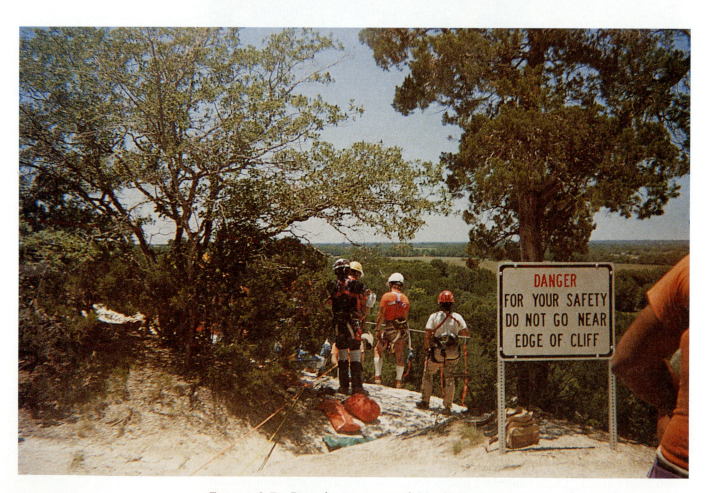

DANGER
FOR YOUR SAFETY
DO NOT GO NEAR
EDGE OF CLIFF

FIGURE 3-7 Even the most peaceful-looking scene can pose potential dangers.

scenes. Potential hazards include fire, structural collapse, traffic, unstable surfaces, and broken glass or jagged metal. Other risks involve hazardous materials—chemical spills, radiation, or gas leaks that might ignite or explode. A simple spark can set off a gas leak or oil spill. Electric wires threaten both fire and electric shock. Look around to determine the possibility of lightning, avalanche, rock slides, cave-ins, or similar dangers. Other potential hazards include poisonous or caustic substances; biological agents; germ-infested materials; confined spaces such as vessels, trenches, mines, silos, or caves; and extreme heights. In every case, let common sense dictate scene management.

Crime scenes pose a special threat. When responding to a call in which the initial dispatch includes words such as *shooting, stabbing,* or *domestic dispute,* wait for law enforcement personnel to secure the scene before entering (Figure 3-8). In fact, do not even enter the neighborhood, as sitting in your ambulance on the scene may undermine an already unstable environment. If possible, turn off your lights and siren and stage your vehicle a few blocks away, where it cannot be seen from the scene. Refer to the crime scene awareness chapter in Volume 5, *Special Considerations/Operations* for more information on this topic.

Crash scenes requiring heavy-duty rescue procedures, scenes where toxic substances are present, crime scenes with a potential for violence, or scenes with unstable surfaces like slippery slopes, ice, or rushing water all call for specialized crews, additional medical supplies, and sophisticated equipment (Figure 3-9). Do not even consider entering such situations unless you have the proper clothing, equipment, and training to work in them. Because getting backup requires extra time, this phase is critical. A prompt call to your dispatch center can save critical minutes in a life-threatening situation.

Without the appropriate protective gear, you will jeopardize your safety and your patient's. To participate in a rescue operation, you should have at least the following equipment immediately available: four-point suspension helmets, eye goggles or industrial safety glasses, high-quality hearing protection, leather work gloves, high-top steel-toed boots, insulated coveralls, and turnout gear (Figure 3-10). Only personnel thoroughly trained in hazardous material (haz-mat) suits or self-contained breathing apparatus (SCBA) should use them (Figure 3-11). These items are often supplied on specialty support vehicles such as haz-mat response units and heavy-rescue trucks (Figure 3-12).

After you ensure that responding personnel have adequate safety equipment to manage the rescue scene, consider patient safety. Many considerations for rescuer safety also apply to patients. Additionally, patient safety equipment should at least include construction-type hard hats, eye goggles, hearing and respiratory

In every case, let common sense dictate scene management.

Do not even consider entering hazardous scenes unless you have the proper clothing, equipment, and training to work in them.

A prompt call for backup can save critical minutes in a life-threatening situation.

Content Review

MINIMUM RESCUE-OPERATION EQUIPMENT

Four-point suspension helmets
Eye goggles and industrial safety glasses
High-quality hearing protection
Leather work gloves
High-top steel-toed boots
Insulated coveralls
Turnout gear

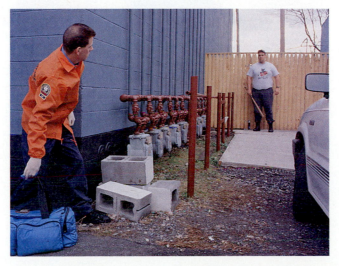

FIGURE 3-8 Wait for the police before entering a potentially hazardous scene.

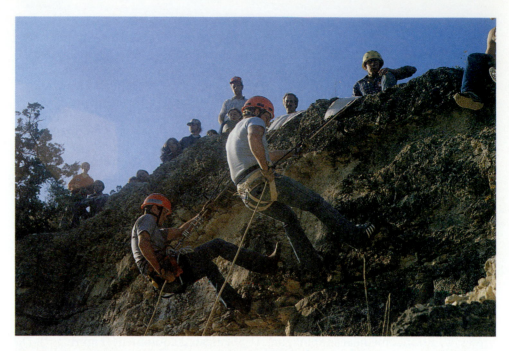

FIGURE 3-9 Never enter a specialized rescue situation without proper training and equipment.

FIGURE 3-10 Full protective gear, including eye protection, helmet, turnout gear, and gloves.

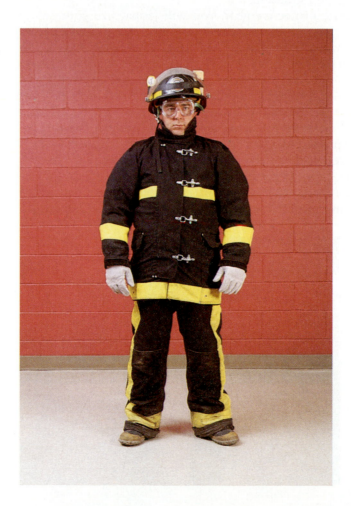

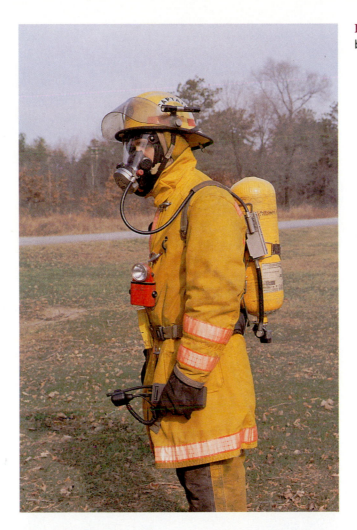

FIGURE 3-11   Self-contained breathing apparatus (SCBA).

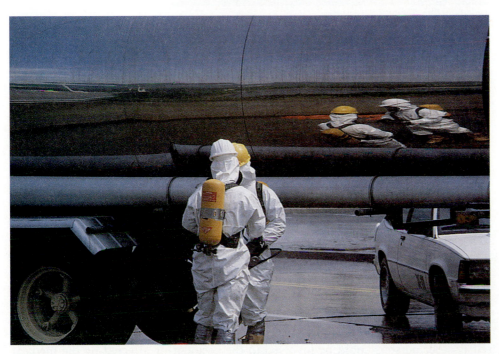

FIGURE 3-12   Hazardous materials responses require special training and equipment.

FIGURE 3-13 Protect the patient from hazards at the scene.

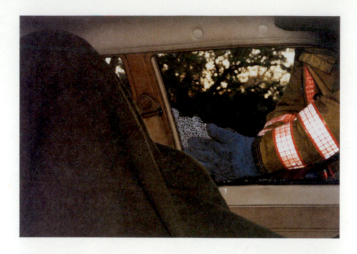

FIGURE 3-14 Tape lines help to keep bystanders out of hazardous scenes.

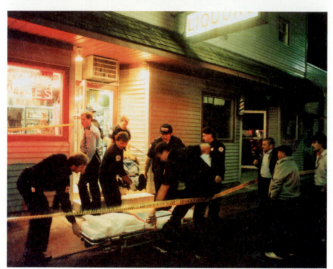

Source: In the Dark Photography/Craig Jackson

Safe, orderly, and controlled incident management is essential for everyone's safety.

protection, protective blankets, and protective shielding. You will need these to protect your patient during rescue operations (Figure 3-13). Patient safety also includes simple measures such as removing them from unstable environments such as temperature extremes, smoky rooms, or hostile crowds. For example, the simplest way to begin managing a patient suffering from hypothermia is to move him into a warm environment.

Safe, orderly, and controlled incident management is essential for everyone's safety. Call for specialty personnel to stabilize wreckage or turn off electrical power. Make sure someone routes traffic safely around a vehicle collision. Control bystanders and spot potential human hazards. Be certain that a hostile crowd or someone who assaulted your patient is not ready to attack you. Scenes involving toxic exposures, environmental hazards, and violent patients are especially worrisome. When possible, have law enforcement personnel establish a tape line to cordon off the hazard zone to protect bystanders who do not realize the potential dangers of watching operations (Figure 3-14).

LOCATION OF ALL PATIENTS

Scene size-up also includes a search of the area to locate all of the patients. Ask yourself if other persons could be involved in the accident or affected by the medical problem. Determine where you are most likely to find the most seriously affected patients and how many patients will need transport. The mechanism of injury or the nature of the illness can help you determine the number of patients. For example, a two-car accident must include at least two drivers. Clues such as diaper bags, child auto seats, toys, coloring books, clothing, or twin spider-web impact marks in the windshield should lead you to search for more patients, especially children, than those who may be readily apparent. Some medical situations such as carbon monoxide poisoning can affect an entire household. A hazardous liquid spill in the chemistry lab can affect students and staff in an entire wing of a school.

If you find more patients than you can safely and effectively manage, call for assistance early. If possible, you should do this before you make contact with any patients, because you are less likely to call for help once you become involved with patient care. Often, as you proceed into a scene, more patients become apparent. It is wise to overestimate when asking for help at the scene.

Initiate the mass casualty plan according to your local protocols (Figure 3-15). Again, try not to become involved in patient care, for two important functions must occur in the initial stages of any mass casualty incident—command and triage. If you and your partner find yourselves in a situation that overwhelms your resources, one of you should establish command while the other begins triaging patients. The command person performs a scene size-up, determines the needs of the incident, makes a radio report requesting the necessary additional help, and directs on-coming crews to their duties (Figure 3-16). The triage person performs a triage exam on every patient and prioritizes them for immediate or delayed transport (Figure 3-17). He may perform simple life-saving procedures such as opening the airway or controlling bleeding, but as a rule he should not stop to provide intensive care for any one patient.

Searching the area to locate all patients.

Call for assistance early; it is wise to overestimate when asking for help.

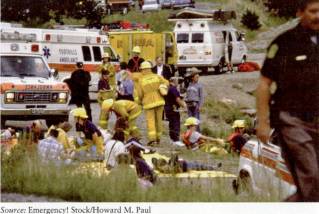

Source: Emergency! Stock/Howard M. Paul

FIGURE 3-15 Follow local protocols when you respond to a mass-casualty incident.

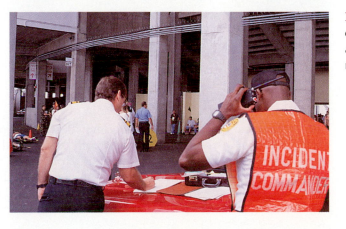

FIGURE 3-16 The incident commander directs the response and coordinates resources at a multiple-casualty incident.

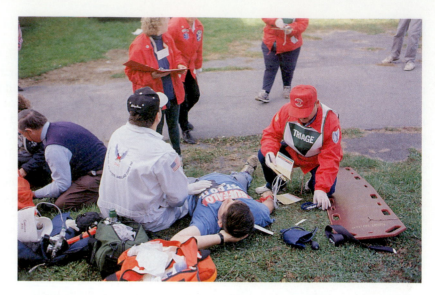

FIGURE 3-17   The triage person examines and prioritizes patients.

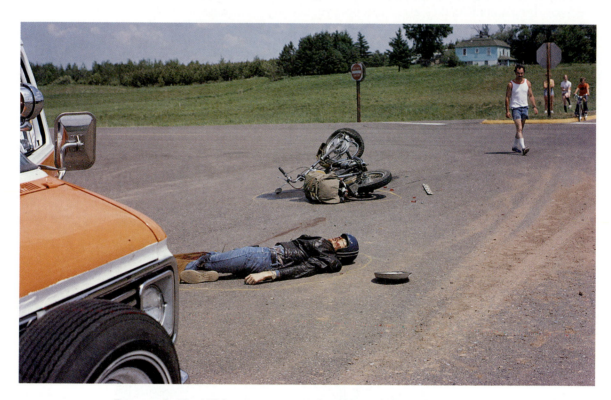

FIGURE 3-18   With trauma, try to determine the mechanism of injury during scene size-up.

MECHANISM OF INJURY

* mechanism of injury combined strength, direction, and nature of forces that injured your patient.

The **mechanism of injury** is the combined strength, direction, and nature of forces that injured your patient. It is usually apparent through careful evaluation of the trauma scene and can help you anticipate both the location and the seriousness of injuries. Identify the forces involved, the direction from which they came, and the bodily locations affected (Figure 3-18). For example, in a fall injury, how high was the patient, what did he land on, and what part of his body hit first? If your patient jumped from a height and landed on his feet, expect lower extremity, pelvic, and lumbar spine injuries.

In an automobile accident, the mechanism of injury is the process by which forces are exchanged between the automobile and what it struck, between your patient and the automobile's interior, and among the various tissues and organs as they collide with one another within the patient. Close inspection of the automobile and the forces, or various collisions, can lead to an **index of suspicion** (a prediction of injuries based on the mechanism of injury) for possible injuries. What does the car look like? If the windshield is cracked, expect head and neck injuries. If the steering wheel is bent, expect chest and abdominal injuries. With a major intrusion into the passenger compartment, expect major trauma.

Expect a pedestrian struck by a car to have fractures of the lower extremities. If the auto was moving at 20 miles per hour, expect less severe fractures than if it were moving at 55 miles per hour. Also, internal injuries are less likely at lower speeds than at higher speeds. By evaluating the strength and nature of impact, you can anticipate which organs are injured and the degree of their damage.

For a gunshot patient, determine the type of gun used, the range of the shot, and if an exit wound exists. This information will enable you to estimate the damage along the bullet's path and to formulate an index of suspicion for your patient's possible injuries. Expect the internal injuries from serious blunt trauma to be more extensive and severe than those you see externally. Often the mechanism of injury is the only clue to the possibility of serious internal injury. The chapters on blunt and penetrating trauma in Volume 4, *Trauma Emergencies*, describe the mechanisms of these injuries in depth.

NATURE OF THE ILLNESS

Determine the nature of the illness from bystanders, family members, or your patient himself. If he is alert and oriented, he is usually the best source of information about his problem. If he is unresponsive, disoriented, or otherwise unable to provide information, rely on family members, bystanders, or visual cues for this information.

The scene can give additional clues to your patient's condition. How is he positioned? Does he sit bolt upright gasping to breathe? Are pill bottles or drug paraphernalia nearby? Is medical-care equipment such as an oxygen tank, a nebulizer, or a glucometer in the room? For example, if you respond to a "difficulty breathing" call and your patient is using his nebulizer when you arrive, suspect a history of pulmonary disease such as asthma, emphysema, or chronic bronchitis. If your patient is an agitated 17-year-old with a rapid pulse and you notice crack cocaine ampules on the floor, suspect a substance abuse problem.

Sometimes the nature of the illness is not readily apparent. Your patient with severe difficulty breathing, for instance, may be suffering from respiratory disease, a cardiac problem, an allergic reaction, or a toxic exposure. Remember that the nature of your patient's illness may be very different from his chief complaint.

THE INITIAL ASSESSMENT

The **initial assessment** exemplifies the basis of all prehospital emergency medical care. Its goal is to identify and correct immediately life-threatening patient conditions of the <u>A</u>irway, <u>B</u>reathing, or <u>C</u>irculation (**ABCs**). If you find these conditions during this part of your assessment, treat them at once. For example, open a closed airway, provide ventilation, or control hemorrhage before moving on. Immediately following the initial assessment, decide priority regarding immediate

* **index of suspicion** your anticipation of possible injuries based upon your analysis of the event.

Often the mechanism of injury is the only clue to the possibility of serious internal injury.

Remember that the nature of your patient's illness may be very different from his chief complaint.

* **initial assessment** prehospital process designed to identify and correct life-threatening airway, breathing, and circulation problems.

STEPS OF INITIAL ASSESSMENT

1. Form general impression
2. Stabilize cervical spine as needed
3. Assess baseline level of response
4. Assess airway
5. Assess breathing
6. Assess circulation
7. Assign priority

The initial assessment should take less than one minute, unless you have to intervene with life-saving measures.

* **general impression** your initial, intuitive evaluation of your patient.

transport or further on-scene assessment and care. The initial assessment consists of the following steps:

- Forming a general impression
- Stabilizing the cervical spine as needed
- Assessing a baseline mental status
- Assessing the airway
- Assessing breathing
- Assessing circulation
- Determining priority

The initial assessment should take less than one minute, unless you have to intervene with life-saving measures. Perform the initial assessment as part of your ongoing assessment throughout the patient contact, especially after any major intervention or whenever your patient's condition changes.

FORMING A GENERAL IMPRESSION

The **general impression** is your initial, intuitive evaluation of your patient. It will help you determine his general clinical status (stable vs. unstable) and priority for immediate transport. Base your first impression on the information you gather from the environment, the mechanism of injury, the nature of the illness, the chief complaint, and your instincts.

Your patient's age, gender, and race often influence your index of suspicion. Very old and very young patients are more apt to have severe complications from injury or illness. For example, age is a factor in burn mortality, along with degree and body percentage. A 25-year-old patient with third degree burns over 50% of his body will have a 75% chance of mortality. A 45-year-old patient with the same burns will have a 95% chance of mortality. Suspect a female of child-bearing age with lower abdominal pain and vaginal bleeding to have a life-threatening gynecological emergency known as ruptured ectopic pregnancy. Black Americans have a higher incidence of hypertension and cardiovascular disease than members of other races.

Determine whether your patient's problem results from trauma or from a medical problem. Sometimes this will not be readily apparent. For example, did your patient slip and fall or get dizzy and fall? Note your patient's face and his posture and decide whether rapid intervention or a more deliberate approach is warranted. With experience you will be able to recognize even the most subtle clues of a patient in critical condition. Generally, the more serious the condition, the quieter your patient will be. Look at, listen to, and smell the environment. Gather as many clues as possible as you enter the scene.

Take the necessary body substance isolation precautions with every patient. Then, if your patient is alert, identify yourself and begin to establish a rapport. For example, "Hello, I'm Jen Stevens, a paramedic with ALS Ambulance Service. I'm here to help you." This establishes your level of training, authority, and reason for being at your patient's side. It also allows your patient to refuse care. As discussed in the chapter on medical/legal aspects of advanced prehospital care (Volume 1, *Introduction to Advanced Prehospital Care*) you cannot provide care without either implied or informed consent.

Reassure your patient. Listen to him and do not trivialize his complaints. Frequently we forget how significant an injury or illness, even a minor one, seems to a patient. With your experience, his problem may seem small, but for your patient it is a real concern. The ill or injured patient may worry about the long-term

Listen to your patient and do not trivialize his complaints.

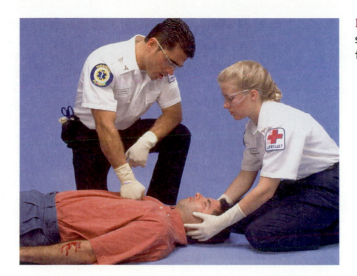

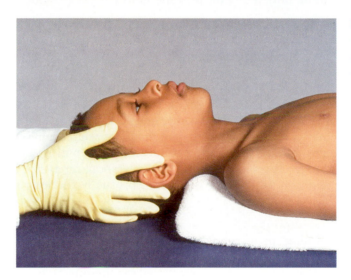

FIGURE 3-19b Place a folded towel under your young patient's shoulders to keep the airway aligned.

consequences for work, child care, and finances. Understand these fears and support your patient psychologically as well as physiologically.

If the mechanism of injury is significant or if your patient is unresponsive, have your partner manually stabilize your patient's head and neck (Figure 3-19a). Do this before establishing his mental status and continue manual stabilization until you fully immobilize him to a long spine board. If your patient is awake, explain what you are doing and ask him not to move his neck. You do not want him to turn his head when you try to assess mental status. Ask your partner to maintain your patient's head in a neutral position as you begin your assessment. If your patient is a small child, place a small towel or pad beneath the shoulders to maintain proper alignment of the cervical spine (Figure 3-19b). This will compensate for the large occiput of the child's head, which normally would flex his neck when he was placed on a flat surface.

MENTAL STATUS

Your assessment of baseline mental status is crucial for all patients. For example, when you deliver your head injury patient to the emergency department, the neurosurgeon will want a chronological report of your patient's mental status from the

Your assessment of baseline mental status is crucial for all patients with serious head trauma.

time you arrived on the scene. This vital information helps the surgical team diagnose a deteriorating brain injury. If the patient was alert and oriented when you arrived, then became sleepy en route, and within 30 minutes was responsive only to deep pain stimuli, the suspicion for epidural hematoma is high. Rapid surgical intervention can save lives in most cases if the diagnosis is made quickly. Your baseline mental status documentation is critical to these patients' emergency care. Establishing a baseline mental status is also crucial in assessing the variety of medical situations that cause altered levels of response. Drug overdoses, poisonings, diabetic emergencies, sepsis, hypoxia, and hypovolemia are just a few of the many conditions that result in altered mentation. For the stroke patient, identifying the time of the symptoms' onset is critical for the emergency physician to consider administering clot-dissolving drugs within the three-hour window of opportunity. This is possible only with your accurate assessment of your patient's change in mental status.

To record your patient's mental status, use the acronym *AVPU*. Your patient either is <u>A</u>lert, responds to <u>V</u>erbal stimuli, responds only to <u>P</u>ainful stimuli, or is <u>U</u>nresponsive. Perform this exam by starting with verbal, then moving to painful stimuli only if he fails to respond to your verbal cues.

Alert An alert patient is awake, as evidenced by open eyes. He may be oriented to person (who he is), place (where he is), and time (day, month, and year) and give organized, coherent answers to your quetions. He also may be disoriented and confused. For example, the patient with a suspected concussion will often present as dazed and confused. The hypoxic or hypoglycemic patient may present as combative. The shock patient may be restless and anxious. If his eyes are open and he appears awake, he is categorized as alert. Children's responses to your questions will vary with their age-related physical and emotional development. Infants and young children usually will be curious but cautious when a stranger approaches. Their level of response may not indicate the gravity of their condition. In fact, the quiet child is usually the seriously injured or ill child.

Verbal If your patient appears to be sleeping but responds when you talk to him, he is responsive to verbal stimuli. He can respond by speaking, opening his eyes, moaning, or just moving. Note the level of his verbal response. Does he speak clearly, mumble inappropriate words or make incomprehensible sounds? Children may respond to your verbal commands by turning their heads or stopping activity. For infants you may have to shout to elicit a response.

Pain If your child or adult patient does not respond to verbal stimuli, try to elicit a response with painful stimuli. Pinch his fingernails or rub your knuckles on his sternum and watch for a response. Again, he may respond by waking up, speaking, moaning, opening his eyes, or moving. Note the type of his motor response to the painful stimuli. Is his response purposeful or nonpurposeful? If he tries to move your hand away or to move himself away from the pain, it is purposeful. **Decorticate** (arms flexed, legs extended) or **decerebrate** (arms and legs extended) posturing is nonpurposeful and suggests a serious brain injury. For the infant, flick the soles of the feet and expect crying as the appropriate response.

Unresponsive The unresponsive patient is comatose and fails to respond to any noxious stimulus. The AVPU scale describes your patient's general mental status. Avoid using terms such as *semi-conscious, lethargic,* or *stuporous* since they are broadly interpreted and you have not had a chance to conduct a comprehensive neurological exam at this point. Your patient's response to stimulation will tell you a great deal about his condition. Any alteration or deterioration in mental status may indicate an emergent or already serious problem. A patient with an impaired mental status may have lost, or be in danger of losing, the ability to protect his airway. Take immediate steps to protect your patient's airway by proper positioning, use of

✱ **decorticate** arms flexed, legs extended.

✱ **decerebrate** arms and legs extended.

Any alteration in mental status may indicate an emergent or already serious problem.

airway adjuncts, or intubation, as appropriate. Provide oxygen to any patient with diminished mental status and seek out its cause.

AIRWAY ASSESSMENT

If your patient is responsive and can speak clearly, you can assume that his airway is patent. If your patient is unconscious, however, his airway may be obstructed. The supine unconscious patient's tongue often obstructs his upper airway. Because the mandible, tongue, and epiglottis are all connected, gravity allows these structures to block your patient's upper airway as his facial muscles relax (Figure 3-20a).

You can open your patient's airway with one of two simple manual maneuvers, the jaw thrust and the head-tilt/chin-lift. For the trauma patient with a suspected cervical spine injury, use the jaw thrust, to avoid movement of the cervical spine. Place your thumbs on your patient's cheeks and lift up on the angle of the jaw with your fingers (Figure 3-20b). For all other patients, use the head-tilt/chin-lift. Place

You must constantly adjust infants' and young children's airways to maximize patency.

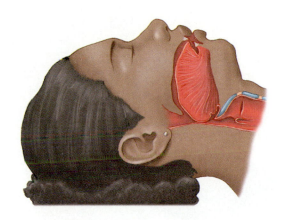

FIGURE 3-20a   Your unconscious patient's tongue may fall and close the upper airway.

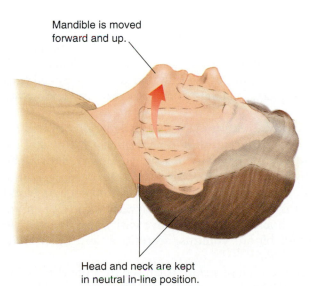

FIGURE 3-20b   Use the jaw thrust to open your patient's airway if you suspect a cervical spine injury.

FIGURE 3-20c The head-tilt/chin lift maneuver in an adult.

ADULT

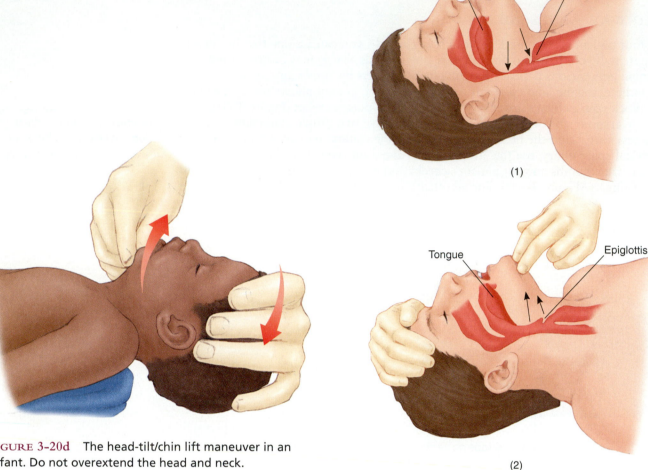

Tongue

Epiglottis

(1)

Tongue

Epiglottis

(2)

FIGURE 3-20d The head-tilt/chin lift maneuver in an infant. Do not overextend the head and neck.

one hand on your patient's forehead and lift up under the chin with the fingers of your other hand (Figure 3-20c). To open the airways of infants and young children, apply a gentle and conservative extension of the head and neck (Figure 3-20d). These patients' upper airway structures are very flexible and are easily kinked when their necks are flexed or hyperextended. You must constantly readjust their airways to maximize patency.

To assess your patient's airway, look for chest rise while you listen and feel for air movement. If the airway is clear, you should hear quiet air flow and feel free air movement. A noisy airway is a partially obstructed airway. Snoring occurs when the tongue partially blocks the upper airway. In this case, reposition the head and neck and reevaluate. Gurgling indicates that fluid such as blood, secretions, or gastric contents is blocking the upper airway. Gently open and examine the mouth for foreign bodies you can remove easily and quickly. Use aggressive suctioning to remove blood, vomitus, secretions, and other fluids (Figure 3-21).

The high-pitched inspiratory screech of stridor is caused by a life-threatening upper airway obstruction that may be due to a foreign body, severe swelling, allergic reaction, or infection. If you suspect a foreign body obstruction and your patient exhibits poor air movement, a weak cough, or a diminishing mental sta-

Stridor signals a potentially life-threatening airway obstruction.

FIGURE 3-21   Suction fluids from your patient's airway.

tus, immediately deliver abdominal thrusts (Heimlich maneuver) to dislodge the object. If your patient is less than one year old, use back blows and chest thrusts instead of abdominal thrusts. If these maneuvers are ineffective, remove the object under direct laryngoscopy with Magill forceps.

Other causes of stridor require vastly differently approaches. Upper respiratory infections such as croup or epiglottitis call for blow-by oxygen and a quiet ride to the hospital; respiratory burns demand rapid endotracheal intubation; and anaphylaxis necessitates vasoconstrictor medications. Since these vastly different management techniques are potentially life-threatening when applied inappropriately, your correct field diagnosis is critical. If your patient presents with stridor, take time to evaluate the history and clinical signs and symptoms for foreign body obstruction (sudden onset while eating), epiglottitis (fever, illness, drooling, inability to swallow), respiratory burns (history of facial burns, hoarseness), and anaphylaxis (hives, history of allergies).

The softer, expiratory whistle of wheezing is caused by constricted bronchioles, the smaller, lower airways. You will hear it in cases such as asthma, bronchitis, emphysema, or other causes of bronchospasm. Bronchiolitis, a lower respiratory infection, often causes these sounds in infants and young children. Wheezing patients require a bronchodilator medication to dilate the bronchioles and reduce airway resistance.

If your patient is not moving air, he is in respiratory arrest. Immediately provide ventilation with a bag-valve mask (Figure 3-22). Ventilate adult patients at a minimum of 12 breaths per minute and all children at a minimum of 20 breaths per minute. If you cannot ventilate the lungs, reposition the head and neck and try again. If there is still no air movement, assume a complete obstruction and begin measures to correct it.

Once you have cleared the airway, keeping it open may require constant attention. In these cases, insert a basic airway adjunct to help keep the tongue from blocking the upper airway. If your patient is unconscious and lacks a gag reflex, insert an oropharyngeal airway (Figure 3-23). If he has a gag reflex or significant oro-facial trauma, insert a nasopharyngeal airway (Figure 3-24). Be cautious using a nasopharyngeal airway if you suspect a basilar skull fracture. If he has no gag reflex and cannot protect his airway, you will need to use advanced techniques

Once you have cleared the airway, keeping it open may require constant attention.

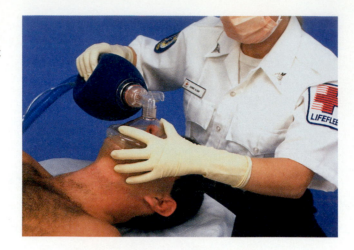

FIGURE 3-22 Immediately use a bag-valve mask to ventilate patients who are not moving air.

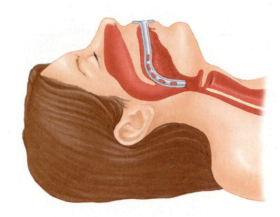

FIGURE 3-23 Use an oropharyngeal airway for unconscious patients without a gag reflex.

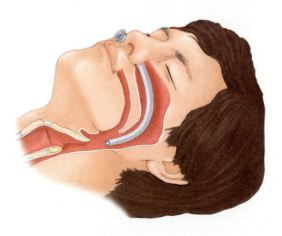

FIGURE 3-24 The nasopharyngeal airway rests between the tongue and the posterior pharyngeal wall.

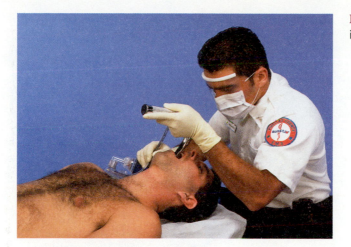

FIGURE 3-25   Endotracheal intubation.

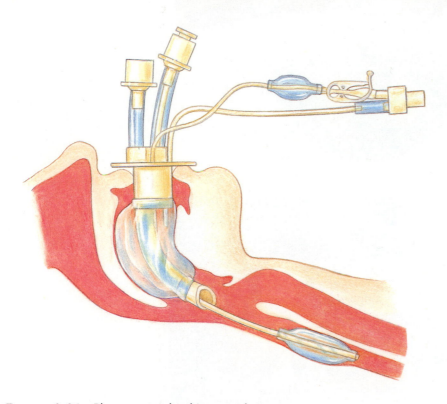

FIGURE 3-26   Pharyngotracheal Lumen airway.

to maintain airway patency. These include endotracheal intubation, multi-lumen airways such as the Pharyngotracheal Lumen (PL) airway and the Esophageal Tracheal CombiTube (ETC), and transtracheal techniques such as needle or surgical cricothyroidotomy (Figures 3-25 through 3-28). The multi-lumen airways are not appropriate for use in children. All of these devices for maintaining upper airway patency are described in detail in the airway management and ventilation chapter of Volume 1, *Introduction to Advanced Prehospital Care*. If your patient has an airway problem or an altered mental status, administer high concentration oxygen by nonrebreather mask.

FIGURE 3-27 Esophageal Tracheal CombiTube.

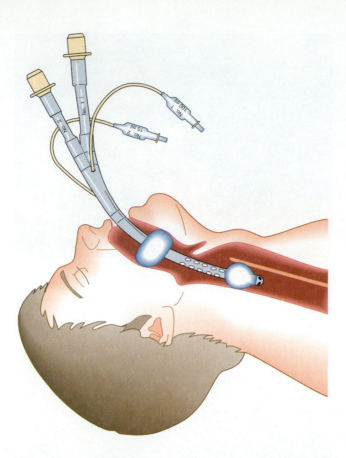

FIGURE 3-28 Needle cricothyrotomy.

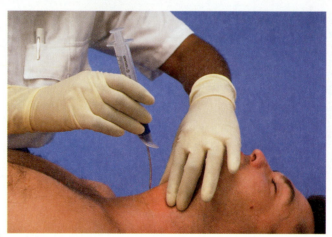

Content Review

SIGNS OF INADEQUATE BREATHING

Altered mental status
Shortness of breath
Retractions
Asymmetric chest wall movement
Accessory muscle use
Cyanosis
Audible sounds
Abnormal rate or pattern
Nasal flaring

BREATHING ASSESSMENT

Assess your patient for adequate breathing. Immediately note any signs of inadequate breathing. These include:

- Altered mental status, confusion, apprehension, or agitation
- Shortness of breath while speaking
- Retractions (supraclavicular, suprasternal, intercostal)
- Asymmetric chest wall movement
- Accessory muscle use (neck, abdominal)
- Cyanosis

Table 3-1	RESPIRATORY RATES		
Age		Low Rate	High Rate
Newborn		30	60
Infant (<1 year)		30	60
Toddler (1–2 years)		24	40
Preschooler (3–5 years)		22	34
School age (6–12 years)		18	30
Adolescent (13–18 years)		12	26
Adult (>18 years)		12	20

- Audible sounds
- Abnormally rapid, slow, or shallow breathing
- Nasal flaring

Assess the respiratory rate and quality. Normal respiratory rates vary according to your patient's age. Abnormally fast or slow rates (Table 3-1) actually decrease the amount of air that reaches the alveoli for gas exchange. For patients with abnormally fast or slow respiratory rates and decreased tidal volumes, provide positive pressure ventilation with, for example, a bag-valve mask and supplemental oxygen, to ensure full lung expansion and maximum oxygenation. Note the respiratory pattern. Rapid (tachypneic), deep (hyperpneic) respirations are a compensatory mechanism and suggest the body is attempting to rid itself of excess acids. They may indicate a diabetic problem, severe acidosis, or head injury. They also may result from hyperventilation syndrome or from simple exertion. Kussmaul's respirations (deep, rapid breathing) accompanied by a fruity breath odor are a classic sign of a patient in a diabetic coma. In either case, always ensure an adequate inspiratory volume and administer high-flow oxygen. Cheyne-Stokes respirations, a series of increasing and decreasing breaths followed by a period of apnea, most likely result from a brain stem injury or increasing intracranial pressure. Biot's respirations, identified by short, gasping, irregular breaths, may signify severe brain injury. Again, ensure adequate inspiratory volume and provide ventilation with supplemental oxygen as needed.

If your trauma patient's breathing is inadequate, immediately conduct a rapid trauma assessment of the neck and chest before moving on to circulation. Identify and correct any life-threatening conditions such as a sucking chest wound, a flail chest, or a tension pneumothorax. If your patient exhibits adequate breathing, move directly to circulation.

CIRCULATION ASSESSMENT

The **circulation assessment** consists of evaluating the pulse and skin and controlling hemorrhage. Go directly to the wrist and feel for a radial pulse (Procedure 3-1a on page 196). Its presence suggests a systolic blood pressure of at least 80 mmHg. If the radial pulse is absent, check for a carotid pulse (Procedure 3-1b). The carotid pulse's presence suggests a systolic blood pressure of at least 60 mmHg. In the infant, palpate the brachial pulse (Procedure 3-1c) or, if necessary, auscultate the apical pulse. If the pulse is absent in the adult patient, begin chest compressions immediately, evaluate the cardiac rhythm, and provide prompt defibrillation as needed. In the child, immediately begin cardiopulmonary resuscitation (CPR).

Assess your patient's pulse for rate and quality as detailed in Chapter 2. The normal heart rate varies with your patient's age (Table 3-2). Very fast rates

If your patient's breathing is inadequate, immediately conduct a rapid trauma assessment of the neck and chest and provide positive pressure ventilation with supplemental oxygen.

* **circulation assessment** evaluating the pulse and skin and controlling hemorrhage.

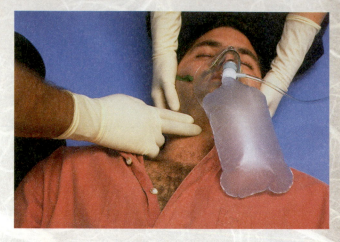

3-1a To assess an adult's circulation feel for a radial pulse.

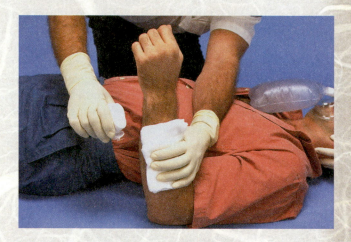

3-1b If you cannot feel a radial pulse, palpate for a carotid pulse.

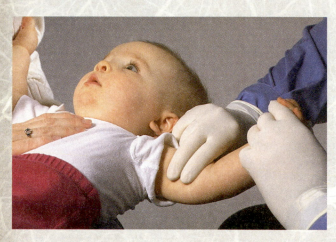

3-1c To assess an infant's circulation, palpate the brachial pulse.

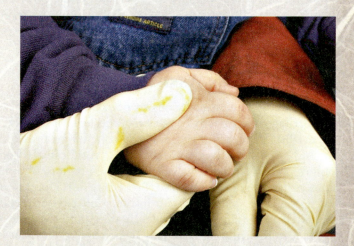

3-1d Control major bleeding.

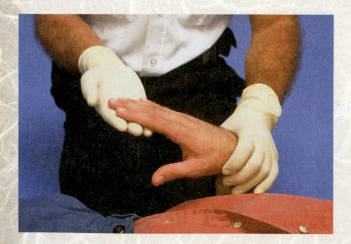

3-1e Assess the skin.

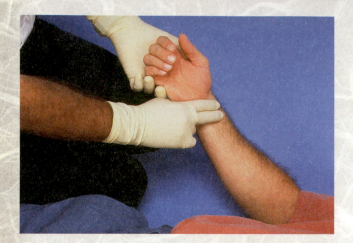

3-1f Capillary refill time provides important information about the circulatory status of infants and young children.

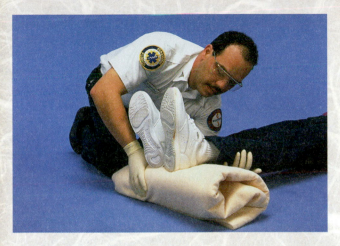

3-1g   Elevate your patient's feet if you suspect circulatory compromise.

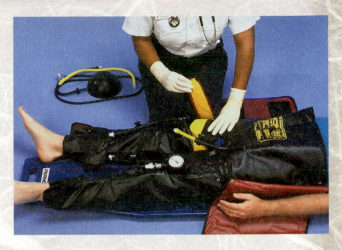

3-1h   Apply a pneumatic antishock garment according to your local protocol.

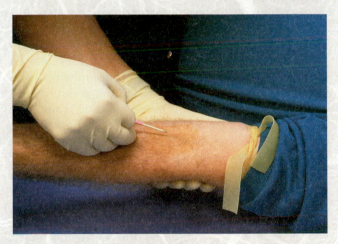

3-1i   En route to the hospital, establish an IV.

Table 3-2	NORMAL PULSE RATE RANGES	
Age	**Low Rate**	**High Rate**
Newborn	100	180
Infant (<1 year)	100	160
Toddler (1–2 years)	80	110
Preschooler (3–5 years)	70	110
School age (6–12 years)	65	110
Adolescent (13–18 years)	60	90
Adult (>18 years)	60	100

(tachycardia) and very slow rates (bradycardia) may indicate a life-threatening cardiac dysrhythmia. Note the quality of the pulse. The normal pulse should be regular and strong. An irregular pulse may indicate a cardiac dysrhythmia requiring advanced cardiac life support procedures. In head injury, heat stroke, or hypertension, you will often find a strong, bounding pulse. A weak, thready pulse usually indicates poor perfusion due to fluid loss, pump failure, or massive vasodilation.

Stop your patient's bleeding if you haven't already done so (Procedure 3-1d). Major bleeding usually originates with trauma, but it also can result from a medical emergency. For example, vaginal bleeding, rectal bleeding, and even a nosebleed associated with hypertension can result in life-threatening blood loss. For external bleeding, employ any appropriate measures for hemorrhage control, including direct pressure and elevation, pressure dressings, pressure points, and the last-resort tourniquet. Internal bleeding is not easily controlled in the prehospital setting and demands initiating transport as soon as possible.

Assess the skin for temperature, moisture, and color (Procedure 3-1e). Peripheral vasoconstriction decreases peripheral perfusion to the skin early in shock. The skin may appear mottled (blotchy), cyanotic (bluish), pale, or ashen. It may also feel cool and moist (clammy). This often indicates that warm, circulating blood has been shunted away from the skin to the core of the body to maintain perfusion of vital organs. If you find any of these signs, suspect conditions related to or caused by poor perfusion. In infants and young children capillary refill is a reliable indicator of circulatory function (Procedure 3-1f). In adults, smoking, medications, cold weather, or chronic conditions of the elderly may affect capillary refill, so you should always also consider the other indicators of circulatory function.

If your patient shows signs of circulatory compromise, consider elevating his legs to support venous return to the vital organs (Procedure 3-1g). Keep him warm, and on adult patients only, apply and inflate the pneumatic antishock garment as indicated by your local protocol (Procedure 3-1h). The chapter on hemorrhage and shock in Volume 4, *Trauma Emergencies,* explains this procedure fully. Consider starting large-bore intravenous lines en route to the hospital and infusing fluids to augment your patient's circulating blood volume (Procedure 3-1i). Also consider using vasoconstricting drugs and antidysrhythmic medications for other specific causes of poor perfusion.

Internal bleeding is not easily controlled in the prehospital setting and demands initiating transport as soon as possible.

PRIORITY DETERMINATION

Once you have conducted an initial assessment, determine your patient's priority. If his initial assessment suggests a serious illness or injury, conduct a rapid head-to-toe assessment to identify other life threats and transport him immediately to the near-

Do not delay transport for detailed assessments and procedures that you can provide en route to the hospital.

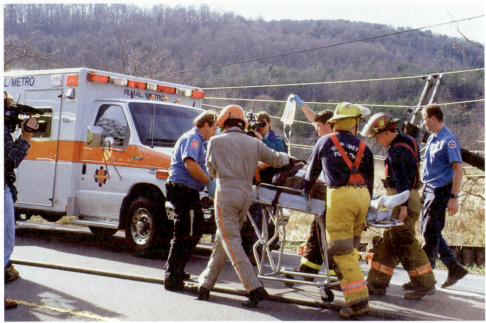

Source: Glen Jackson

FIGURE 3-29   Expedite transport for a high priority patient and continue assessment and care en route.

est appropriate facility that can deliver definitive care (Figure 3-29). Do not delay transport for detailed assessments and procedures that you can provide en route to the hospital. Consider top priority and rapid transport for the following patients:

- Patients with a poor general impression
  – Apnea
  – Pulselessness
  – Obvious severe distress
- Patients with altered mental status
- Patients with airway compromise
  – Obstructive sounds such as gurgling, snoring, or stridor
  – Vomitus, secretions, blood, or foreign bodies obstructing the airway
  – Inability to protect the airway (absence of a gag reflex)
- Patients with abnormal breathing
  – Rates less or greater than normal for age
  – Absent or diminished air movement and breath sounds
  – Retractions
  – Accessory muscle use
- Patients with poor circulation
  – Weak or absent peripheral pulses
  – Pulse rates less or greater than normal for age
  – Irregular pulse
  – Pale, cool, diaphoretic skin
  – Uncontrolled bleeding
- Obvious serious or multiple injuries

In these cases, decide whether to stabilize your patient on the scene or expedite transport and initiate advanced life support procedures en route. On the way to the hospital you can conduct a detailed history and physical exam and provide additional care as time allows. If your patient is stable, before transport you can conduct a focused history and physical exam—a problem-oriented patient assessment—followed by a detailed physical exam either at the scene or during transport as the situation requires, if time allows.

The initial assessment is the crucial first-step in providing life-saving measures to seriously ill or injured patients. It should take you less than one minute to perform, yet it will provide you with enough vital information to confirm your priority determination.

THE FOCUSED HISTORY AND PHYSICAL EXAM

The **focused history and physical exam** is the second stage of patient assessment. It is a problem-oriented process based on your initial assessment and your patient's chief complaint. How you conduct the focused history and physical exam will depend on which of four general categories your patient's initial presentation falls under:

* Trauma patient with a significant mechanism of injury or altered mental status
* Trauma patient with an isolated injury
* Responsive medical patient
* Unresponsive medical patient

Each type of patient requires a vastly different approach.

THE MAJOR TRAUMA PATIENT

The **major trauma patient** is one who has sustained a significant mechanism of injury or has an altered mental status from the incident. For serious trauma patients, you will conduct an initial assessment followed by a rapid trauma assessment, package your patient, provide rapid transport to the emergency department, and perform an ongoing assessment en route, in that order. If time allows, you can also perform a detailed assessment.

Mechanism of Injury

Begin the focused history and physical exam for major trauma patients by reconsidering the mechanism of injury (Figure 3-30). Although trauma poses a serious threat to life, its appearance often masks your patient's true condition. Extremity injuries, for example, are frequently obvious and grotesque, yet they rarely cause death. Conversely, life-threatening problems such as internal bleeding and rising intracranial pressure often occur with only subtle signs and symptoms. Your assessment of trauma patients must look beyond obvious injuries to the mechanism of injury for evidence that suggests life-threatening situations. Certain mechanisms predictably cause serious internal injury:

* Ejection from a vehicle
* Fall from higher than 20 feet
* Rollover of vehicle

✱ **focused history and physical exam** problem-oriented assessment process based on initial assessment and chief complaint.

✱ **major trauma patient** person who has suffered significant mechanism of injury.

Content Review

ORDER OF FOCUSED HISTORY AND PHYSICAL EXAM FOR MAJOR TRAUMA PATIENTS
Initial assessment
Rapid trauma assessment
Packaging
Rapid transport and
  ongoing assessment

Content Review

PREDICTORS OF SERIOUS INTERNAL INJURY
Ejection from vehicle
Death in same passenger
  compartment
Fall from higher than 20 feet
Rollover of vehicle
High-speed vehicle collision
Vehicle-passenger collision
Motorcycle crash
Penetration of head, chest,
  or abdomen

Your assessment of trauma patients must look beyond obvious injuries to the mechanism of injury.

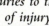

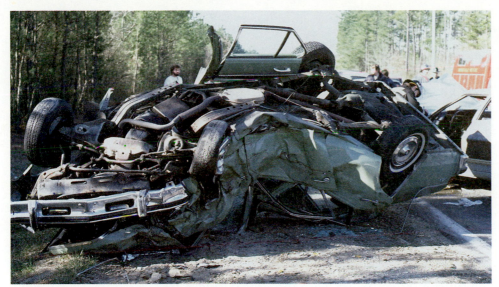

Source: Robert J. Bennett

FIGURE 3-30 Evaluate the trauma scene to determine the mechanism of injury.

- High-speed vehicle collision with resulting severe vehicle deformity
- Vehicle-passenger collision
- Motorcycle crash
- Penetration of the head, chest, or abdomen

Additional considerations for infants and children include:

- Fall from higher than ten feet
- Bicycle collision
- Medium-speed vehicle collision with resulting severe vehicle deformity

These mechanisms' presence suggests a high index of suspicion for serious injury. Quickly transport patients to a trauma center when either the mechanism of injury or your patient's clinical presentation indicates a likelihood of internal injury.

Other significant mechanisms of injury can result from seat belts, airbags, and child safety seats. Do not rule out serious injury just because your patient wore a seat belt. Seat belts can actually cause injuries, even when worn properly. Always ask your patient if he wore a seat belt and look for bruises across the chest or around the waist. If present, expect hidden internal injuries.

In general, airbags have been effective devices in preventing serious injury by protecting passengers from hitting the windshield, steering wheel, and dashboard. They deploy only when the front of the car hits another object. But they are not without complication. For example, they are designed to cushion the chests of large adults. If the passenger is a child or a short adult, the airbag will hit him in the face, causing injury. Also, airbags are designed to deflate automatically within seconds after inflation, which may allow passengers to be propelled into the steering wheel or dashboard. For this reason, they may not be effective without the seat belt. Always lift the deployed bag and inspect the steering wheel for deformity. If you discover a bent steering wheel, suspect serious internal injury (Figure 3-31).

A child safety seat, when used appropriately, also can save a life. But if the safety seat is not securely fastened to the car seat, it can come loose and be thrown when the collision occurs, causing severe head, neck, and body cavity

> **Content Review**
>
> **ADDITIONAL PREDICTORS OF SERIOUS INTERNAL INJURY FOR INFANTS AND CHILDREN**
> Fall from higher than ten feet
> Bicycle collision
> Medium-speed vehicle collision

Quickly transport patients with a high likelihood of internal injury to an appropriate medical facility.

Do not rule out serious injury just because your patient wore a seat belt.

Always lift a deployed airbag and inspect the steering wheel for deformity.

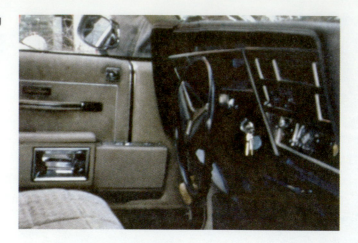

trauma to its occupant. If the safety seat is used in the car's front seat, the child can suffer a serious injury when the airbag deploys.

If your initial assessment rules out any immediate life threat, examine the suspected area of trauma. Physical signs of trauma such as abrasions or contusions confirm your index of suspicion. If you do not identify any physical evidence, reexamine the mechanism of injury and evaluate your patient's vital signs. You will miss many serious injuries if your index of suspicion is too low.

Usually you will distinguish between those patients who need on-the-scene stabilization and those who need rapid transport after your initial assessment and rapid trauma assessment. Whether to transport your patient immediately or to attempt more extensive on-the-scene assessment and care is among your most difficult decisions, but the care you provide will be more effective if you decide quickly. As a rule, patients who experience the mechanisms of injury listed earlier or who display serious clinical findings should be transported quickly with intravenous access and other procedures attempted en route. Remember, you often arrive at the patient's side only minutes after the accident. He may not yet have lost enough blood internally to demonstrate signs of shock or progressive head injury. If in doubt, transport to an appropriate medical facility without delay. It is always best to err on the side of precaution.

It is always best to err on the side of precaution.

Rapid Trauma Assessment

After you finish your initial assessment, conduct a rapid trauma assessment to identify all other life-threatening conditions. Every trauma patient with a significant mechanism of injury, altered mental status, or multiple body-system trauma should receive a rapid trauma assessment. If your patient is responsive, ask him about symptoms as you proceed with your exam. Do not, however, focus totally on the areas your patient identifies as his chief problem. A patient with multiple injuries usually complains about his most painful injury. Sometimes, this may not be his most serious problem. Assess your patient systematically and avoid the tunnel-vision invited by dispatch information, first responders' reports, and your patient's chief complaint.

Assume that any trauma patient has a spinal injury if he has injuries above the shoulders, has a significant mechanism of injury, or complains of weakness, numbness, or spinal pain. Maintain spinal immobilization throughout your rapid trauma exam.

As you proceed through the exam and discover additional information about your patient, reconsider your decision to transport. Things can change unexpectedly, especially with children. For example, your child patient who appeared stable

Avoid the tunnel vision invited by dispatch information, first responder's reports, and your patient's chief complaint.

suddenly deteriorates, requiring you to expedite transport to the closest appropriate facility. The hallmark of an experienced paramedic is the ability to improvise, adapt to new situations, and overcome obstacles that hinder good patient care.

The **rapid trauma assessment** is not a detailed physical exam but a fast, systematic assessment for other life-threatening injuries. Since you perform it before packaging your patient for transport, you must conduct it quickly. First, reassess your patient's mental status using the AVPU mnemonic and compare your findings with the baseline mental status from your initial assessment. Pay special attention to the head, neck, chest, abdomen, and pelvis. Injuries in these areas can occur with limited signs and symptoms, yet they may rapidly lead to patient deterioration and death. When inspecting an area for injury, keep in mind that the discoloration of contusions will develop over time and may not be apparent at first. Remember, your major concern may not be the injury you see but the internal injuries beneath the superficial wounds. Palpate to identify other signs such as tenderness, deformity, crepitation, symmetry, subcutaneous emphysema, or paradoxical movement. Compare muscle tone and tissue compliance from one side of the body or from one limb to another.

The mnemonic DCAP-BTLS may be helpful. The letters represent eight common signs of injury for which you are looking during most of this assessment: <u>D</u>eformities, <u>C</u>ontusions, <u>A</u>brasions, <u>P</u>enetrations, <u>B</u>urns, <u>T</u>enderness, <u>L</u>acerations, and <u>S</u>welling.

Head Assess the head for DCAP-BTLS and crepitation (Procedure 3-2a on page 206). The scalp is extremely vascular and lacks the protective vasospasm mechanism that helps control bleeding. Thus even the most minor lacerations tend to bleed profusely. Inspect the scalp for lacerations that are hidden under hair matted with clotted blood. Look for blood flowing into the hair, and examine your gloved fingers periodically for blood or other body fluids (Procedure 3-2b). If you detect uncontrolled bleeding from the scalp, apply a direct pressure dressing immediately. A simple scalp laceration can cause a life-threatening hemorrhage.

Palpate the skull for open wounds, depressions, protrusions, lack of symmetry, and any unusual warmth. Use cupped hands and do not probe with your fingers. If you feel a depression, stop palpating it, as this risks pushing a broken piece of bone into the brain. If you find an impaled object, stabilize it in place with bulky dressings. If your patient presents with an altered mental status and any abnormality in the structure of the skull, consider this a serious emergency and expedite transport while you continue your assessment and treatment.

Neck Inspect and palpate the neck for DCAP-BTLS and crepitation (Procedure 3-2c). Immediately cover any lacerations that may involve the major blood vessels such as the carotid arteries and jugular veins with an occlusive dressing. This is a high pressure area and your patient can suffer significant blood loss quickly. Because inspiration generates negative pressures in the chest, the jugular veins may draw in air. This can result in a massive air embolus that prevents the heart from pumping blood.

Examine the jugular veins for abnormal distention. In a patient lying supine without circulatory compromise, these veins should distend slightly. If they do not, your patient may be hypovolemic. In the **semi-Fowler's position** (sitting up at 45°), the veins should not distend. Distention beyond 45° is significant because something is inhibiting blood return to the chest. In the trauma patient, this may be the result of cardiac tamponade or tension pneumothorax.

Inspect and palpate the position of the trachea. It should lie midline and remain fixed during the breathing cycle. Tugging to one side during inspiration suggests a pneumothorax on that side. Displacement to one side may indicate a tension pneumothorax on the opposite side as the entire mediastinum is pushed away from the injury.

* **rapid trauma assessment** quick check for signs of serious injury.

Content Review

DCAP-BTLS

Deformities
Contusion
Abrasions
Penetration
Burns
Tenderness
Lacerations
Swelling

Immediately cover any neck lacerations that may involve the major blood vessels.

* **semi-Fowler's position** sitting up at 45°.

* **subcutaneous emphysema**
crackling sensation caused by
air just underneath the skin.

Finally, inspect and palpate the neck for **subcutaneous emphysema**, the crackling sensation caused by air just underneath the skin. This condition is the result of air leaking from the respiratory tree into the tissues of the neck. It strongly indicates a serious neck or chest injury.

Now palpate the posterior neck for evidence of spinal trauma (Procedure 3-2d). Gently feel the spinous processes and note any deformities, swelling, and tenderness. If you feel a muscle spasm, consider it a reflex sign following injury somewhere along the spinal column. When a corroborating mechanism of injury is present, suspect a significant spinal injury requiring immobilization. At this point you can apply a cervical spinal immobilization collar (CSIC). Have someone maintain head and neck stabilization even after applying the collar until your patient is fully fastened to the long board.

Chest Look for signs of acute respiratory distress. If your patient has an upper airway obstruction, he may need to create tremendous negative pressures within his chest just to draw in air. To do so he will use accessory muscles in his neck and chest to help lift the chest wall. These negative pressures may cause suprasternal, supraclavicular, and intercostal retractions. A patient with a lower airway obstruction may have difficulty moving air out. To do so, he may use his abdominal muscles to force the diaphragm upward and inward. He also may purse his lips during exhalation in an attempt to maintain a back pressure to keep the airways open. Infants and small children grunt to maintain this back pressure. Accessory muscle use always indicates a patient in respiratory distress due to a difficulty in moving air. Assist these patients with positive pressure ventilation and supplemental oxygen as needed.

Quickly inspect and then palpate the chest. Begin palpating at the clavicles and work down and around the rib cage, checking for stability. Palpate the clavicles over their entire length, bilaterally (Procedure 3-3a on page 207). These bones, which fracture more frequently than any other bone in the human body, are located directly over the subclavian artery and vein and the superior-most aspect of the lung. Their fracture and displacement may lacerate the vessels or puncture lung tissue, leading to hemothorax, pneumothorax, hypovolemia, or all three.

Be especially careful when palpating the ribs. Beneath each rib lie an artery, a vein, and a nerve that overaggressive palpation can easily damage. Classical soft-tissue injury signs may not be present because the ecchymotic coloration of bruising likely will not have had time to develop. Look for erythema caused by impact to the ribs. The first three ribs are well supported by muscles, ligaments, and tendons. Because of the energy required to fracture them, you should suspect major damage to the underlying organs, especially vascular structures, when they are broken.

If you notice the crackling of subcutaneous emphysema during chest palpation, suspect pneumothorax or a tracheo-bronchial tear. This condition results when air collects in the soft tissues. Subcutaneous air will normally flow from the upper chest to the neck and head. In some cases, it will drastically change your patient's facial features before your eyes.

Observe for equal, symmetrical, effortless chest rise. The chest should rise with inhalation and fall with exhalation. An abnormality in the chest wall may inhibit this process. For example, a patient with a rib fracture hesitates to expand his chest because it hurts. The fracture of two or more adjacent ribs in two or more places causes an unstable flail (floating) segment which may be evidenced by paradoxical chest wall movement. Paradoxical movement may not appear early in a flail segment because the muscles surrounding the fractured ribs may contract spasmodically, securing the ribs in place. As the muscles fatigue and relax, the flail segment becomes obvious in the paradoxical movement. A flail chest greatly reduces air movement. The underlying lung contusion and subsequent decreased tidal volume limit the air available for gas exchange. To ensure enough air movement for adequate gas exchange, assist ventilation with a bag-valve mask and supplemental oxygen. If the flail segment is loose, stabilize it to the chest wall with a large pad and tape (Procedure 3-3b).

Inspect your patient's chest front and back for open wounds. The lungs expand because they adhere to the inner chest wall. This adherence is made possible by the presence of two thin membranes, the visceral pleura, which covers the lungs, and the parietal pleura, which covers the inner chest wall. A film of liquid between these two layers creates a negative-pressure bond that forces the lungs to expand with the chest wall. Any opening in this system can disrupt adherence and cause the lung to collapse. Since air follows the path of least resistance, it may enter the chest cavity through the hole instead of through the respiratory tract. Thus, you should seal any open wounds with an occlusive dressing such as Vaseline gauze at the end of exhalation. Tape the dressing on three sides only to create a "one-way valve" effect, allowing air to escape but not be drawn in (Procedure 3-3c). Remember to check carefully under the armpits and back for knife and small-caliber gunshot wounds. You can easily miss these because the elastic skin closes quickly over the wound and limits external bleeding.

Auscultate both lungs quickly at each mid-axillary line for equal and adequate air movement. Unequal air movement may indicate the presence of a collapsed lung from a pneumothorax or hemothorax. Absent sounds on one side and diminished sounds on the other may suggest a life-threatening condition known as tension pneumothorax. This condition also presents with severe respiratory distress, accessory muscle use, retractions, tachycardia, hypotension, narrowing pulse pressure, and distended neck veins. Tracheal deviation may be a late sign of tension pneumothorax. If authorized, perform needle decompression immediately. Insert a large-bore IV catheter into the pleural space at the second intercostal space over the tip of the rib, midclavicular line, allowing the trapped air to escape and release the tension (Procedure 3-3d). Only through practice and repetition will you gain the confidence to recognize the difference between adequate and diminished lung sounds. Again, for patients with inadequate lung sounds, administer 100% oxygen and assist ventilation with a bag-valve mask as needed.

Abdomen Inspect and palpate the abdomen for DCAP-BTLS and crepitation. Note any areas of bruising and guarding. Exaggerated abdominal-wall motion to assist respiration may result from spinal injury, airway obstruction, or respiratory muscle failure. Solid organs such as the kidneys, liver, and spleen can bleed enough blood into the abdominal cavity to cause profound shock.

Two characteristic areas for bruising are over the umbilicus (**Cullen's sign**) and over the flanks (**Grey-Turner's sign**). Both signs indicate intra-abdominal hemorrhage but usually will not occur until hours after the injury. Perform deep palpation over each quadrant and note any tenderness, rigidity, and guarding. Be careful, because deep palpation sometimes can aggravate the problem. Avoid spending time needlessly trying to make a specific diagnosis. You need only to recognize the possibility that an intra-abdominal hemorrhage exists and that your patient requires immediate transport to an appropriate medical facility for surgery.

Hollow organs such as the stomach and intestines spill their toxic contents into the abdomen, irritating the peritoneum, the inner-abdominal lining. Testing for rebound tenderness will help you determine if your patient's peritoneum is irritated. Gently palpate an area and let your hand up quickly. If your patient experiences pain with this release, it is likely due to peritoneal irritation. If you suspect intra-abdominal hemorrhage, provide oxygen and expedite transport. En route to the hospital, provide IV fluid resuscitation as needed.

* **Cullen's sign** bruising over the umbilicus.

* **Grey-Turner's sign** bruising over the flanks.

Avoid spending time needlessly trying to make a specific diagnosis during rapid trauma assessment of the abdomen.

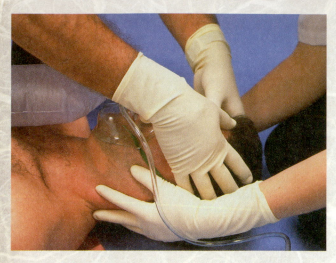

3-2a The first step in the rapid trauma assessment is to palpate the head.

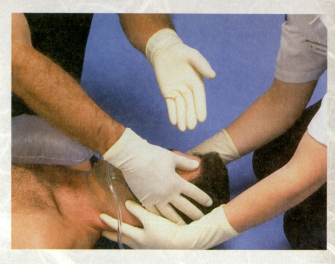

3-2b Periodically examine your gloves for blood.

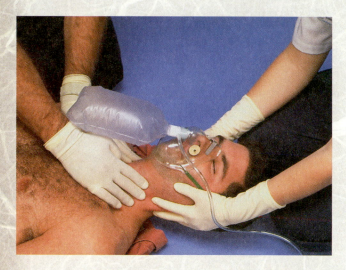

3-2c Inspect and palpate the anterior neck. Pay particular attention to tracheal deviation and subcutaneous emphysema.

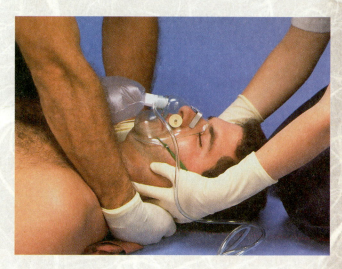

3-2d Inspect and palpate the posterior neck. Note any tenderness, irregularity, or edema.

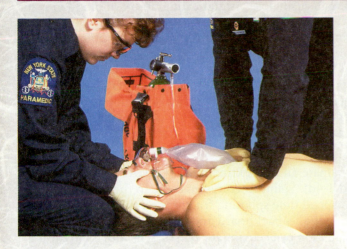

3-3a   Palpate the clavicles.

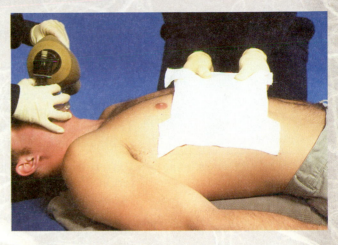

3-3b   Stabilize flail chest.

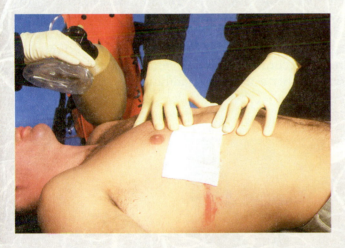

3-3c   Seal any sucking chest wound with tape on three sides.

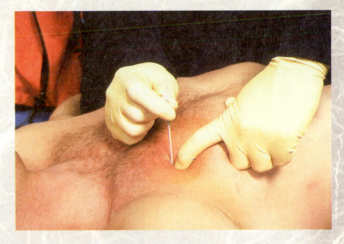

3-3d   Perform needle decompression to relieve tension pneumothorax if authorized.

Pelvis Examine the pelvis for DCAP-BTLS and crepitation. The importance of a stable pelvic ring cannot be overemphasized. A patient with a pelvic fracture or dislocation risks lacerating the iliac arteries and veins, major blood vessels running through that area. He can easily lose a significant amount of blood into the pelvic cavity.

Evaluate the pelvic ring at the iliac crests and symphysis pubis. With the palms of your hands, direct pressure medially and posteriorly (Procedure 3-4a and 3-4b on next page). Then press posteriorly on the symphysis pubis, being careful not to entrap the penis or cause injury to the urinary bladder. Any pain, instability, or crepitus suggests a pelvic fracture. Always immobilize the pelvis before transport to prevent movement and a possible circulatory catastrophe. The pneumatic antishock garment may be used as a splint to immobilize an unstable pelvic fracture.

Extremities Inspect and palpate all four extremities for DCAP-BTLS and crepitation (Procedure 3-4c and 3-4d). Splint fractures en route to the hospital if your patient is unstable. Do not spend time splinting fractures on the scene.

Before placing your patient on a backboard and immobilizing his spine, evaluate distal neurovascular function by checking for pulses, sensation, and the ability to move (Procedure 3-4e and 3-4f). If you cannot locate a pulse, determine the adequacy of perfusion by assessing the temperature, color, and condition of the skin of the extremity. Assume vascular compromise if pulse is absent, the extremity is cool, or the skin is ashen or cyanotic. The inability to feel and move both legs indicates complete spinal cord disruption. Diminished sensation or diminished motor ability may indicate a partial disruption. Weakness or disability on only one side of the body suggests brain injury due to a stroke or head injury. Evaluate these functions again after spinal immobilization to make certain they have not changed. Report and record all extremity function tests. Check for Medic Alert tags, which will identify a medical condition that may complicate the injury (Figure 3-32).

Do not spend time splinting an unstable patient's fractures on the scene.

FIGURE 3-32 Medic alert tags can give important information about the patient's condition and medical history.

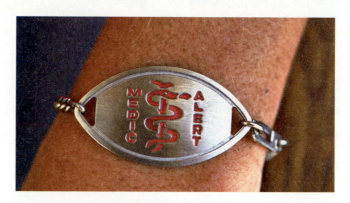

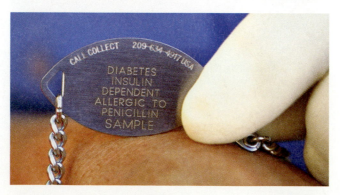

Procedure 3-4 · Rapid Trauma Assessment—The Pelvis and Extremities

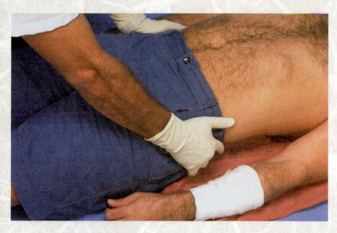

3-4a   Assess the integrity of the pelvis by gently pressing medially on the pelvic ring.

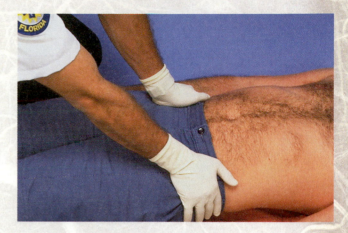

3-4b   Compress pelvis posteriorly.

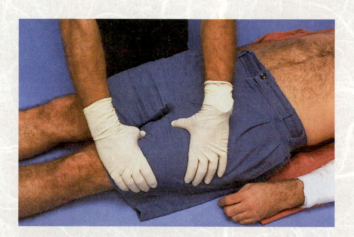

3-4c   Palpate the legs.

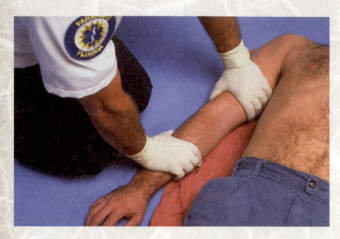

3-4d   Palpate the arms.

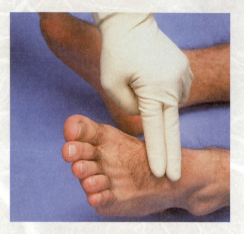

3-4e   Palpate the dorsalis pedis pulse to evaluate distal circulation in the leg.

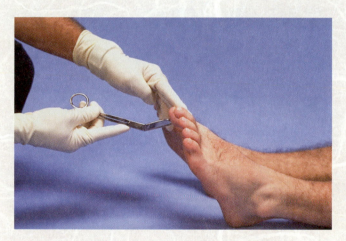

3-4f.   Assess distal sensation and motor function.

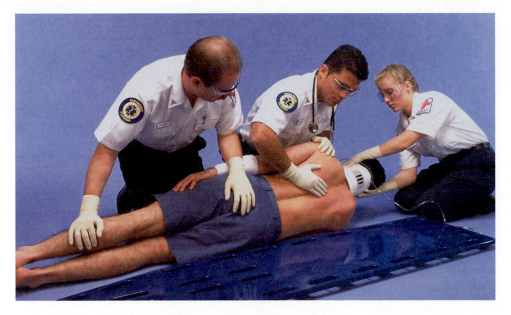

FIGURE 3-33   Inspect and palpate the posterior body.

Posterior Body If you suspect a spinal injury, carefully maintain manual stabilization of the head and spine as you log-roll the patient onto his side. Then inspect and palpate the posterior trunk for DCAP-BTLS and crepitation (Figure
3-33). Particularly note any tenderness in the spinal area. Palpate the buttocks to
rule out hemorrhage, contusion, or other injury. Though predominantly soft tissue, this area is a large mass and can conceal considerable internal blood loss.
Next place the long spine board snugly against your patient's body and maintain
alignment of the head and spine as you log-roll him into a supine position on the
spine board. He is now ready to be secured to the spine board and transported.

Vital Signs

Take a baseline set of vital signs, either at the scene or during transport, as your
patient's condition and circumstances allow. These vital signs include pulse rate
and quality, blood pressure, respiration rate and quality, and skin temperature
and condition. During your EMT-B training, you may have learned to include
pupils as part of your vital sign check. Including a basic pupil response check (direct response to light) as part of your baseline and serial vital sign assessment is
acceptable; however, during the detailed physical exam you may perform an expanded assessment of the pupils (consensual response, near-far response, and accommodation) as outlined in Chapter 2.

History

The history consists of four elements: the chief complaint, the history of present
illness, the past history, and the current health status. (Refer to Chapter 1 for a
detailed description of taking a history.) For major trauma cases when time is
critical, use an abbreviated format that forms the acronym SAMPLE: **S**ymptoms,
Allergies, **M**edications, **P**ast medical history, **L**ast oral intake, and **E**vents preceding the incident. This handy mnemonic is especially useful for eliciting a quick
history from your trauma patient. If your patient cannot provide this information, elicit it from family, friends, and bystanders.

Content Review

BASELINE VITAL SIGNS

Pulse rate and quality
Blood pressure
Respiration rate and quality
Skin condition

Content Review

SAMPLE HISTORY

Symptoms
Allergies
Medications
Past medical history
Last oral intake
Events preceding the
   incident

THE ISOLATED-INJURY TRAUMA PATIENT

Focus your minor-trauma assessment on the specific injury and conduct a DCAP-BTLS exam in that area.

Some trauma patients sustain an isolated injury such as a cut finger or sprained ankle. These patients have no significant mechanism of injury and show no signs of systemic involvement such as poor peripheral perfusion, altered mental status, tachycardia, or breathing problems. They do not require an extensive history or comprehensive physical exam. To treat the trauma patient with an isolated injury, first ensure his hemodynamic status via the initial assessment. Then conduct your focused history and physical exam on the specific isolated injury. Use the mnemonic DCAP-BTLS to evaluate the injured area and take a full set of vital signs. Then, if time allows, this is an excellent opportunity to use some of the advanced assessment techniques you learned in Chapter 2. After your exam of the isolated injury, take a SAMPLE history. Remember that some trauma patients may complain of an isolated problem but actually have more significant injuries. Avoid tunnel vision and develop a low threshhold for suspecting other injuries based on the mechanism of injury and your patient's story.

IN THE FIELD

1. Your patient is a young football player who twisted his knee and lies on the ground, complaining loudly of knee pain. After a quick initial assessment and DCAP-BTLS assessment, you conclude that your patient is in stable condition with no signs or symptoms of systemic involvement and good distal neurovascular function. Before splinting your patient's leg, you decide to elicit more information through a detailed exam of the knee. You inspect the normal concavities for evidence of excessive fluid in the joint by "milking the knee joint" on one side and looking for a fluid wave on the opposite side. Next you palpate the medial and lateral collateral ligaments for tenderness. Then, if doing so does not cause your patient undue pain, you examine the stability of the collateral ligaments with the "side-to-side" test and the cruciate ligaments with the "drawer test." Finally, you assess the knee's passive range of motion (flexion and extension) and note any limitations.

2. Your patient sustains a laceration to the palm of his hand from a breadknife. After you have controlled the bleeding and ensured no systemic involvement or major loss of blood, you decide to examine the hand further before bandaging it. You conduct a DCAP-BTLS exam and note that distal neurovascular function is intact. Knowing that the flexor tendons all run through the palm of the hand, you examine each tendon's function through a full range of motion exam. You ask your patient to make a fist, then open his hand and extend all of his fingers. You note any abnormalities, pain, or limitations in the range of motion.

3. Your patient is a teenager who was punched in the eye during a minor altercation with a classmate. After determining that he had no loss of consciousness and that he is alert and oriented with stable vital signs, equal and reactive pupils, and no signs or symptoms of serious head injury, you may conduct a more detailed exam of the injured eye. First you inspect the external structures for discoloration, deformity, or swelling and find all three. You palpate the orbit of the eye for tenderness and deformity. You look for evidence of hyphema (blood in the anterior chamber), indicating severe blunt trauma. You then examine your patient's visual acuity with a visual acuity card. With a penlight, you check for direct and consensual response to light and for the near-far reflex and accommodation. Finally, you assess the integrity of the extraocular muscles with the H test.

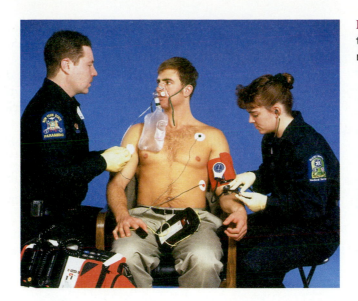

THE RESPONSIVE MEDICAL PATIENT

Assessing the responsive patient with a medical emergency is entirely different from assessing the trauma patient for two reasons. First, the history takes precedence over the physical exam. This is because, in the majority of cases, you will formulate your field diagnosis from your patient's story. The physical exam serves mostly to support your diagnostic impression. Second, your physical exam is aimed at identifying signs of medical complications such as inflammation, infection, and edema rather than signs of injury. The focused physical exam evaluates pertinent areas suggested by the history. Remember that you will begin treatment as you conduct your assessment. For example, while interviewing your patient who complains of chest pain, simultaneously take vital signs, administer oxygen, provide cardiac monitoring, and start an IV if appropriate (Figure 3-34). The following focused history and physical exam pertains to the responsive medical patient. For a more detailed description of the information and techniques outlined here, refer to Chapters 1 and 2.

Listen to your patient; he will tell you what is wrong.

The History

Conscious, alert patients can usually tell you a great deal about their illness. Remember the old medical adage, "Listen to your patient; he will tell you what is wrong." Ask questions and then listen intently to your patient's answers. Since children may not be able to describe their illness and medical history clearly, look to their parents for this information. Elderly patients may pose several obstacles to the clear communication of medical information. They are more likely to be confused, to have poor short-term and long-term memory, and to have hearing, speech, or sight difficulties. Obtaining an accurate history from such patients requires patience, empathy, and outstanding communication skills.

The history consists of four elements: the chief complaint, the history of the present illness, the past history, and the current health status.

The Chief Complaint The **chief complaint** is the pain, discomfort, or dysfunction that caused your patient to request help. Ask your patient, "What seems to be the problem?"

✱ **chief complaint** the pain, discomfort, or dysfunction that caused your patient to request help.

The Focused History and Physical Exam **213**

Let the diagnostic impression you formed during the history guide your examination of a responsive medical patient.

The History of Present Illness Discover the circumstances surrounding the chief complaint, following the acronym OPQRST—ASPN:

Onset	What was your patient doing when the problem/pain began? Did emotional or environmental factors contribute to the problem?
Provocation/**P**alliation	What makes the problem/pain worse or better?
Quality	Can your patient describe the problem/pain?
Region/**R**adiation	Where is the problem/pain and does it radiate anywhere?
Severity	How bad is the problem/pain? Can your patient rate it on a scale of 10?
Time	When did the problem/pain begin? How long does the pain last?
Associated **S**ymptoms	Is your patient having any other problems?
Pertinent **N**egatives	Are any likely associated symptoms absent?

Past Medical History The past medical history may provide significant insights into your patient's chief complaint and your field diagnosis. It includes your patient's general state of health, childhood and adult diseases, psychiatric illnesses, accidents and injuries, surgeries and hospitalizations. If your history taking reveals significant medical problems, investigate in more detail. Note when your patient first recognized the problem and how it affected him. How frequently did it happen and what medical care did he seek? Was the treatment effective or did the problem recur?

Current Health Status The current health status assembles all of the factors regarding your patient's medical condition. It tries to gather information that will complete the puzzle surrounding your patient's primary problem. The elements of the current health status include current medications, allergies, tobacco use, alcohol and substance abuse, diet, screening exams, immunizations, sleep patterns, exercise and leisure activities, environmental hazards, the use of safety measures, and any pertinent family or social history. Look for clues and correlations among the various sections of this part of the history. If your patient is critical and your time is limited, use the abbreviated SAMPLE format to elicit the history.

Focused Physical Exam

Once you have obtained the history, begin a focused physical exam based on the information you elicited from your patient. Let the diagnostic impression you formed during the history guide your examination. For example, if you suspect a myocardial infarction, examine areas pertinent to a patient having a heart attack—cardiac and respiratory systems, chest, neck, and peripheral perfusion. It would be pointless and impractical to test deep tendon reflexes, extraocular movements, or the elbow's range of motion. Use those exam techniques presented in Chapter 2 that pertain to your patient's special situation and clinical status.

Three common presentations among your responsive medical patients will be cardiac chest pain/respiratory distress, altered mental status, and acute abdomen. The following sections outline problem-oriented physical exams for those complaints. Note that for each of these cases, the focused physical exam is different. As you gain clinical experience you will be able to quickly assess your patient's pertinent areas according to your suspected field diagnosis. Likewise, clinical judgment and the seriousness of your patient's condition will determine which exam techniques you use on the scene and which you use en route to the hospital.

Chest Pain/Respiratory Distress For a patient complaining of chest pain or respiratory distress, assess the following:

HEENT (head, eyes, ears, nose, and throat) Note the color of the lips. Lip cyanosis is an ominous sign of central circulatory hypoxia. For a patient complaining of chest pain or respiratory distress, assess the following: Examine the oral mucosa for pallor suggesting decreased circulation as in shock. Inspect any fluids in the mouth. Pink, frothy sputum (the result of plasma proteins' mixing with air and red blood cells in the alveoli) is a classic sign of acute pulmonary edema. Always keep the mouth clear of any fluids that may block the upper airway by aggressive suctioning. Note any swelling, redness, or hives, suggesting an allergic reaction.

Neck Observe the neck for accessory muscle use and retractions, signs of acute respiratory distress. Retractions in the supraclavicular (above the clavicles) and suprasternal (above the sternum) notches indicate your patient is having difficulty inhaling. Palpate the carotid arteries for rate, quality, and equality; if you detect weak or unequal pulses, auscultate for bruits. Examine the jugular veins for abnormal distention. In a patient lying supine without circulatory compromise, these veins should distend slightly. This is normal. If the jugular veins do not distend in the supine position, your patient may be hypovolemic. In the semi-Fowler's position (sitting up at 45°), the veins should disappear. Distention beyond 45° is significant because something is inhibiting blood return to the chest. This may be the result of cardiac tamponade, tension pneumothorax, or right heart failure. Inspect and palpate the position of the trachea. It should lie midline and remain fixed during the breathing cycle. Tugging to one side during inspiration suggests a pneumothorax on that side. Displacement to one side may indicate a tension pneumothorax on the opposite side as the entire mediastinum is displaced.

Chest Assess the respiratory rate and pattern again and administer oxygen or ventilation as needed. Note the length of the inspiratory and expiratory phases. A prolonged inspiratory phase suggests an upper airway obstruction. A prolonged expiratory phase suggests a lower airway obstruction such as in asthma and emphysema. Inspect and palpate the chest wall for symmetry of movement and intercostal retractions. A barrel chest suggests a history of emphysema. Look for the classic midline scar from open heart surgery or the typical bulge of an implanted pacemaker or defibrillator.

Auscultate all lung fields (anterior to posterior, apices to bases) and compare side-to-side. Report and record the sounds you hear (crackles, wheezes), where you hear them (in the bases, apices, diffuse), and when they occur during the respiratory cycle (inspiratory, expiratory). For example, if your patient has bilateral inspiratory rales, you might suspect congestive heart failure or pulmonary edema. If he has diffuse expiratory wheezing, you might suspect the bronchospasm associated with asthma or chronic obstructive pulmonary disease. The presence of both would suggest acute pulmonary edema. A localized wheeze might indicate a pulmonary embolism, a foreign body aspiration, or an infection. Patients with unilateral (one-sided) decreased breath sounds require further testing such as tactile fremitus, bronchophony, egophony, or whispered pectoriloquoy. Percuss the chest and back for hyperresonance (asthma, emphysema, pneumothorax) and dullness (pulmonary edema, pleural effusion, pneumonia).

Cardiovascular Inspect for signs of arterial insufficiency or occlusion in your patient's trunk and extremities. Look for skin pallor and other signs of decreased perfusion. Inspect and palpate the chest for the PMI. Assess central and peripheral pulses for equality, rate, regularity, and quality. Auscultate for heart sounds, identifying S1, S2, and any additional sounds.

Always keep the mouth clear of any fluids that may block the upper airway by aggressive suctioning.

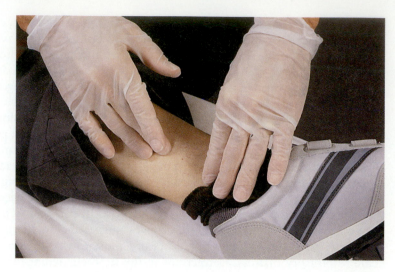

FIGURE 3-35   Check for peripheral edema.

Abdomen   Look for exaggerated abdominal muscle use during exhalation, a sign of lower airway obstruction as seen in asthma and emphysema. Inspect and palpate the abdomen for distention due to air or fluid. Ascites is an accumulation of fluid within the abdominal cavity caused by increased pressure in the systemic circulation as seen in patients with right heart failure. It is also common in patients with cirrhosis of the liver, where portal circulation (to and from the liver) is increased. This is often seen in patients with right heart failure or cirrhosis of the liver. Inspect and palpate the flanks and presacral area for edema in bedridden patients suspected of having congestive heart failure. Check for unusual pulsation of the descending aorta, just left of the umbilicus. Palpate for liver enlargement or upper quadrant tenderness suggesting ulcer disease, gall bladder disease, or pancreas problems, all of which can be confused as chest pain.

Extremities   Perform neurovascular checks on both hands and feet. These consist of checking for pulses, sensation, and the ability to move. Pay special attention to the equality of pulses in all extremities. Unequal pulses in the upper extremities suggest a thoracic aneurysm; unequal pulses in the lower extremities suggest an abdominal aneurysm. Assume vascular compromise if the pulse is absent, the limb is cool, or the skin is cyanotic or ashen. In cardiac and respiratory emergencies, evaluate the lower extremities for pitting edema. Depress the skin on the tibial plateau (Figure 3-35). If the depression remains after you remove your finger, pitting edema exists. This is a sign of chronic fluid retention as seen in heart and renal failure. Examine the fingernails for pitting. Check the wrists for Medic Alert identification.

Altered Mental Status   For a patient with an altered mental status, assess the following:

HEENT   Inspect and palpate the head to rule out any evidence of trauma. For example, your stroke patient may have suffered a skull fracture from falling on the floor. Palpate the fontanels of the infant for sunkenness (dehydration) and bulging (increasing intracranial pressure). Examine the face for symmetry. Unilateral facial drooping may indicate a stroke or inflammation of the facial nerve (Bell's Palsy). Examine the pupils for direct and consensual response to light. One pupil's getting larger or reacting more slowly to light could indicate a deteriorating brain pathology such as a stroke. A small portion of the population, however, has unequal pupils, a benign condition known as anisocoria. Bilaterally sluggish pupils usually suggest decreased blood flow to the brain and hypoxia. Fixed and dilated pupils indicate severe brain anoxia. Your patient's pupils also may dilate from sympathomimetic or anticholinergic drug use. Pinpoint pupils suggest a narcotic drug overdose or pontine hemmorhage (bleeding within the pons). Next, test for near response and accommodation. Test the integrity of the extraocular muscles with the "H" test. Normally your patient will move his eyes conjugately (together) to follow your finger. He may exhibit a nystagmus, a fine jerking of the eyes. At the far extremes of the test, nystagmus may be normal, but if you observe it during all extraocular movements it suggests a pathology. Examine the conjunctiva for redness (irritation), pallor (hypoperfusion), or cyanosis (hypoxia). Inspect the sclera for jaundice.

Chest Inspect, palpate, and auscultate the chest for any signs of cardiorespiratory involvement.

Abdomen Look for evidence of trauma or internal bleeding. Listen for bowel sounds that are absent in anticholinergic drug ingestions.

Pelvis Look for evidence of incontinence.

Extremities Perform neurovascular checks on both hands and feet. These consist of checking for pulses, sensation, and the ability to move. Assume vascular compromise if the pulse is absent, the limb is cool, or the skin is cyanotic or ashen. Since the motor and sensory nerves run along different pathways in the spinal cord, you must check your patient's extremities both for mobility and for sensation of light touch and pain. As with trauma patients, the inability to feel and move both legs indicates complete spinal cord disruption. Diminished sensation or diminished motor ability indicates a partial disruption. Weakness or disability on only one side suggests brain dysfunction such as a stroke. Report and record all extremity function tests.

Posterior Body Inspect the posterior body for deformities of the spine. Also check for evidence of incontinence. In the supine patient, inspect the flanks for presacral edema.

Neuro Reassess your patient's level of consciousness and compare his response to your earlier findings. Note his speech pattern and any deficits in speech or language. Observe mood swings or behaviors that suggest anxiety or depression. Determine your patient's person, time, and place orientation. Does he know his name, the day of the week, and where he is? Perform the one-minute cranial nerve exam outlined in Table 3-3. Inspect general body structure, muscle development, positioning, and coordination. Note any obvious asymmetries, deformities, or involuntary movements. Assess muscle tone by feeling the muscle's resistance to passive stretching in the extremities. Note the degree of resistance. Test for muscle strength by applying resistance during the range of motion evaluation. Check for pronator drift and watch for any drifting sideways or upward. Assess for coordination and cerebellar function, using rapid alternating movements and point-to-point testing. Note seizure activity tremors.

Table 3-3	ONE-MINUTE CRANIAL NERVE EXAM
Cranial Nerves	**Test**
I	Normally not done.
II, III	Direct response to light.
III, IV, VI	"H" test for extraocular movements.
V	Clench teeth; palpate massiter and temporal muscles. Test sensory to forehead, cheek, and chin.
VII	Show teeth.
IX, X	Say "aaaahhhh"; watch uvula movement. Test gag reflex.
XII	Stick out tongue.
VIII	Test balance (Romberg test) and hearing.
XI	Shrug shoulders, turn head.

Acute Abdomen For a patient complaining of abdominal pain, assess the following:

HEENT Notice any unusual odors coming from your patient's mouth. The smell of alcohol does not rule out a serious medical condition. The sweet smell of ketones suggests diabetes. A fecal odor may indicate a lower-bowel obstruction. The acidic smell of gastric contents means that your patient has vomited and may again. Inspect any fluids in the mouth. Coffee-ground emesis (vomiting) results from blood's mixing with stomach acids and suggests an upper GI bleed. Fresh blood usually means recent hemorrhage from the upper gastrointestinal tract.

Chest Listen to breath sounds. Crackles may indicate pneumonia, a cause of upper abdomen pain.

Abdomen Look for discoloration over the umbilicus (Cullen's sign) or over the flanks (Grey-Turner's sign) suggesting intra-abdominal bleeding. Check for any visible pulsation, peristalsis, or masses. If you notice a bounding or exaggerated pulsation, suspect an aortic aneurysm. Visible peristalsis may indicate a bowel obstruction. Auscultate for bowel sounds and renal bruits. Percussing the abdomen produces different sounds based on the underlying tissues. Percuss the abdomen in the same sequence you used for auscultation. Note the distribution of tympany and dullness. Expect tympany in most of the abdomen; expect dullness over the solid abdominal organs such as the liver and spleen.

Palpate the abdomen last to detect tenderness, muscular rigidity, and superficial organs and masses. The normal abdomen is soft and non-tender. Abdominal pain upon light palpation suggests peritoneal irritation or inflammation. If you feel rigidity or guarding while palpating, determine whether it is voluntary (patient anticipates the pain or is not relaxed) or involuntary (peritoneal inflammation). Then palpate the abdomen deeply to detect large masses or tenderness. If the peritoneum is inflamed, your patient will experience pain when you let go.

Posterior Body Inspect the posterior body for evidence of rectal bleeding.

Baseline Vital Signs

Prehospital medicine employs four basic vital signs: blood pressure, pulse, respiration, and temperature. As mentioned earlier, you may add a basic pupil assessment to this list. Your patient's vital signs are your windows to what is happening inside his body. They provide a unique, objective capsule assessment of his clinical status. Vital signs indicate severe illness and the urgency to intervene. Subtle alterations in these vital signs are often the only indication that your patient's condition is changing. They can warn you that your patient is deteriorating, or they can reassure you that he is responding to therapy.

Of the physical assessment techniques, taking accurate sets of vital signs reveals the most important information. As a paramedic you must assess these signs on every patient you evaluate. If your patient is with you for an extended time, measure and record his vital signs at intervals as his clinical condition dictates. Always reevaluate the vital signs after invasive procedures such as endotracheal intubation or fluid resuscitation and after any sudden change in your patient's condition. Accurate records of these numbers are invaluable when documenting your patient assessment.

If you suspect your patient of being hypovolemic, consider performing an orthostatic vital sign exam, commonly known as the tilt test. Take your patient's pulse and blood pressure while he is supine. Then have him sit up and dangle his feet. Finally, tell him to stand. Then in 30–60 seconds retake the vital signs. They should not change in the healthy patient. An increase in the pulse rate of 10–20 beats per minute or a drop in blood pressure of 10–20 mmHg, is a positive tilt test. This is a common finding in patients suspected of hypovolemia. Chapter 2 describes vital sign evaluation in detail.

Always reevaluate vital signs after invasive procedures and after any sudden change in your patient's condition.

Additional Assessment Techniques

Additional techniques include pulse oximetry, cardiac monitoring, and blood glucose determination. Refer to Chapter 2 for detailed descriptions of these techniques.

Pulse Oximetry The pulse oximeter is a noninvasive device that measures the oxygen saturation of your patient's blood. It is usually a good indicator of cardiorespiratory status because it tells you how well your patient is oxygenating the most distal ends of his circulatory system. It also quantifies the effectiveness of your interventions such as oxygen therapy, medications, suctioning, and ventilatory assistance. Normal oxygen saturation at sea level should be between 96% and 100%. Generally, if the reading is below 95%, suspect shock, hypoxia, or respiratory compromise. Provide your patient with the appropriate airway management, supplemental oxygen, and watch him carefully for further changes. Any reading below 90% requires aggressive airway management, positive pressure ventilation, or oxygen administration.

Cardiac Monitoring The cardiac monitor, which measures electrical activity, is essential in assessing and managing the patient who requires advanced cardiac life support (**ACLS**) measures. You should apply it to any patient you suspect of having a serious illness or injury. Its one major disadvantage, however, is that it cannot tell you if the heart is pumping efficiently, effectively, or at all. Always assess your patient and compare what you see on the monitor with what you feel for a pulse. If available, perform 12-lead ECG monitoring to identify the presence and location of a possible myocardial infarction.

Blood Glucose Determination In cases of altered mental status, such as diabetic emergencies, seizures, and strokes, measure your patient's blood sugar level. The arrival of inexpensive, hand-held glucometers makes this test simple and easy to perform in the field.

Emergency Medical Care

After conducting your physical exam, provide the necessary emergency medical care authorized by your medical director via standing orders. Then contact the on-line medical direction physician to request further orders. For example, you may administer 50 percent dextrose to an adult patient (25 percent dextrose to a pediatric patient) with documented hypoglycemia (Figure 3-36), intubate a patient in severe respiratory distress, or apply external cardiac pacing to a patient with third degree heart block. Always base your emergency care on your patient's signs and symptoms as obtained through a thorough focused history and physical exam. Finally, en route to the hospital conduct an ongoing assessment as described later in this chapter.

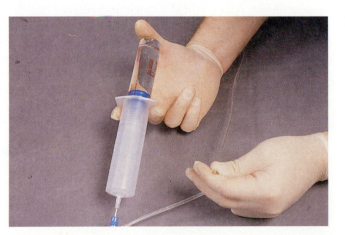

Apply the cardiac monitor to any patient you suspect of having a serious illness or injury.

Always base care of responsive medical patients on your patient's signs and symptoms as obtained through a thorough focused history and physical exam.

FIGURE 3-36 Administer 50 percent dextrose to a patient in insulin shock.

Again, if time allows, in certain situations you may wish to selectively use some of the advanced assessments described in Chapter 2. For example, en route to the hospital you might conduct a complete neurological exam for your patient who complains of stroke-like symptoms. This would comprise a full mental status assessment including orientation, appearance and behavior, speech and language, mood, thoughts and perceptions, insight and judgment, and memory and attention; a cranial nerve exam; a motor system assessment including muscle bulk, tone, and strength; a sensory exam including sharp and dull identification, temperature discrimination, position and vibration sense, and discriminative sensation; and deep tendon, as well as superficial, reflex tests. For your patient with upper respiratory distress and flu symptoms you may decide to examine the posterior pharynx and tonsils for redness and exudate; palpate the cervical lymph nodes for presence and tenderness; and thoroughly assess the lungs through tactile fremitus, egophony, bronchophony, and whispered pectoriloquoy. For your patient suspected of having acute appendicitis, you may wish to use the psoas test. Ask your patient to bring his right knee to his chest, contracting the iliopsoas muscle group. This motion usually causes pain as the muscles rub against the inflamed appendix. Your clinical experience and judgment will guide these types of decisions. The scope of paramedic practice is changing, not in procedures but in assessment capabilities. You will learn much more than your predecessors about anatomy and physiology, pathophysiology, and patient assessment. In time, you will learn which exam techniques yield the most relevant information and use them in your daily practice.

THE UNRESPONSIVE MEDICAL PATIENT

Since he cannot tell you what is wrong, the unresponsive medical patient requires an entirely different approach than the responsive patient. Assess the unresponsive medical patient much as you would a trauma patient. Begin with the initial assessment; then conduct a rapid head-to-toe exam known as the rapid medical assessment; and finally take a brief history from family or friends. This approach to the unresponsive medical patient also will help you to detect whether trauma may be involved.

After conducting the initial assessment, position your patient so that his airway is protected. If the cervical spine is not involved, place your patient in the recovery position—laterally recumbent. This will prevent secretions from obstructing his airway. Now begin the rapid medical assessment. The rapid medical assessment is similar to the rapid trauma assessment, except that you will look for signs of illness, not injury. Assess the head, neck, chest, abdomen, pelvis, extremities, and posterior aspect of the body. Perform the entire exam with the unresponsive patient. Then, assess baseline vital signs: pulse, blood pressure, respiration, and temperature. Finally, obtain a history from bystanders, family members, friends, or medical identification devices or services. If possible it should include the chief complaint, history of the present illness, past medical history, and current health status.

Evaluate your data and provide emergency medical care while performing additional tests such as cardiac monitoring, blood glucose determination, and pulse oximetry as needed. Consider your unresponsive patient unstable and expedite transport to the hospital, performing an ongoing assessment every five minutes en route.

Expedite transfer of unresponsive medical patients to the hospital and perform an ongoing assessment every five minutes en route.

IN THE FIELD

The rapid assessment is not a comprehensive history and physical exam, but a practical, systematic assessment aimed at quickly identifying the cause of your patient's unresponsive condition. Your care for a patient with a coma of unknown origin, for example, might go something like this:

You are dispatched to an "unresponsive person" in a residential neighborhood. Your patient is an elderly man who presents laterally recumbent on the floor of his bathroom. You conduct an initial assessment while your partner elicits information from the patient's wife:

General: Your patient appears pale and diaphoretic, moaning unintelligibly. You find no apparent signs of trauma, and he appears to have slumped to the floor from the toilet.

Mental Status: You establish your patient's mental status with the AVPU mnemonic. He responds to your voice but cannot answer your questions.

Airway: You open your patient's airway with a head-tilt/chin-lift maneuver and observe his breathing. His airway is clear. His breathing is rapid and shallow, but not labored. You ask another rescuer to administer positive pressure ventilation with supplemental oxygen while you continue with your assessment.

Circulation: You palpate his radial pulse, and note its absence. His carotid pulse is slow, irregular, and weak. His skin is pale, cool, and clammy, indicating poor peripheral perfusion.

You prioritize this patient high because of his altered mental status; his rapid, shallow breathing; and his poor peripheral perfusion. You suspect shock and begin a rapid medical assessment.

HEENT: You note lip cyanosis, a sign of central hypoxia. You see no lip pursing, nasal flaring, or other signs of increased breathing effort such as retractions or accessory muscle use. You smell no unusual odors or fluids from the mouth. The face is symmetrical; the pupils are equal and round, but react to light sluggishly. The trachea is midline, there is no JVD.

Chest: You note symmetrical chest wall movement and an equal and adequate rise and fall of the chest with each ventilation. You note some crackles in the lung bases. Your patient has no surgical scars.

ABD: You see no ascites or abdominal distention, no rigidity or guarding, no rebound tenderness, no renal or carotid bruits, no needle marks, no surgical scars or pulsating masses.

Pelvis: You see no evidence of bladder or bowel incontinence or of rectal bleeding.

Extremities: No finger clubbing, no medical identification, no needle marks. Peripheral circulation is poor with no radial or pedal pulses. You note no needle marks, but some pitting edema in lower extremities.

Posterior: You note some edema in your patient's flanks.

Vitals: Heart rate, 46 and regular; BP, 78/38; respirations, 36 and shallow.

Additional: ECG monitor shows third-degree AV block; pulse oximetry, 92% on room air, 99% with oxygen; blood glucose, 110.

Your patient's wife reveals his long history of heart disease and a long list of cardiac medications. Your field diagnosis is cardiogenic shock due to the bradycardic rate of the third-degree block. While your partner initiates an IV, you set up for immediate external cardiac pacing.

THE DETAILED PHYSICAL EXAM

The **detailed physical exam** uses many components of the comprehensive evaluation presented in the previous two chapters. It is a careful, thorough process of eliciting the history and conducting a physical exam. The detailed physical exam is a luxury, designed for use en route to the hospital, if time allows, for patients with significant trauma or serious medical illnesses. Ironically, with critical patients you usually will not have time to perform this in-depth exam because you will be preoccupied with performing ongoing assessments and providing emergency care. So you will seldom, if ever, perform a complete exam in the field. In fact, physicians in the emergency department rarely perform a detailed exam on their critical patients. It is too comprehensive and time-consuming and yields little relevant information.

In the emergency setting, individualize the exam to your patient's particular situation.

In the emergency setting, use a modified approach. You can individualize the exam to your patient's particular situation in many ways. For example, for the multi-trauma patient, perform a head-to-toe survey that is more detailed and slower than the rapid trauma assessment yet focuses on injury. For the 17-year-old football player who presents with shoulder pain, you may perform the entire portion of the shoulder exam. Palpating the abdomen and auscultating heart sounds would yield little useful information. For your stable patient who complains of abdominal pain, you may conduct an extensive history as detailed in Chapter 1, instead of the abbreviated SAMPLE history. Often you will elicit vital information from a seemingly obscure question during the review of systems. Again, clinical experience and your patient's condition will determine how you proceed with the detailed exam.

When you conduct the detailed exam you will use components of the comprehensive exam presented in Chapters 1 and 2. Refer to those chapters for a complete description of the components outlined in this section. Interview your patient to ascertain the history, then conduct a systematic head-to-toe physical exam. Place special emphasis on those areas suggested by your patient's chief complaint and present problem. Remember that the physical exam can be an anxiety-provoking experience for both the patient and the examiner. Using a professional, calm demeanor will minimize this anxiety. The following example illustrates how you might conduct a detailed physical exam for a multi-trauma patient en route to the hospital.

Aggressively suction patients with facial fractures to keep the upper airway clear.

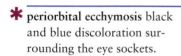

Head Palpate the cranium from front to back for symmetry and smoothness (Procedure 3-5a on page 224). Note any tenderness, deformities, and areas of unusual warmth. Inspect and palpate the facial bones for stability and note any crepitus or loose fragments (Procedure 3-5b). Any instability or asymmetry of the eye orbits, nasal bones, maxilla, or mandible suggests a facial bone fracture. In these cases, pay careful attention to the upper airway for obstruction from blood, bone chips, and teeth. Suction these patients aggressively to keep the upper airway clear.

When the base of the skull is fractured, blood and fluid from the brain can seep into the soft tissues around the eyes and ears and can drain from the ears or nose. Observe the bony orbits of the eye and the mastoid process behind the ears for discoloration. **Periorbital ecchymosis** (raccoon's eyes) is a black and blue discoloration surrounding the eye sockets. **Battle's sign** is a similar discoloration over the mastoid process just behind the ears (Procedure 3-5c). They are both late signs and usually are not visible on the scene unless a previous injury exists. Evaluate the temporomandibular joint for tenderness, swelling, and range of motion.

Eyes Examine the external structure of the eyes for symmetry in size, shape, and contour. Inspect the sclera and conjunctiva for discoloration, swelling, and exudate. Inspect the eyes for discoloration, foreign bodies, or blood in the anterior chamber (hyphema). Hyphema suggests that a tremendous blunt trauma to the anterior part of the eye has occurred. Check the pupils for equality in size and reaction to light (Procedure 3-5d). Bilaterally sluggish pupils usually suggest decreased cerebral perfusion and hypoxia. Fixed and dilated pupils indicate severe cerebral anoxia. Unequal pupils may indicate a variety of pathologies, including brain lesions, meningitis, drug poisoning, third-nerve paralysis, and increasing intracranial pressure.

Examine the eyes for conjugate movement, their ability to move together. Muscle or nerve damage to the eyes and certain drugs can cause dysconjugate gaze, in which the eyes seem to look in different directions. Check for extraocular movements. Note any inability of the eyes to follow your finger as you draw a large imaginary "H" in front of them; this indicates either nerve damage or an orbital fracture impinging on the extraocular muscles (Procedure 3-5e). Test for visual acuity and peripheral vision, if appropriate.

Ears Examine the external ears and observe the surrounding area for deformities, lumps, skin lesions, tenderness, and erythema. Examine the ear canal for drainage (Procedure 3-5f). A basilar skull fracture can cause blood and clear cerebrospinal fluid to leak into the auditory canals and flow to the outside. Do not try to block this flow; just cover it with sterile gauze to prevent an easy route for infection. Check for hearing acuity as appropriate.

Nose and Sinuses Check your patient's nose from the front and from the side and note any deviation in shape or color. Palpate the external nose for depressions, deformities, and tenderness. Examine the nares for flaring, a sign of respiratory distress, especially in small children. Pay special attention to infants less than three months old. They are mainly nose breathers and need a clear, unobstructed nasal cavity for respiration. Examine the nasal mucosa for evidence of drainage and note the color, quantity, and consistency of the discharge (Procedure 3-5g). A clear, runny discharge may indicate leaking cerebral spinal fluid (CSF) from a basilar skull fracture. Test for nasal obstruction.

The nasal cavity has a rich blood supply to warm the inspired air. Unfortunately, this can make bleeding in the nasal cavity severe and very difficult to control. If unconscious, these patients require aggressive suctioning. The patient who swallows this blood may complain later of nausea and vomiting.

Mouth and Pharynx Note the condition and color of the lips. Lip cyanosis is an ominous sign of central circulatory hypoxia. Examine the oral mucosa for pallor suggesting poor perfusion as in shock (Procedure 3-5h). Ask your patient to extend his tongue straight out and then move it from side to side. Press a tongue blade down on the middle third of the tongue and have your patient say "aaaahhhh." Examine the movement of the uvula. Asymmetrical movement of the uvula suggests a cranial nerve lesion. Note any odors or fluids coming from your patient's mouth; they can provide clues to infection, poisoning, and metabolic processes such as diabetic ketoacidosis.

Lip cyanosis is an ominous sign of central circulatory hypoxia.

Neck Briefly inspect the neck for general symmetry. Note any obvious deformity, deviation, tugging, masses, surgical scars, gland enlargement, or visible lymph nodes. Examine any penetrating injuries to the neck closely for injury to the trachea or major blood vessels. Look for jugular vein distention while your patient is sitting up and at a 45° incline. Palpate the trachea for midline position (Procedure 3-5i). Then, palpate the carotid arteries and note their rate and quality.

Chest and Lungs Observe your patient's breathing. Look for signs of acute respiratory distress. Count his respiratory rate and note his breathing pattern. Inspect the anterior and posterior chest walls for symmetrical movement. Note the use of neck muscles (sternocleidomastoids, scalene muscles) during inhalation or abdominal muscles during exhalation. Accessory muscle use suggests partial

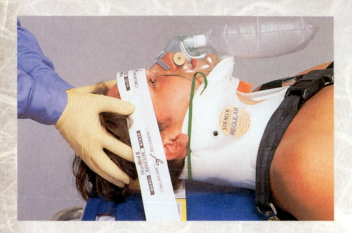

3-5a Inspect and palpate the cranium from front to back.

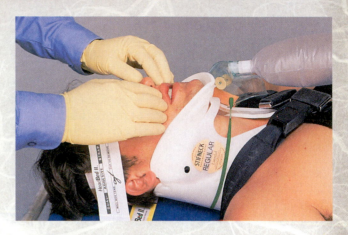

3-5b Inspect and palpate the facial bones.

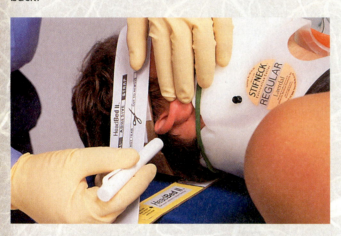

3-5c Inspect the mastoid process for Battle's sign.

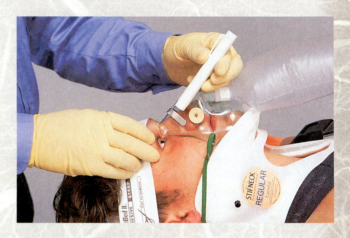

3-5d Check the pupils for reaction to light.

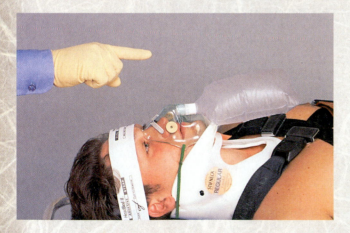

3-5e Check for extraoccular movement.

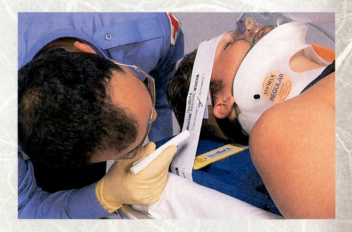

3-5f Inspect the ear canal for drainage.

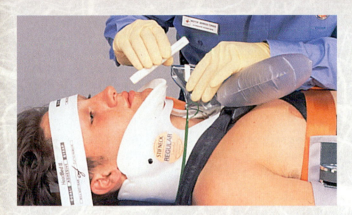

3-5g   Examine the nasal mucosa for drainage.

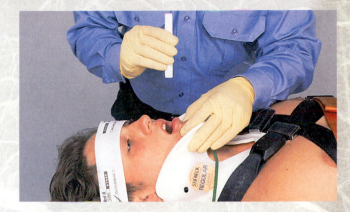

3-5h   Examine the oral mucosa for pallor.

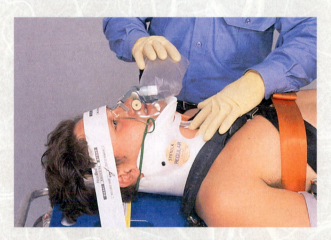

3-5i   Palpate the trachea for midline position.

airway obstruction and difficulty moving air. Inspect the intercostal spaces for retractions or bulging.

Palpate the rib cage for rigidity (Procedure 3-6a on next page). Feel for tenderness, deformities, depressions, loose segments, asymmetry, and crepitus. Evaluate for equal expansion. Percuss the chest symmetrically from the apices to the bases. Identify and note any area of abnormal percussion. Auscultate all lung fields and compare side-to-side (Procedure 3-6b).

Percussion can also provide evidence regarding chest pathology. If the region is hyperresonant, the thorax may contain air under pressure (tension pneumothorax). If the region is dull to percussion, it may be filled with blood (hemothorax) or other fluid (pleural effusion). Be sure to compare the sounds left-to-right and, during examination of the posterior body, front-to-back to confirm your evaluation.

Cardiovascular System Look for skin pallor and other signs of decreased perfusion. Inspect and palpate the carotid arteries for rate, rhythm, and quality or amplitude. Inspect and palpate the chest for the PMI. Auscultate for normal, abnormal, and extra heart sounds.

Abdomen Inspect the skin of the abdomen and flanks for scars, dilated veins, stretch marks, rashes, lesions, and pigmentation changes. Look for Cullen's sign or Grey-Turner's sign suggesting intra-abdominal bleeding. Assess the size and shape of your patient's abdomen and note its symmetry. Palpate the abdomen last to detect tenderness, muscular rigidity, and superficial organs and masses (Procedure 3-6c). Assess for rebound tenderness, a classic sign of peritoneal irritation, by pushing down slowly and then releasing your hand quickly off the tender area.

Pelvis Reevaluate the pelvic ring at the iliac crests and symphysis pubis (Procedure 3-6d). With the palms of your hands, direct pressure medially and posteriorly. Then press posteriorly on the symphysis pubis, being careful not to entrap the penis or cause injury to the urinary bladder. Any pain, instability, or crepitus suggests a pelvic fracture. Always immobilize the pelvis before transport to prevent movement and a possible circulatory catastrophe. If your patient presents in shock with an unstable pelvis, apply and inflate the pneumatic antishock garment.

Genitalia The external genitalia are extremely vascular and can bleed profusely when lacerated. Control hemorrhage in this area with direct pressure. Examine the male organ for priapism, a painful, prolonged erection usually caused by spinal cord injury or blood disturbances. Suspect a major spinal cord injury in any patient with a priapism. The female genitalia are somewhat well-protected from all but penetrating injury.

If you suspect your patient may have been raped or sexually abused, limit your assessment and management to only those techniques that are essential to patient stabilization. If possible, have a member of the same sex treat these patients. This may relieve any hostilities and anxiety that might be directed toward a caregiver of the opposite sex. Encourage the patient not to bathe. One of your most important tasks is to provide emotional support and reassurance. (For more on this subject, see the abuse and assault chapter in Volume 5, Special Considerations/Operations.)

Anus and Rectum Examining the anus is normally not a prehospital assessment practice. If your patient presents with severe rectal bleeding apply direct pressure to the area with sterile pads and be prepared to treat him for shock. You will have no other reason to examine this area.

Peripheral Vascular System Inspect all four extremities, noting their size and symmetry. Palpate the peripheral arteries for pulse rate and quality. Assess the skin for temperature, moisture, color, and capillary refill.

One of your most important tasks for possible victims of rape or sexual abuse is to provide emotional support and reassurance.

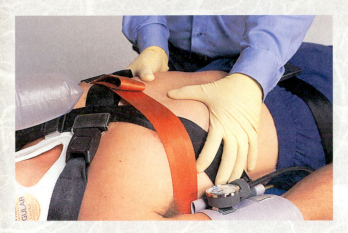

3-6a   Palpate the ribcage.

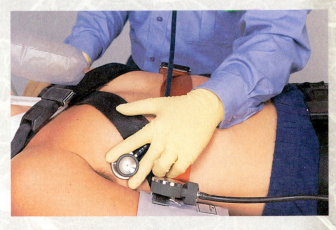

3-6b   Auscultate the lungs.

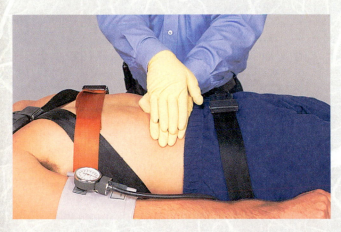

3-6c   Palpate the abdomen.

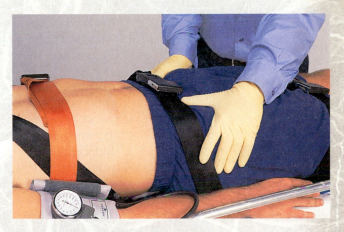

3-6d   Evaluate the pelvis.

Musculoskeletal System Reinspect and palpate all four extremities. Inspect and palpate your patient's joints, their structure, their range of motion, and the surrounding tissues. Inspect for swelling in or around joints, changes in the surrounding tissue, redness of the overlying skin, deformities, and symmetry of impairment. Compare both sides for equal size, shape, color, and strength. Palpate for tenderness in and around the joint. Try to identify the specific structure that is tender, such as a ligament, or tendon.

Test for range of motion passively and against gravity and resistance. Difficulty during passive range of motion tests suggests a joint problem. Difficulty with gravity or against resistance suggests a muscular weakness or nerve problem. Listen for crepitation, the crunching sounds of unlubricated parts rubbing against each other, while you manipulate the joint. Perform distal neurovascular checks.

Nervous System A nervous system exam covers five areas: mental status and speech; the cranial nerves; the motor system; the reflexes; and the sensory system.

Mental Status and Speech First, assess your patient's level of consciousness and compare his response to your earlier findings. Observe his posture and motor behavior and his grooming and personal hygiene. Note his speech pattern and use of language. Observe your patient's mood from his verbal and nonverbal behavior. Assess his thought content, perceptions, insight and judgment, memory, attention, and learning ability.

Cranial Nerves Test any cranial nerves that you have not already checked. (Review Table 3-3 for a quick, reliable, practical, cranial nerve exam that should take no longer than one minute to perform.)

Motor System Inspect your patient's general body structure, muscle development, positioning, and coordination. Note any obvious asymmetries, deformities, or involuntary movements. Assess muscle tone by feeling the muscle's resistance to passive stretching in the extremities. Test for muscle strength by applying resistance during the range of motion evaluation. Check for pronator drift and watch for any drifting sideways (laterally) or upward (superiorly). Assess for coordination and cerebellar function, using rapid alternating movements and point-to-point testing.

Reflexes Test your patient's deep tendon reflexes with a reflex hammer and note any hyperactive or diminished response. Check the biceps, triceps, brachioradialis, quadriceps, and Achilles reflexes. Test the superficial abdominal reflexes and plantar response.

Sensory System Test for pain, light touch, temperature, position, vibration, and discriminative sensations. Compare distal areas to proximal areas, symmetrical areas bilaterally, and scatter the stimuli to assess most of the dermatomes. Assess your patient's ability to distinguish sharp from dull sensations.

VITAL SIGNS

Take another set of vital signs and compare them to earlier sets to detect any trends, patterns that indicate either an improvement or deterioration in your patient's condition. These trends include a rising or falling pulse rate and blood pressure; an increasing or decreasing respiratory rate and effort; changing skin temperature, color, and condition; and changing pupillary equality and response to light. Such trends may suggest specific pathologies that you will learn in Book 3, *Medical Emergencies,* and Volume 4 of *Trauma Emergencies,* of *Paramedic Emergency Care.*

RECORDING EXAM FINDINGS

Record all exam findings on the appropriate run sheet or chart. Remain objective and nonjudgmental when recording the data. Chapter 6, "Documentation," gives detailed instructions on writing patient care reports.

Content Review

AREAS OF NERVOUS SYSTEM EXAM
Mental status and speech
Cranial nerves
Motor system
Reflexes
Sensory system

Content Review

REFLEX TESTS
Biceps
Triceps
Brachioradialis
Quadriceps
Achilles
Abdominal plantar

Content Review

SENSORY SYSTEM TESTS
Pain
Light touch
Temperature
Position
Vibration
Discriminative

ONGOING ASSESSMENT

En route to the hospital, conduct an ongoing series of assessments to detect trends, determine changes in your patient's condition, and assess the effectiveness of your interventions. Patient condition can change suddenly. You must steadfastly reassess mental status, airway patency, breathing adequacy, circulation, and any deterioration in areas already compromised (Procedure 3-7a on next page). Conduct your ongoing assessment every fifteen minutes for stable patients, every five minutes for unstable patients. Compare your findings to the baseline findings and note any trends.

MENTAL STATUS

Recheck your patient's mental status by performing the AVPU exam frequently during transport. Any deterioration in mental status is cause for great concern. The brain demands a constant supply of oxygen and glucose and a constant elimination of waste products. When it is deprived of either, even briefly, expect rapid mental status changes. A falling level of response indicates either a direct or indirect brain pathology. For example, following a head injury, your patient who was alert and oriented at the scene gradually becomes sleepy and eventually unarousable. You should suspect a life-threatening increase in intracranial pressure (pressure inside the enclosed skull) and expedite transport to the appropriate medical facility. Or your patient with an intra-abdominal hemorrhage becomes increasingly less arousable due to the decreased oxygenated blood flow to the brain (indirect pathology). Or sometimes patients improve following your interventions. After you administer 50% dextrose to your hypoglycemic diabetic patient, for instance, he becomes alert and begins talking.

AIRWAY PATENCY

The patency of your patient's airway can change instantly. Bleeding, vomiting, and even secretions can suddenly obstruct the upper airway. Be prepared to suction your patient quickly. Respiratory burns and anaphylaxis can cause life-threatening swelling in a matter of minutes. Croup and epiglottitis also can quickly deteriorate into total upper airway occlusion.

Endotracheal intubation is the best way to secure the airway in patients with no gag reflex. But endotracheal tubes can become dislodged easily during transport. Recheck for tube placement frequently during transport and every time you move your patient onto a back board, onto the stretcher, or onto the hospital gurney.

The price of proper airway management is eternal vigilance and a pessimistic outlook— anything that can go wrong will go wrong. Be prepared for the worst.

BREATHING RATE AND QUALITY

A change in respiratory rate or quality might indicate improvement or deterioration. A sudden increase in rate or respiratory effort suggests deterioration. For example, if your patient suddenly begins to gasp for air, has retractions, and uses his accessory neck muscles, he has a serious problem. Sometimes the signs are not so obvious. Subtle increases in respiratory rate can suggest a developing problem. A decrease in rate and effort could mean that your treatments are effective and your patient is improving. For example, after you administer an albuterol treatment, your patient breathes easier and his lung sounds improve. In infants and young children, however, a decrease in rate and effort may mean that your patient is exhausted and requires aggressive intervention. If, while assisting ventilation with a bag-valve mask, your partner suddenly complains that squeezing the bag is becoming more difficult, consider the possibility that a tension pneumothorax is developing or that bronchospasm or laryngospasm may be occurring. Airway and breathing management require constant reevaluation.

Content Review

ONGOING ASSESSMENT

Detects trends
Determines changes
Assesses interventions' effects

You must steadfastly reassess mental status, ABCs, and any areas already compromised.

Any deterioration in mental status is cause for great concern.

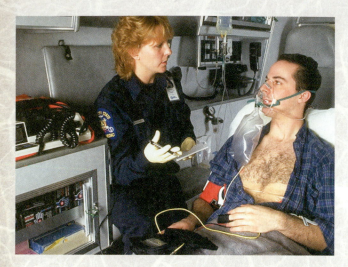

3-7a   Reevaluate the ABCs.

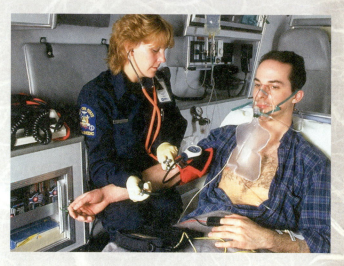

3-7b   Take all vital signs again.

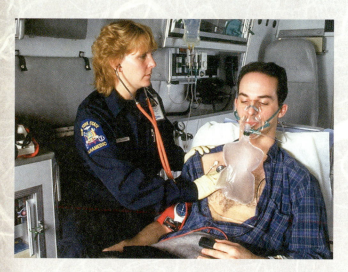

3-7c   Perform your focused assessment again.

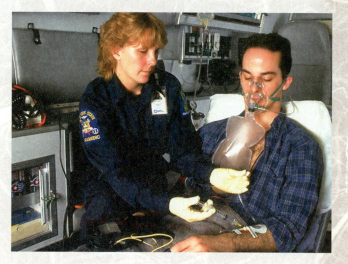

3-7d   Evaluate your interventions' effects.

PULSE RATE AND QUALITY

Check central and peripheral pulses and compare the findings to earlier measurements. A rising pulse rate could indicate shock, hypoxia, or cardiac dysrhythmia. A falling rate could mean the terminal stage of shock or a rise in intracranial pressure. A sudden change in rate or regularity may suggest a cardiac dysrhythmia. The loss of peripheral pulses could mean decompensating shock.

SKIN CONDITION

Similar to mental status, the skin quickly reflects the body's hemodynamic status. Reevaluate your patient's skin color, temperature, and condition. Cyanosis suggests decreased oxygenation. Lip cyanosis indicates central hypoxia (overall oxygen status), while peripheral cyanosis indicates decreased oxygen to the tissues. Pallor and coolness suggest decreased circulation to the skin, as seen in shock. If your patient suddenly develops hives after you administer a medication, suspect an allergic reaction. A localized redness and warmth could indicate bleeding under the skin or vasodilation. Cyanosis and coolness in a lower extremity suggest a peripheral vascular problem such as an arterial occlusion. A deep vein thrombosis will result in redness, swelling, and warmth in the lower leg.

TRANSPORT PRIORITIES

Sometimes stable patients suddenly deteriorate en route to the hospital. For example, the formerly conscious and alert head-injury patient now responds only to pain. Or your stable cardiac patient suddenly develops a life-threatening dysrhythmia. Or your patient suddenly cannot breathe because his simple pneumothorax has developed into a tension pneumothorax. In these cases, while you provide life-saving treatments, change your transport decision to a higher priority. By the same token, if your unstable patient becomes stable, you may wish to downgrade your priority transport decision and decrease the danger and liability of driving with lights and siren on.

VITAL SIGNS

Reassessing vital signs reveals trends clearly (Procedure 3-7b). A rising pulse rate combined with a falling blood pressure indicates shock. A decreasing pulse rate combined with a rising blood pressure, associated with an irregular respiratory pattern, suggests a rise in intracranial pressure. Any change in heart rate could indicate a cardiac dysrhythmia. A narrowing pulse pressure with a weakening pulse indicates cardiac tamponade, a tension pneumothorax, or hypovolemic shock. Reevaluate your critical patient's vital signs every five minutes and look for changes.

Reevaluate your critical patient's vital signs every five minutes.

FOCUSED ASSESSMENT

Elicit your patient's chief complaint again to determine if the problem still exists or if other problems have arisen. Often following trauma your patient will develop more complaints en route to the hospital as the excitement of the incident begins to wear off. Patients often focus on their major injuries and might not even be aware of other problems. Repeat your focused assessment as your patient's chief complaint dictates (Procedure 3-7c).

EFFECTS OF INTERVENTIONS

Evaluate the effects of any interventions (Procedure 3-7d). Did the albuterol treatment help open the lower airways? Did the oxygen and nitroglycerin relieve the chest pain? What are the affects of the fluid challenge? Is the pneumatic anti-shock garment inhibiting your patient's breathing? Did your intervention help or harm your patient? Is he getting better or worse? Know the expected therapeutic benefits of your interventions, and then evaluate whether they worked. For example, you administer lidocaine to convert ventricular tachycardia. Following administration, observe your patient's electrocardiogram for changes while noting any harmful side effects such as nausea, vomiting, or seizures.

MANAGEMENT PLANS

Have the courage to admit it if your plan is not working and the flexibility to change it.

Evaluate whether your care is working. If it is not, consider another management plan. Develop the courage to admit when your plan is not working and the flexibility to change your course of action. For example, your patient, an elderly man with a history of congestive heart failure (CHF) and chronic obstructive pulmonary disease (COPD), presents with severe difficulty breathing and audible wheezing. You suspect he is having an exacerbation of his COPD and administer two nebulizer treatments and begin transporting. En route, however, he is not improving, and now you also can hear crackles bilaterally. At this point, you suspect he is in CHF and change your management to administering nitroglycerin, furosemide, and morphine.

Your ability to reassess your patient, reevaluate your field diagnosis, and alter your management plan will optimize patient care.

Patients often present with multiple complaints, symptoms, and histories. Formulating a definitive diagnosis is difficult without the hospital's labs, X-rays, and other assessment tools. Your ability to reassess your patient, reevaluate your field diagnosis, and alter your management plan will optimize patient care.

SUMMARY

Patient assessment is the key to providing effective prehospital emergency medical care. Its components include the initial assessment, the focused history and physical exam, vital signs, ongoing assessment, and the detailed physical exam. The initial assessment is designed to identify life-threatening airway, breathing, and circulation problems. The focused history and physical exam is designed to identify the signs and symptoms surrounding your patient's chief complaint. It is a problem-oriented approach that is easily modified to match your patient's clinical situation. The ongoing assessment is designed to reevaluate your patient for changes in status en route to the hospital. The detailed physical exam is a comprehensive head-to-toe evaluation designed to identify any conditions not already found. Although more suited to a clinical setting, it is intended to be done en route to the hospital if time allows.

The four general types of patients require distinctly different assessment approaches. The trauma patient with a significant mechanism of injury should receive an initial assessment, a rapid trauma assessment, and rapid transport. The patient with isolated, minor trauma, such as a cut finger or sprained ankle, should receive a physical exam focused on his particular problem or area. The responsive medical patient requires an initial assessment, a history and physical exam that focuses on his chief complaint, and vital signs. The unresponsive medical patient requires an initial assessment, followed by a rapid head-to-toe medical assessment and rapid transport. You will perform detailed history and physical exam techniques en route to the hospital if time and your patient's condition allow.

The assessment templates in this chapter are only guidelines. They do not dictate an exact procedure for assessing every patient. Instead, they provide general chronological guides to help you make critical transport and management decisions. As a paramedic you will be expected to use clinical judgment when deciding which assessment tools to use for your particular patient and situation. With time and experience, you will become adept at assessing real patients in crisis. The more effective and efficient you become with this process, the better your patient care will be.

YOU MAKE THE CALL

You are sitting at the station reading the latest EMS journals when the call comes in for "difficulty breathing" at the VFW post on Wheatley Drive. You quickly recognize the address as a club where your unit responds at least once a week to a variety of medical problems among its membership of elderly veterans. Preliminary dispatch information reveals a man in his 80s with a history of "breathing problems" in severe distress. Because the patient is in acute respiratory distress, prearrival instructions are in progress.

En route to the scene, you begin to formulate a list of differential field diagnoses for acute respiratory distress. As you arrive on the scene you notice nothing unusual and no potential hazards. The scene appears safe to enter. As you walk through the door you can hear obvious wheezing coming from the barroom. Mentally you begin to modify your differential field diagnosis. When you finally meet your patient, he sits upright on a barstool with his elbows on the bar. He appears very thin, with pursed lips, and is struggling to breathe effectively. He is in obvious distress, as evidenced by bulging neck muscles, retractions, and noisy respirations.

1. Outline each phase of your patient assessment for this patient.

See Suggested Responses at the back of this book.

FURTHER READING

Bates, Barbara, Lynn S. Bickley, and Robert A. Hoekelman. *A Guide to Physical Examination and History Taking.* 6th ed. Philadelphia: J. B. Lippincott, 1995.

Bledsoe, Bryan E., Richard A. Cherry, and Robert S. Porter. *Intermediate Emergency Care.* 2nd ed. Upper Saddle River, N.J.: Brady, 1998.

Campbell, John E. *Basic Trauma Life Support for Paramedics and Advanced EMS Providers.* 3rd ed. update. Upper Saddle River, N.J.: Brady, 1995.

Dalton, Alice, et al. *Advanced Medical Life Support.* Upper Saddle River, N.J.: Brady, 1999.

Dickinson, Edward. *Fire Service Emergency Care.* Upper Saddle River, N.J.: Brady, 1999.

Eichelberger, Martin R., et al. *Pediatric Emergencies: A Manual for Prehospital Care Providers.* 2nd ed. Upper Saddle River, N.J.: Brady, 1998.

Foltin George, et al. *Teaching Resource for Instructors in Prehospital Pediatrics.* New York: Center for Pediatric Medicine, 1998.

Hafen, Brent Q., et al. *Prehospital Emergency Care.* 5th ed. Upper Saddle River, N.J.: Brady, 1996.

O'Keefe, Michael F., et al. *Emergency Care.* 8th ed. Upper Saddle River, N.J.: Brady, 1998.

ON THE WEB

Visit Brady's Paramedic Website at www.brady books.com/paramedic.

CHAPTER 4

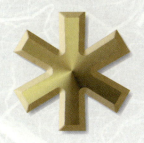

Clinical Decision Making

Objectives

After reading this chapter, you should be able to:

1. Compare the factors influencing medical care in the out-of-hospital environment to other medical settings. (p. 237)

2. Differentiate between critical life-threatening, potentially life-threatening, and non-life-threatening patient presentations. (pp. 237-238)

3. Evaluate the benefits and shortfalls of protocols, standing orders, and patient care algorithms. (pp. 238-240)

4. Define the components, stages, and sequences of the critical thinking process for paramedics. (pp. 240–246)

5. Apply the fundamental elements of critical thinking for paramedics. (pp. 244–246)

6. Describe the effects of the "fight or flight" response and its positive and negative effects on a paramedic's decision making. (p. 243)

7. Summarize the "six *R*s" of putting it all together: *R*ead the patient, *R*ead the scene, *R*eact, *R*eevaluate, *R*evise the management plan, *R*eview performance. (p. 247)

8. Given several preprogrammed and moulaged trauma and medical patients, demonstrate clinical decision making. (pp. 236–247)

CASE STUDY

On a hot, muggy Friday evening the call comes in for a car vs. pedestrian accident. Reports from the scene are that a 14-year-old girl was struck by a car while in-line skating and lies in the street with blood coming from her mouth. First to arrive, Assistant Chief Tom Shoemaker secures the scene, confirms the initial report, and calls for Air-One, the county medevac helicopter. As the fire department rescue rolls out the door, the ambulance follows with paramedic Sue Bauer and EMT-Basic Jim Parent.

Upon arrival, Sue instructs Carl Coffee from the rescue to immobilize the patient's head and neck while she begins an initial assessment. Her patient's name is Marcie. She is alert and oriented but does not remember what happened to her. She presents with obvious trauma to the mouth—all of her front teeth are missing or loose and she has minor bleeding. After the initial assessment and a rapid trauma assessment, Marcie appears hemodynamically stable. Sue decides to transport her by ground to a local community hospital. The rescue team immobilizes Marcie on a full backboard and quickly transports her.

En route to the hospital, Carl rides along to maintain verbal contact with Marcie and evaluate her mental status for changes. Sue begins her ongoing assessment and notes a declining mental status. Within minutes, Marcie becomes sleepy but is easily arousable by verbal stimuli. Sue decides to transport

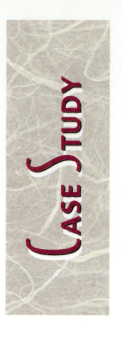

her to University Hospital, a level-1 trauma center with a specialized pediatric emergency department. This is a longer transport, but Sue believes her patient may be developing increasing intracranial pressure.

Marcie begins complaining of wanting to vomit. Sue and Carl quickly log roll her onto her side, but her nausea subsides. In the ED, Marcie vomits the frank blood she swallowed from her dental trauma, and her level of consciousness deteriorates further. Within minutes she becomes responsive only to deep pain. The emergency physician, Dr. Olsson, asks Sue for a chronological report on Marcie's mental status. Sue reports that she was alert and oriented 30 minutes earlier, then became responsive only to verbal commands approximately 15 minutes ago. They quickly transfer Marcie for a computerized tomography (CT) scan, which reveals an epidural hematoma from lacerating the middle meningeal artery and some minor bleeding from the middle cerebral artery.

INTRODUCTION TO CRITICAL THINKING

As a paramedic you inevitably will face your moment of truth—a critical decision that can mean the difference between life and death.

As a paramedic you eventually will face your "moment of truth." You will confront a situation that requires you to make a critical decision. Often, you will have several options, but choosing the best one may mean the difference between life and death. And you will be all alone. Others may be at the scene, but as the paramedic, you will be responsible for that decision. That you someday will have to make a decision on which your patient's life hinges is a sobering thought.

In the 1970s, with rare exceptions the first paramedics made few critical decisions. They usually worked under rigidly-written protocols developed by their medical director. Mostly, they were required to contact the medical direction physician who, after hearing their report, would diagnose the patient's problem and order treatment. They were no more than technicians who needed only good psychomotor skills to conduct patient assessments and follow orders. As prehospital care has evolved, paramedics now do much more than collect data for the physician to evaluate. You not only will have to gather information, but analyze it, form a field diagnosis, and devise a management plan. In most cases you will do these things before contacting your medical direction physician.

Twenty-first-century paramedics are prehospital practitioners of emergency medicine—not field technicians.

Twenty-first-century paramedics are prehospital practitioners of emergency medicine—not field technicians. To fill this role, you will need to develop your critical decision making skills—to be able to think rationally about what you are doing. Because patients seldom present with the classic textbook signs and symptoms, you will encounter situations that appear totally unfamiliar. These cases will call for you to use sound judgment in devising a management plan that meets your patient's needs. Making such decisions requires **clinical judgment**, using your knowledge and experience to make critical decisions regarding patient care. No one can teach you clinical judgment; you must develop it from experience. Unfortunately, experience often includes making bad decisions. We learn from our mistakes, if someone points them out and explains them to us. Your hospital and field preceptors will do this for you during this program.

✱ **clinical judgment** the use of knowledge and experience to diagnose patients and plan their treatment.

During this program, your instructors also will place you in as many problem-solving situations as possible to begin developing your clinical judgment. The number and type of supervised patient contacts you make during this program will determine how much clinical judgment you develop as a student. The more types of cases you see during your clinical rotations, the more clinically competent you will be when you complete your education.

PARAMEDIC PRACTICE

As a paramedic, you must gather, evaluate, and synthesize much information in very little time. You will obtain this information using your senses (sight, smell, hearing, and touch) during the history and physical exam. Analyzing these data will involve the total of your education, training, and clinical experience. For example, as you enter a patient's home, the sound of his gasping for breath with audible wheezes startles you. Having heard wheezing before and having learned in class that it results from a variety of problems will help you to make what is called a differential diagnosis. The differential diagnosis is a preliminary list of possible causes for your patient's problem. For example, a differential diagnosis for diffuse wheezing might include asthma, emphysema, bronchitis, and acute pulmonary edema. Now you conduct a history and physical exam and arrive at a **field diagnosis,** or impression.

> * **field diagnosis** prehospital evaluation of the patient's condition and its causes.

Your next step will involve applying your clinical experience and exercising independent decision making as you develop and implement a management plan. For example, your gasping and wheezing patient is an elderly male who presents with severe difficulty breathing. He has a history of cardiac and pulmonary disease, and you are not sure which problem precipitates this episode. You gather information and make an initial field diagnosis of congestive heart failure. You immediately administer medications (nitroglycerin, furosemide, morphine) to reduce cardiac preload, ease the workload of the heart, and increase urine production. You also decide to intubate and ventilate your patient to ease his respiratory effort. This decision to administer potentially life-threatening drugs requires you to think clearly and work effectively under pressure. Few prehospital situations create more pressure than a patient struggling to breathe.

The prehospital emergency medical setting is unlike any other medical care environment. Paramedics carry out the same tasks as other clinicians. They assess patients, obtain vital signs, start IVs, manage airways, and perform many other invasive procedures. The difference is that paramedics perform these procedures in various uncontrolled and unpredictable environments under circumstances that do not exist in other clinical settings and without information gathered from laboratory results and X-ray. For example, starting an IV line in a well lit, quiet hospital room is not a major challenge. Starting one while balancing yourself in the back of a rapidly moving ambulance is. Often you will use your skills in seemingly unmanageable circumstances. The key is to block out the distractions and focus on the task. Experienced paramedics do this better than anyone.

PATIENT ACUITY

Not everyone who calls 911 has a life-threatening emergency. Just the opposite is true. The vast majority of our patients are people who want transportation to the hospital for non-life-threatening problems. For others, the emergency department is their only health care option, even for a sore throat. The spectrum of care in the prehospital setting includes three general classes of patient **acuity:** those with obvious critical life threats, those with potential life threats, and those with non-life-threatening presentations. Patients with obvious life-threatening

> * **acuity** the severity or acuteness of your patient's condition.

Content Review

CLASSES OF PATIENT
ACUITY

- Critically life-threatening
- Potentially life-threatening
- Non-life-threatening

conditions include major multisystem trauma; devastating single system trauma; end stage disease presentations such as liver or renal failure when the patient is in the last days of his terminal illness and is close to death; and acute presentations of chronic diseases such as asthma or emphysema. These patients present with serious airway, breathing, circulation, or neurological problems and often require aggressive resuscitation. Potential life-threatening conditions include serious multisystem trauma and multiple disease etiologies such as a diabetic with cardiac complications. Non-life-threatening presentations include isolated minor illnesses and injuries. You will be expected to manage cases in all three categories. In a typical twelve-hour shift you may manage a patient in cardiac arrest; deliver a baby; control a lacerated, spurting artery; and transfer an elderly woman back to her nursing home. The wide range of patient types, degrees of severity, and complicating environmental factors makes out of hospital care a unique form of emergency medicine.

Arriving at a management plan for patients with minor medical and traumatic events requires little critical thinking or clinical judgment. For example, if your patient has a fractured tibia, you will splint the leg and transport him to the emergency department for X-rays and casting. You have no real life-saving decisions to make. On the opposite end of the acuity spectrum, patients with obvious life-threats such as cardiac arrest and major trauma also require few critical decisions because caring for them is largely rote and standardized. For cardiac arrest, you perform CPR and work through the protocol associated with your patient's cardiac rhythm. For major trauma, you manage the ABCs while providing rapid transport to a trauma center.

Patients who fall between minor medical and life-threatening on the acuity spectrum pose the greatest challenge to your critical thinking abilities. These patients might become unstable at any moment. For example, if your patient is an infant with signs of respiratory distress, you must recognize the signs of early respiratory failure and take precautionary measures to keep him from deteriorating to respiratory arrest. In these cases, you use your knowledge of pediatric respiratory assessment, your skills in airway and breathing management, and your clinical judgment to determine how and when to intervene. You will constantly reassess and revise your interventions as needed.

Patients who fall between minor medical and life-threatening on the acuity spectrum pose the greatest challenge to your critical thinking abilities.

PROTOCOLS AND ALGORITHMS

Paramedics function in an emergency medical services system under the license of a medical director. Every state has enacted legislation allowing paramedics to practice medicine in the field and describing the scope of their practice. Within these laws, state and local EMS medical directors devise **protocols** that detail exactly what paramedics can do. Protocols are standards that include general and specific procedures for managing certain patient conditions. For example, every system will develop standards for managing asthma, congestive heart failure, and tension pneumothorax. Each will also develop protocols for special situations such as physician-on-scene, radio failure, and termination of resuscitation. **Standing orders** authorize you to perform certain procedures before contacting your medical direction physician. For example, you may administer oxygen, start an IV, and administer aspirin and nitroglycerin to a patient with cardiac chest pain. For repeat nitro orders, you may have to consult the physician. Patient care **algorithms** are flow-charts with arrows, lines, and boxes arranged schematically (Figure 4-1). To use them, you simply start at the top and follow wherever your patient's signs and symptoms lead.

Protocols, standing orders, and patient care algorithms provide a standardized approach to emergency patient care. However, they address only "classic patients." Unfortunately, many patients present with atypical signs and symp-

* **protocol** standard that includes general and specific principles for managing certain patient conditions.

* **standing orders** treatments you can perform before contacting the medical control physician for permission.

* **algorithm** schematic flow chart that outlines appropriate care for specific signs and symptoms.

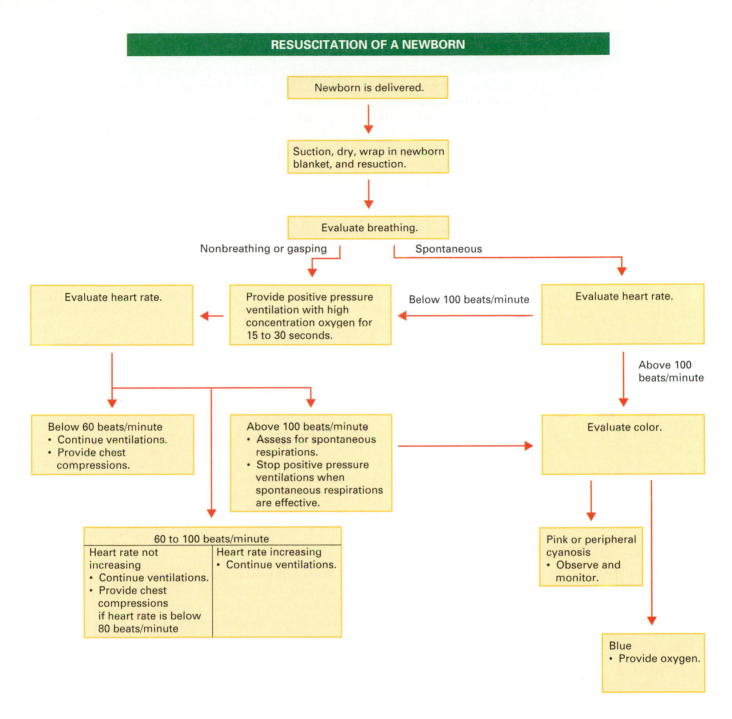

RESUSCITATION OF A NEWBORN

Newborn is delivered.

Suction, dry, wrap in newborn blanket, and resuction.

Evaluate breathing.

Nonbreathing or gasping | Spontaneous

Evaluate heart rate.

Provide positive pressure ventilation with high concentration oxygen for 15 to 30 seconds.

Below 100 beats/minute

Evaluate heart rate.

Above 100 beats/minute

Below 60 beats/minute
• Continue ventilations.
• Provide chest compressions.

Above 100 beats/minute
• Assess for spontaneous respirations.
• Stop positive pressure ventilations when spontaneous respirations are effective.

Evaluate color.

60 to 100 beats/minute	
Heart rate not increasing • Continue ventilations. • Provide chest compressions if heart rate is below 80 beats/minute	Heart rate increasing • Continue ventilations.

Pink or peripheral cyanosis
• Observe and monitor.

Blue
• Provide oxygen.

FIGURE 4-1   To use a patient care algorithm, follow the arrows to your patient's symptoms and provide care as indicated.

toms, often requiring you to use clinical judgment and instinct to develop a management plan. Patients frequently present with nonspecific complaints that do not match any specific algorithm. Sometimes your patients just do not clearly describe what is bothering them. Another limitation of protocols is that they cannot adequately cover multiple disease etiologies such as the patient with chronic obstructive pulmonary disease and congestive heart failure. When your patient with this multiple history presents with severe difficulty breathing, you must quickly identify the underlying condition that is causing the present problem and follow the appropriate protocol. Nor do protocols deal with managing more than one patient problem at a time in possible multiple treatment situations. For example, your stroke patient also presents with shock and with bilateral Colles' fractures and a fractured hip from the fall. Protocols are standards designed to promote consistent patient care in common situations. They are written also to allow you, in consultation with the medical direction physician, to use clinical judgment to provide optimum care in unusual situations. The linear thinking, or "cookbook medicine," that protocols promote should not restrict you from consulting with your medical direction physician in difficult or unusual cases.

CRITICAL THINKING SKILLS

The ability to think under pressure and make decisions cannot be taught; it must be developed. As a paramedic, you will be a team leader on emergency scenes. In that role you must make sound, reasonable decisions regarding your patient's care. Several aspects of this program will help you to develop this essential skill. In the classroom you will work on case histories. In the labs you will practice patient scenarios on moulaged victims. In the hospital you will assess and help manage real patients in the emergency department and critical care units. In the field internship, you will assess and manage patients in the streets. In all of these settings you will begin developing clinical judgment.

FUNDAMENTAL KNOWLEDGE AND ABILITIES

First, you must have an excellent working knowledge of anatomy and physiology and of the pathophysiology of your patient's disease or injury. To assess and manage a patient with difficulty breathing, for instance, you must know which organs and body systems are involved in breathing. You must understand the process of normal breathing and each body system's role in that effort. You must recall the factors that inhibit normal breathing and recognize the signs and symptoms of respiratory distress. For example, a patient might wheeze because of lower airway obstruction from secretions, bronchoconstriction, edema, or any combination of these conditions. All reduce the inner diameter of the airways, restricting airflow and making moving air in and out of the lungs difficult. Managing this patient would require a knowledge of the respiratory and cardiovascular causes of wheezing, because their treatments are vastly different. Respiratory causes for generalized wheezing include asthma and bronchitis, which you would manage with bronchodilators. Cardiac causes for wheezing include congestive heart failure, which you would manage with vasodilators and diuretics. Without a good working knowledge of these diseases, you might make a mistaken and potentially devastating field diagnosis.

You also must be able to focus on many specific data. When you conduct a patient assessment, you will evaluate all relevant information while focusing on specific important findings. You will be inundated with information requiring you to establish relationships and form conclusions. Your patient who presents with difficulty breathing and wheezing in the previous example would require an in-depth history and focused examination of his cardiac and respiratory systems. You also would assess other systems relative to his chief complaint (HEENT, musculoskeletal, neurological, and lymphatic), while remaining focused on the primary problem (cardiorespiratory). Although his chief complaint is difficulty breathing, his primary problem might be cardiac, muscular, infectious, allergic, or neurologic.

You must be able to organize the information you obtain and form concepts from it. Initially you elicit your patient's chief complaint and begin to formulate a **differential field diagnosis.** As you conduct the history and a clearer picture of your patient's problem emerges, you narrow your differential field diagnosis to the most probable disease. For example, your patient has severe difficulty breathing and inspiratory stridor. Your differential field diagnosis might include foreign body obstruction, epiglottitis, respiratory burns, anaphylaxis, laryngeal trauma, and throat cancer. Then you learn that he is hoarse and febrile, has had a sore throat for two days, and in the past six hours has had increasing difficulty swallowing. You now suspect epiglottitis. This ability to formulate a working field diagnosis is essential for paramedics.

You must be able to identify and deal with medical ambiguity. Many patients present with vague signs and symptoms. It is not unusual for a patient to complain of "just not feeling right." He will provide you with an imprecise story and you will be unable to arrive at a specific field diagnosis. In these cases, your field diagnosis will have to be generalized: "abdominal pain" or "general illness." Often it will be almost impossible to definitively diagnose your patient without laboratory results, X-rays, and other tests.

You must be able to differentiate between relevant and irrelevant data. You will have to sift the important data from the many bits of information you receive during your patient assessment. A positive family history for sudden cardiac death is relevant for your patient with chest pain; for your patient with a fractured arm it is not. Pupil and extraocular movement exams are relevant for trauma and for patients with an altered mental status; for a patient with asthma or arthritis they are not. When you radio the medical direction physician, you will report critical information only. Likewise, in your written documentation you will record relevant information and omit the rest.

You must be able to analyze and compare similar and contrasting situations. What were the similarities between your last three stroke patients? Did all three have facial drooping, slurred speech, and unilateral paralysis? Did they all have a history of hypertension? Can you depend on any patterns of presentation for future calls like this? Have some patient presentations been unusual? Have any patients presented with signs of stroke but had a different diagnosis? For example, your patient is a 45-year-old woman who presents with right-sided facial drooping. Your initial impression may be stroke, but further investigation reveals no other neurological deficits. You now change your impression to Bell's Palsy, caused by inflammation of the facial nerve (CN-VII). You must be able to recall the factors that help rule in or rule out a particular disease or injury.

You must be able to explain your decisions and construct logical arguments. Often, the emergency physician will want to know what you were thinking when you made your field diagnosis. You must be able to express yourself rationally while you make your case. These are the times when you demonstrate your professionalism to other health care providers. Observe the following conversation:

Physician: Why did you think your patient had Bell's Palsy and not a stroke? How can you rule out a stroke in the field?

Paramedic: Well, she had paralysis on the entire right side of her face, indicating a lesion of the seventh cranial nerve, rather than the lower facial paralysis of a stroke. All other neuro tests were negative.

Physician: OK, I agree, good job!

Through interactions such as this, you establish credibility with the emergency physician. The next time you contact him regarding a patient, he is more apt to trust your assessment and judgment.

* **differential field diagnosis** the list of possible causes of your patient's symptoms.

USEFUL THINKING STYLES

As a paramedic, you will face confusing emergencies that would challenge even the most knowledgeable, analytical care provider. You must be able to stay calm and not panic. Your self-control in the face of extreme chaos will set the example for other team members to follow. Even when you are struggling to maintain your composure—especially then—never let others know. The key is focusing on the task and blocking out the distractions. Be like the duck—cool and calm on the water's surface, while paddling feverishly underneath.

Assume and plan for the worst, and always err on the side of benefitting your patient. For example, if you are deliberating whether to immobilize your patient, initiate advanced life support procedures, or administer oxygen, just do it! It is better to err by providing care than by withholding it. Be pessimistic! Anticipate all potential bad side effects of your treatments and prepare "plan B." For example, as you deliver a bronchodilating drug to your severe asthmatic patient, anticipate that it will not work and mentally prepare to intubate him and perform positive pressure ventilation. Or while you are administering atropine to your patient with symptomatic bradycardia, plan ahead for external cardiac pacing and dopamine, if atropine therapy fails to restore adequate circulation.

Establish and maintain a systematic assessment pattern. Practice your assessments until they become second nature, and you will avoid skipping and missing steps. Be disciplined and stay focused, especially when you are confronted with a complex emergency scene. For example, your patient lies moaning on the ground in a pool of blood. Bystanders are screaming at you to help him; others are trying to tell you what happened. The police are gathering the story and trying unsuccessfully to talk with your patient. You must gain control of this scene. You do so by focusing on your patient and performing a systematic assessment. Use common acronyms (MS-ABC, OPQRST, SAMPLE) or make up your own to help you remember the key elements of your assessment. Except for safety concerns, never allow anything to distract you from your most important job—assessing and caring for your patient.

The different situations you encounter will require a variety of management styles. Adapting your styles of situation analysis (reflective vs. impulsive), data processing (convergent vs. divergent), and decision making (anticipatory vs. reactive) to each situation will enable you to provide the best possible care in every case.

Reflective vs. Impulsive Some situations call for you to be **reflective,** take your time, and figure out what is wrong with your patient. You have a patient who complains of "not feeling well." She has a long history of cardiac, renal, respiratory, and diabetic problems. Since she is in no real distress and is hemodynamically stable, you can take your time to determine her primary problem. Other situations call for immediate action. They require you to make an instinctive, **impulsive** decision and manage your patient's life-threatening condition. For example, if your patient presents apneic and pulseless, you will immediately begin CPR and prepare for rapid defibrillation. If he presents with a spurting artery, you will at once take measures to control the hemorrhage. If he is choking and has a weak, ineffective cough, you will quickly perform the Heimlich maneuver. You have to think fast in these situations.

Divergent vs. Convergent To process the data you receive from your patient and the scene, you can use either a divergent approach or a convergent approach. The **divergent** approach considers all aspects of a situation before arriving at a solution. It is insightful and works well when you are confronted with complex

FACILITATING BEHAVIORS
- Stay calm
- Plan for the worst
- Work systematically
- Remain adaptable

Be like the duck—cool and calm on the water's surface, while paddling feverishly underneath.

Except for safety concerns, never allow anything to distract you from your most important job—assessing and caring for your patient.

✱ **reflective** acting thoughtfully, deliberately, and analytically.

✱ **impulsive** acting instinctively without stopping to think.

✱ **divergent** taking into account all aspects of a complex situation.

scenarios. For example, your emotionally distraught, stable patient presents with multiple problems and a long, complicated medical history. You need to consider the physical, emotional, and psychological aspects of his condition before making a field diagnosis and management plan. Likewise, extricating a victim from a wooded scene requires you to weigh a variety of environmental and medical factors before selecting a mode of transport.

On the other hand, the **convergent** approach focuses narrowly on a situation's most significant aspects. This technically oriented approach relies heavily on step-by-step problem solving and is best suited for simple, uncomplicated situations that require little thought or reflection. For example, you have an unresponsive, apneic, pulseless patient who presents in ventricular fibrillation. Your immediate concern is simple and straightforward—you manage the ABCs and defibrillate him as quickly as possible. Experienced paramedics employ both approaches effectively in the appropriate situations.

Anticipatory vs. Reactive Your decision-making process can be either anticipatory or reactive. You either anticipate the possible ramifications of your actions in a proactive way or you react to events as you encounter them. For example, your patient presents with a severe laceration and severe blood loss. The bleeding is controlled. Now you can either anticipate his going into shock and begin measures before it happens, or you can wait until he shows signs of shock and then act. Unfortunately, by then it is often too late to do anything about it. Whenever possible, it is best to anticipate problems and act before they occur.

THINKING UNDER PRESSURE

When you must make a critical decision, physical influences may help or hinder your ability to think clearly. Your **autonomic nervous system,** which controls your involuntary actions, may respond by secreting "fight or flight" hormones. These hormones will enhance your visual and auditory acuity and will improve your reflexes and muscle strength. However, they may also impair your ability to think critically and diminish your ability to assess and concentrate. In these instances you will revert to your most basic instincts. Many an inexperienced paramedic has been "mentally paralyzed" by a complicated, critical call. With experience, you will learn to manage your nervousness and maintain a steadfast, controlled demeanor.

One way to enhance your ability to remain in control is to raise your technical skills to a **pseudo-instinctive** level. This means that you do not have to concentrate on them to perform them. For example, you do not think about tying your shoes, you just tie them. Such "muscle memory" is essential when performing emergency medical skills. When you set up for an Albuterol nebulizer treatment, for instance, you automatically fit together the pieces of the device and administer the treatment without hesitation. This way you can concentrate on your patient's condition, controlling the scene, and managing the multitude of items that usually complicate any emergency call. Concentrating on more than one thing simultaneously is difficult, if not impossible.

MENTAL CHECKLIST

Thinking under pressure is not easy. Maintaining your composure, especially during a chaotic, complicated call is key to developing a management plan for the best patient outcome. Developing a routine mental checklist is a good way

* **convergent** focusing on only the most important aspect of a critical situation.

Whenever possible, anticipate problems and act before they occur.

* **autonomic nervous system** part of the nervous system that controls involuntary actions.

* **pseudo-instinctive** learned actions that are practiced until they can be done without thinking.

Maintaining your composure, especially during a chaotic, complicated call is key to developing a management plan for the best patient outcome.

Content Review

MENTAL CHECKLIST
- Scan the situation
- Stop and think
- Decide and act
- Maintain control
- Reevaluate

to stay focused and systematic. Pilots work through their preflight checklists routinely before ever turning over their engines. Medical clinicians develop acronyms and mnemonics to remember critical elements during stressful incidents. For example, when conducting an initial assessment, use the acronym MS-ABC. Use OPQRST to elicit your patient's present history, or use SAMPLE when time is critical. You can adopt the following checklist any time you must make a critical decision.

Scan the Situation Stand back and scan the situation. Sometimes you can miss subtle signs if you focus too narrowly on one aspect of your patient's problem. Look for environmental factors and other not-so-obvious clues. For example, your patient lies unconscious and cyanotic on the floor. You rule out any airway, breathing, or circulation problems. No medical history is available and no medication bottles are present. When you detect a fruity odor on your patient's breath, you suspect diabetic ketoacidosis.

Stop and Think Do not do anything without stopping and weighing your actions. Consider all of your options before you act. Remember that for every action there is a reaction. Know what reactions to expect and anticipate their possible harmful effects. For example, after administering lidocaine, monitor your patient closely for the expected benefits (eradication of ventricular tachycardia) and early signs of toxicity (numbness and tingling to the lips, drowsiness, nausea).

Decide and Act Once you have assessed the situation, make your decision and act confidently. Announce your management plan to your crew with a combination of authority, confidence, and respect. Convey the feeling that you know your actions are correct and will work. This confidence helps reassure your patient, his family, your crew, and other responders even in the most stressful situations.

Maintain Control To maintain clear, efficient control of the scene and everyone involved, you must first control yourself. Many situations will challenge your inner strength and self-control. You will eventually be in charge of a scene where everyone seems out of control. These chaotic incidents can occur anywhere and anytime. Your job is to remain steadfast under fire.

Reevaluate Regularly reevaluate your plan's effects and revise it accordingly. Never assume that your plan is working to perfection. Anticipate ways your patient might deteriorate and devise alternate plans. Conduct an ongoing assessment en route to the hospital and be prepared to revise your management plan. For example, if you note increased lung congestion after administering fluids, stop the infusion.

THE CRITICAL DECISION PROCESS

* **critical thinking** thought process used to analyze and evaluate.

Understanding the **critical-thinking** process is essential for a paramedic. Your ability to analyze data effectively and devise a practical management plan optimizes patient care. You can conduct the most comprehensive history and physical exam, but if you cannot analyze the data and devise the proper management plan, your efforts will be fruitless. The critical-thinking process has five steps: forming a concept, interpreting the data, applying the principles, evaluating the results, and reflecting on the incident. To explain the critical decision-making process, we will consider a nineteen-year-old female patient with a sudden onset of sharp pain to her right lower quadrant with some vaginal bleeding.

Form a Concept

The first step in critical decision making is to gather information and form a concept of your patient and the scene. You will get this information by assessing the general environment and the immediate surroundings. Note the mechanism of injury, if applicable. Then observe your patient's mental status, skin color, positioning, and note any deformities or asymmetry. In our sample case, your patient presents at home, sitting on a sofa. At first glance, she appears pale, diaphoretic, and anxious. Next you conduct an initial assessment, focusing on the MS-ABCs. Your initial goal is to identify and manage critical life-threats. In this case, your general impression is of an alert and oriented but anxious young woman in moderate distress who presents with a clear airway; good air movement, as evidenced by her ability to converse in complete sentences; a strong, rapid, regular pulse; and cool, moist skin.

Now you ascertain your patient's chief complaint, history of present illness, past history, and current health status, while observing her affect (her general demeanor and attitude) and her degree of distress. You determine that her chief complaint is lower right quadrant pain that began suddenly 30 minutes ago. She also states she began bleeding at around the same time. She denies any nausea, vomiting, or diarrhea. You learn she has a past history of pelvic inflammatory disease and an active, unprotected sex life with multiple partners. Her last menstrual period was six weeks ago. She has had four pregnancies but no viable births. She appears in moderate distress.

Finally, you conduct a focused physical exam of the appropriate areas. This includes any diagnostic testing, such as an electrocardiogram, pulse oximetry, and blood glucose testing. You take a full set of vital signs, which can help you identify most life-threatening conditions. Remember that your patient's age, underlying physical and medical condition, and current medications can influence her vital signs. For example, the use of beta blockers could cause a general decrease in her pulse and blood pressure. Your patient has some deep palpation tenderness in the lower right quadrant but no rebound tenderness, and the rest of her abdomen is soft and nontender. She has minor bleeding at this time and has used only one sanitary pad since the bleeding began. Her vital signs are: HR—110 and regular; respirations 20, not labored; BP—120/86.

Interpret the Data

After you assess the patient you will interpret all of your data in light of your knowledge and experience. In this case, your knowledge base includes female reproductive anatomy, the physiology of a normal pregnancy, and the pathophysiology of pregnancy complications along with their classic signs and symptoms. It also involves the anatomy, physiology, and pathophysiology of the cardiovascular system and the signs and symptoms of shock. Your experience base includes every patient you have assessed and managed with a similar presentation. Your attitude toward managing patients with these symptoms also becomes a factor, because your experience may prejudice you. Consider all of the data and determine the most common and statistically probable conditions that fit your patient's initial presentation. This is your differential field diagnosis. Then, consider the most serious condition that fits your patient's situation. In our example, a field diagnosis of a ruptured ectopic pregnancy is obvious. When a clear medical diagnosis is elusive, base your treatment on the presenting signs and symptoms.

APPLY THE PRINCIPLES

With your field diagnosis in mind, you devise a management plan that covers all contingencies. You will use written protocols, standing orders, and all the interventions at your disposal to manage your patient's particular problem. Sometimes patients present with atypical signs and symptoms. For example, a patient who presents with a sore throat and cough may actually be having a heart attack and congestive heart failure. Other times a protocol for your patient's problem simply may not exist. For example, your system may not have a protocol for facilitated intubation in head injuries. In these cases, consult with your medical direction physician for guidance in providing optimum care to your patient. The physician's emergency medical expertise and experience can be invaluable to you and your patient in unusual and difficult cases.

In our example, although your patient presents with relatively normal vital signs and is fully alert and oriented, you are very concerned. A basic principle of medicine is that all females of child-bearing age with lower abdominal pain are pregnant until proven otherwise. You initiate advanced life support precautions en route to the hospital, including high-flow oxygen and two large-bore intravenous lines. Her presentation, has led you to expect the worst. If her fallopian tube ruptures and begins to hemorrhage, she will need rapid fluid resuscitation and general shock management. Your experience includes similar patients who suddenly suffered a life-threatening hemorrhage from a ruptured fallopian tube. Again, your attitude becomes a factor in that you will not allow her stable presentation to undermine your initial instinct—that she is potentially in serious trouble.

EVALUATE

During the ongoing assessment you reassess your patient's condition and the effects of your standing order/protocol interventions. In other words, you determine if your treatment is improving your patient's condition and status. For example, has the Albuterol helped your patient's breathing? Did the nitro and oxygen relieve the chest pain? Is the hemorrhage under control? Reflect on your actions and either continue your original plan, discontinue treatment, or take a completely different approach. You may alter your initial impression if your patient's condition worsens or if you discover new information. If time and circumstances allow a detailed exam, you may discover less obvious problems.

In our sample case, your patient remains in potentially unstable condition. Your repeat assessment shows her vital signs are holding with the infusion of IV fluids. She is alert and not as anxious as before, and her skin is becoming warm and normal in color. You deliver her to the emergency department in stable, but guarded, condition.

REFLECT

Make every patient contact a learning experience.

After the call, discuss your field diagnosis and care with the emergency physician. Compare your field diagnosis with his diagnosis. Conduct a run critique with your crew and discuss ways to improve your assessment and management of this case and future cases. Add this data to your information and experience base for future calls. Make every patient contact a learning experience. In this case, the emergency physician confirms your field diagnosis with lab tests and an ultrasound.

PUTTING IT ALL TOGETHER

A helpful mnemonic for the critical decision making process is the "six *R*s":

1. *R*ead the scene—Observe the general environmental conditions, the immediate surroundings, and any mechanism of injury.

2. *R*ead the patient—Observe his level of consciousness, skin color, position, location, and any obvious deformity or asymmetry. Talk to him to determine the chief complaint and whether it is a new problem or a worsening of a preexisting condition. Touch him to evaluate skin temperature and condition, pulse rate and quality. Auscultate for problems with the upper and lower airways. Identify any life threats with the ABCs and take a full set of vital signs.

3. *R*eact—Address any life-threats as found, determine the most common and serious existing conditions, and treat him accordingly.

4. *R*eevaluate—Conduct a focused and detailed physical assessment, note any response to your initial management interventions, and discover other less obvious problems.

5. *R*evise the management plan—Change or stop interventions that are not working or are causing your patient's condition to worsen, or try something new.

6. *R*eview your performance at run critique—Be honest and critically evaluate your performance, always looking for better ways to manage a particular case presentation.

SUMMARY

Clinical decision making is an essential paramedic skill that you will develop with time and experience. The prehospital environment is unlike any other medical care setting and you will have to make decisions in less-than-optimal and sometimes dangerous conditions. Most times you will have the benefit of consulting with your medical direction physician in difficult and unusual situations; other times you may not. Your ability to gather information, analyze it, and make a critical decision may someday be the difference between your patient's life and death. This is inevitable. How well you prepare for that challenge will determine your ultimate success. The process begins in your paramedic training program. You must develop a good working knowledge of anatomy, physiology, pathophysiology, and the principles of emergency medicine. In time, through repeated patient contacts, you will develop the clinical judgment you need to make effective patient care decisions.

Continued

The critical-decision-making process involves a series of steps that experienced clinicians do almost unconsciously. First you gather information (history and physical exam) to form an initial impression and then interpret it against your knowledge and experience to develop a working field diagnosis. You next apply the principles of emergency medicine to devise and implement a management plan and evaluate the effects of your treatments. Then you reevaluate and revise your plan as necessary. Finally you compare your findings with the emergency physician's diagnosis and discuss alternate ways to manage similar patients. With every patient contact, your experience grows and your clinical judgment improves. This is the essence of paramedic practice.

YOU MAKE THE CALL

You are on your lunch break at a local fast-food restaurant when a middle-aged man comes up to you and says, "I have a terrible headache. Do you have any aspirin?" The man fully expects you to simply give him what he asks for. After all, you represent the health care industry and two aspirin seem like a simple request. But you notice that his left hand appears to be shaking. You ask him if this is normal and he replies, "What shaking?" You then ask him his name, and he has trouble remembering it. You also notice a slight slurring of his speech and his gait seems unstable.

1. Would you give him the aspirin?
2. Describe the knowledge base needed to manage this situation.
3. How would you proceed from this point?

See Suggested Responses at the back of this book.

FURTHER READING

Bates, Barbara, Lynn S. Bickley, and Robert A. Hoekelman. *A Guide to Physical Examination and History Taking.* 6th ed. Philadelphia: J.B. Lippincott, 1995.

Dalton, Alice L. "Enhancing Critical Thinking in Paramedic Continuing Education." *Prehospital and Disaster Medicine* 11 (October–December 1996): pp. 246–253.

Farrell, Marian. "Planning for Critical Outcomes." *Journal of Nursing Education* 35 (September 1996): pp. 278–281.

Janing, Judy. "Critical Thinking: Incorporation into the Paramedic Curriculum." *Prehospital and Disaster Medicine* 9 (October–November 1994): pp. 238–242.

Seidel, Henry M., et al. *Mosby's Guide to Physical Examination.* St. Louis: Mosby, 1987.

ON THE WEB

Visit Brady's Paramedic Website at www.bradybooks.com/paramedic.

CHAPTER 5

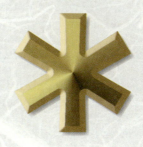

Communications

Objectives

After reading this chapter, you should be able to:

1. Identify the role and importance of verbal, written, and electronic communications in the provision of EMS. (pp. 254–258)
2. Describe the phases of communications necessary to complete a typical EMS response. (pp. 257–258)
3. List factors that impede and enhance effective verbal and written communications. (pp. 254–256)
4. Explain the value of data collection during an EMS response. (pp. 255–256)
5. Recognize the legal status of verbal, written and electronic communications related to an EMS response. (pp. 254–256)
6. Identify current technology used to collect and exchange patient and/or scene information electronically. (pp. 260–264)
7. Identify the various components of the EMS communications system and describe their function and use. (pp. 252–254)

Continued

Objectives Continued

8. Identify and differentiate among the following communications systems:

    - Simplex (p. 261)
    - Multiplex (p. 262)
    - Duplex (pp. 261–262)
    - Trunked (p. 262)
    - Digital communications (pp. 262–263)
    - Cellular telephone (p. 263)
    - Facsimile (p. 263)
    - Computer (pp. 263–264)

9. Describe the functions and responsibilities of the Federal Communications Commission. (p. 268)

10. Describe the role of emergency medical dispatch and the importance of prearrival instructions in a typical EMS response. (pp. 258–259)
11. List appropriate caller information gathered by the emergency medical dispatcher. (p. 258)
12. Describe the structure and importance of verbal patient information communication to the hospital and medical direction. (pp. 267-268)
13. Diagram a basic communications system. (pp. 253–255)
14. Given several narrative patient scenarios, organize a verbal radio report for electronic transmission to medical direction. (pp. 252–268)

CASE STUDY

On a dry, warm Sunday afternoon, a 31-year-old male loses control of his motorcycle and strikes a highway sign. Several people witness the incident. The first bystander to reach the patient rushes to his automobile to dial 911 on his cellular telephone. Emergency medical dispatcher Vern Holland takes the necessary information and dispatches a basic life support engine company and an advanced life support ambulance. As Holland dispatches the emergency units, his partner, paramedic dispatcher Fred Hughes, instructs the caller in basic emergency care. The units receive the call via a computer printout of essential information.

They quickly arrive at the scene and initiate the appropriate care. Because the patient has a severe head injury, the paramedic performs only a limited assessment and immediately initiates transport. As the ambulance departs, he relays the following to Dr. Doyle, the medical direction physician:

Paramedic: Depew Ambulance to Mercy Hospital.

Dr. Doyle: Go ahead, Depew.

Paramedic: We are leaving the scene of a motorcycle accident on I-90. We have one patient, a male who is in his 30s, the rider of a motorcycle that went off the roadway and struck a sign. He responds to pain only, with obvious facial and chest

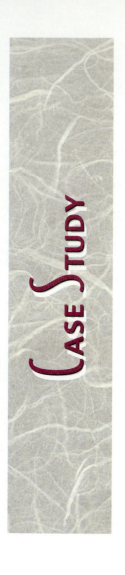

trauma. There is a large laceration above the right eye with an exposed skull fracture. There is also blood draining from the right ear. Vital signs are: blood pressure 110/60, pulse 110 and regular, respirations 10 and labored. Pupils are dilated and minimally reactive, yet equal. Palpation of the cervical spine does not reveal any obvious deformity. There is no tracheal deviation. Breath sounds are symmetrical, yet diminished. There is subcutaneous emphysema on the right side of his chest and several palpable rib fractures. The abdomen is soft, and the pelvis appears stable. There may be some lower-extremity fractures. A rigid C-collar is in place and the spine has been stabilized. An endotracheal tube has been placed. Respirations are being assisted with a BVM using supplemental oxygen. We will attempt an IV en route. Our ETA is 20 minutes.

Dr. Doyle: We copy, Depew. Attempt an IV en route, but expedite transport and notify us of any further problems.

Paramedic: We copy. Attempt an IV en route and we will notify you with any changes.

Dr. Doyle: The patient will be going into Trauma Room 1. The trauma team will be in the ED awaiting your arrival.

Paramedic: Copy that, Mercy. Depew clear.

Upon arrival, the trauma team and a neurosurgeon meet the patient. Despite comprehensive care, the patient dies as a result of his head injury. However, at the family's request, the patient's organs are harvested. They are sent to cities more than 1,500 miles away and used in two transplant operations.

INTRODUCTION TO COMMUNICATION

Knowledge of communications plays an important role in your paramedic training. All aspects of prehospital care require effective, efficient communications. During a routine transfer or a life-threatening emergency run, you will communicate with a wide variety of people. They will include:

- The emergency medical dispatcher (EMD) whose job it is to manage an entire system of EMS response and readiness, not just your call. You will transmit administrative information such as "responding," "arrived," "transporting," and "back-in-service." The EMD must know the location of all his resources to manage the system effectively. On a serious emergency call, the EMD can be your best ally by securing for you the resources you need to manage your incident.

- Your patient, his family, bystanders, and others who may, at times, not understand what you are doing and become obstructive. Quite often, people misconstrue your actions and words. You must try to keep them well-informed.

- Personnel from other responding agencies, such as the police department, fire department, or mutual aid ambulances who may not share your priorities at the scene. You must communicate effectively with other responders to coordinate and implement your treatment plan. You will accomplish this face-to-face and via the radio. These communications require you to exhibit confidence and authority.

- Health care staff from physicians' offices, health care facilities, and nursing homes who usually do not understand the extent of your training or abilities. Often, uninformed staff will call you "ambulance drivers." In these cases, you must exhibit professionalism and a calm demeanor while you ask pertinent questions and discuss the case intelligently.

- The medical direction physician who has extended his license to you in the field. The physician's expertise and advice can be a tremendous resource for you during the call. You will need to communicate patient information and scene assessment effectively to him. He can prepare for your arrival if you have communicated to him the needs of your patient. For example, you are transporting a patient with a serious head injury who exhibits a decreasing level of consciousness. By reporting this information, the emergency department can arrange for the trauma team, including a neurosurgeon, to meet you in the ED upon arrival. In such cases, good communication results in good patient care.

You must interact effectively with everyone involved in the call to coordinate a unified effort resulting in top-quality patient care. EMS is the ultimate team endeavor. Your performance as a paramedic is just one component in a series of interactions that ensure continuous first-rate care. From the call taker to the rehabilitation specialist, every player in this continuum is equally important—only their roles differ. Communication is not merely one aspect of an EMS response; it is the key link in the chain that results in the best possible patient outcome. Effective communication optimizes patient care during every phase of the EMS response.

Communication is the key link in the chain that results in the best possible patient outcome.

BASIC COMMUNICATION MODEL

Communication is the process of exchanging information between individuals. It begins when you have an idea, or message, you would like to convey to someone else. You then encode that information in the language best suited for the situation. This might include words, numbers, symbols, or special codes. For instance, if you wanted to describe an accident scene to the medical direction physician, you would choose words that "paint a clear picture" of what you saw. In some systems, we communicate via code words. For example, 10-80 might mean a motor vehicle crash.

After you have encoded your message, you select the medium for sending it. You can speak face-to-face, send a fax, leave a voice message, send a letter or electronic mail (E-mail), or speak directly via telephone or radio. You might encode your message and send it via a paging system that posts either words or numbers; some pagers allow you to speak your message. Next, the intended receiver must decode and understand your message. Finally, he must give you feedback to confirm that he received your message and understood it. Consider the following example of an effective radio communication:

Dispatcher: Control to Unit 192, respond priority 1 to 483 County Route 22, cross street Canfield Road, on a possible heart.

* **communication** the process of exchanging information between individuals.

Content Review

BASIC COMMUNICATIONS MODEL

1. Sender has an idea, or message.
2. Sender encodes message.
3. Sender sends message.
4. Receiver receives message.
5. Receiver decodes message.
6. Receiver gives feedback to sender.

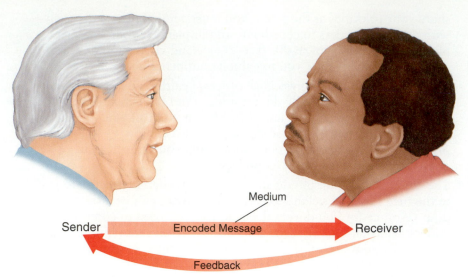

FIGURE 5-1 Communication occurs when individuals exchange information through an encoded message.

> *Unit 192:* Control, Unit 192 copy, responding priority 1 to 483 County Route 22.
> *Dispatcher:* Unit 192 responding, 1228 hours.

In this simple example, the sender (dispatcher) encodes his message in a language that he knows the receiver (Unit 192) will understand. Unit 192 receives the message and acknowledges by repeating the key data. Finally, the sender confirms and concludes the communication (Figure 5-1).

VERBAL COMMUNICATION

✱ **semantic** related to the meaning of words.

✱ **10-code** radio communications system using codes that begin with the word *ten*.

Factors that can enhance or impede effective communication may be either **semantic** (the meaning of words) or technical (communications hardware). Communication requires a mutual language. For example, a city unit and a county unit that use different **10-code** systems will find it difficult to communicate effectively. A 10-10 may mean a working fire in one system and a cardiac emergency in another. Thus, many EMS systems have changed from using 10-codes to plain English.

When reporting your patient's condition to the medical direction physician, you should use terminology that is widely accepted by both the medical and emergency services communities. Using a 10-code system with which the ED staff is unfamiliar would be inappropriate. Telling the medical direction physician that you have a victim of a 10-21-Golf (assault with a gun) may be meaningless. Conversely, if the medical direction physician asks you for your pregnant patient's EDC (due date) or her LMP (last menstrual period) and you do not know those acronyms, you have failed to communicate. The receiver must be able to decode the sender's message.

Your communication network must consist of reliable equipment designed to afford clear communication among all agencies within the system.

Your communication network must consist of reliable equipment designed to afford clear communication among all agencies within the system. This becomes a challenge in systems that cover large geographical areas or where terrain interferes with transmission and reception. If you want to communicate with a unit clear across the county but your radio is not powerful enough to transmit that far, communication will be difficult, if not impossible. A system that covers

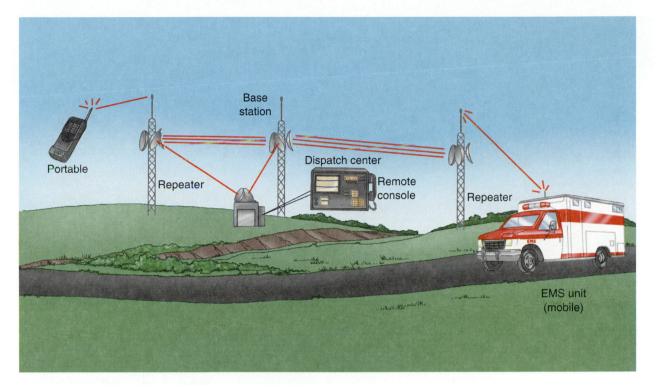

FIGURE 5-2   Example of an EMS system using repeaters.

a large geographical expanse can place repeaters strategically throughout its service area. These devices receive transmissions from a low-powered source and rebroadcast them at a higher power (Figure 5-2).

Your regional EMS system may consist of many agencies that have conducted business for decades on different **radio bands** and **frequencies.** City units may transmit on **ultrahigh frequency** (UHF) radio waves because they penetrate concrete and steel well and are less susceptible to interference. County units may use a low band frequency because those waves travel farther and better over varied terrain. In any event, communicating between agencies will be difficult unless all units share a common frequency. This is rarely the case. The spectrum of communications equipment currently ranges from antiquated radios to mobile data terminals mounted inside emergency vehicles. Geographically integrating communications networks would enable routine and reliable communication among EMS, fire, law enforcement, and other public safety agencies. This would in turn facilitate coordinated responses during both routine and large-scale operations. Developing the necessary hardware (equipment and network) and software (language) will be essential to improving emergency communications.

* **radio band** a range of radio frequencies.

* **radio frequency** the number of times per minute a radio wave oscillates.

* **ultrahigh frequency** radio frequency band from 300 to 3,000 megahertz.

WRITTEN COMMUNICATION

Written records are another important aspect of EMS communications. Your **prehospital care report** (PCR) is a written record of events that includes administrative information such as times, location, agency, and crew, as well as medical information. It will be used by hospital staff, agency administrators, system quality-assurance/improvement committees, insurance and billing departments, researchers, educators, and lawyers. The data collected from your PCR can help to monitor and improve patient care through medical audits, research, education, and system policy changes. Furthermore, your written documentation

* **prehospital care report (PCR)** the written record of an EMS response.

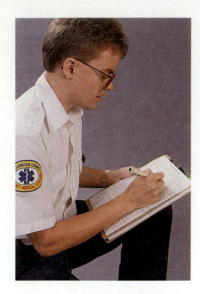

FIGURE 5-3 The prehospital care report is as important as the run itself. Complete it promptly, accurately, and legibly.

Using industry terminology appropriately provides a common means of communicating with other emergency care professionals.

becomes a legal record of the incident and may become part of your patient's permanent medical record. All legal rules regarding confidentiality and disclosure pertain to your PCR.

The same factors that influence verbal communication also affect written communication. Be objective, write legibly, thoroughly document your patient's assessment and care, and use terminology that is widely accepted in the medical community (Figure 5-3). Finally, your PCR illustrates your professionalism. A sloppy, incomplete PCR suggests sloppy, inefficient care. The chapter on documentation deals with PCRs and other written communications in much greater detail.

TERMINOLOGY

Every industry develops its own terminology. Doing so makes communication within the industry more clear, concise, and unambiguous. The airline industry, for example, uses the term *payload* to describe the total weight of everything (passengers, fuel, luggage, and other items) on an airplane. Musical composers and arrangers use words like *fortissimo, allegro,* and *a cappella* to describe a specific tempo or style.

The medical field also uses an extensive list of terms, acronyms, and abbreviations that allow quick, accurate communication of complex information. (The documentation chapter includes an extensive table of standard charting abbreviations.) An emergency physician may request a CBC (complete blood count), ABGs (arterial blood gases), or a CIP (cardiac injury profile)—common terms describing diagnostic tests run on acutely ill patients. The emergency services industry has further developed its own terms for radio communication (Table 5-1). These words or phrases shorten air time and transmit thoughts and ideas quickly. For example, *copy, 10-4,* and *roger* mean "I heard you and I understand what you said." Using industry terminology appropriately is an important part of effective communication. It provides a common means of communicating with other emergency care professionals.

Table 5-1	COMMON RADIO TERMINOLOGY
Term	**Meaning**
Copy, 10-4, roger	I understand
Affirmative	Yes
Negative	No
Stand by	Please wait
Repeat	Please repeat what you said
Land-line	Telephone communications
Rendezvous	Meet with
LZ	Landing zone (helicopter)
ETA	Estimated time of arrival
Over	I am finished with my transmission
Mobile status	On the air, driving around
Stage	Wait before entering a scene
Clear	End of transmission
Unfounded	We cannot find the incident/patient
Be advised	Listen carefully to this

THE EMS RESPONSE

Your ability to communicate effectively during a stressful EMS response will determine the success or failure of your efforts. A brilliant assessment and management plan will be futile if you cannot communicate it to others. Dealing effectively with your patient and bystanders requires a variety of communication skills such as empathy, confidence, self-control, authority, and patience. Your clinical experience will suggest which skills to use in any particular situation. For example, you might use confidence and an authoritative posture when dealing with unruly bystanders. On the other hand, you would need to be gentle and empathetic with a child or an elderly grandmother. If you were in charge of an incident, you would have to communicate your authority within the structure of the emergency scene to providers from other responding agencies. Delegating tasks, listening to initial reports, and coordinating the scene require effective communication and interpersonal skills.

The sequence of an EMS response illustrates the importance of communications in prehospital care. A typical EMS response includes the following chain of events.

Detection and Citizen Access To begin the response to any emergency once it has occurred, someone must detect the problem and summon EMS (Figure 5-4). Any citizen with an urgent medical need should have a simple and reliable mechanism for accessing the EMS system. In the United States, most people access EMS by telephone; thus, a well-publicized universal telephone number such as 911 provides direct citizen access to the communications center. At enhanced 911 (E-911) communication centers, a computer displays the caller's telephone number and location. The centers also have instant call-back capabilities, should the caller hang up too soon. The 911 system has been available since the late 1960s. Currently, 78 percent of households in the United States enjoy a 911 system. Highway call boxes, citizens band (CB) radio, and amateur radio all provide alternate means of accessing emergency help in some regions.

Calls to 911 usually connect the caller to a public safety access point (**PSAP**), which then directs the caller to the appropriate agency for dispatch and response. In some systems, the PSAP call taker will elicit the information and determine the

A brilliant assessment and management plan will be futile if you cannot communicate it to others.

✳ **PSAP** public safety access point.

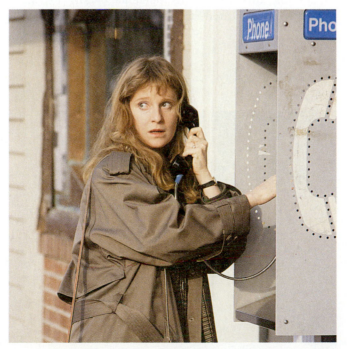

FIGURE 5-4 The response begins when someone detects an emergency and summons EMS support.

nature of the response. In others, he will simply answer with the question, "Is this a police, fire, or medical emergency?" and transfer the caller to the appropriate dispatcher, who will then elicit the information. Many systems use computerized technology at the PSAP to connect the caller automatically with the appropriate agency. Some even provide language translation. Future global positioning systems will allow the dispatcher to pinpoint a cellular-phone caller's location. Additionally, automakers are installing communications computers in some automobiles. When involved in an accident, these "black boxes" automatically will provide the dispatcher with the location, speed, type of collision, projected damage, and suspected severity of injury.

In some systems, all public safety agencies are located within the same facility. In others, they are connected electronically. No one way is best. If the public receives timely, appropriate responses to all emergency calls, the system is effective.

Call Taking and Emergency Response The emergency medical dispatcher (**EMD**) is the public's first contact with the EMS system and plays a crucial role in every EMS response. The most important information the call taker must obtain is the address of the incident, the caller's name, the call-back number, and other pertinent factors. Ideally, he also will ascertain the nature of the emergency and other pertinent factors.

In a coordinated system known as **priority dispatching,** medical dispatchers interrogate a distressed caller using a set of medically-approved questions to elicit essential information about the chief complaint (Figure 5-5). Then, the dispatcher follows established guidelines to determine the appropriate level of response (Figure 5-6). These predetermined guidelines are based on criteria approved by the medical director. For example, an elderly man with a history of heart problems who is complaining of chest pain radiating to his left arm may indicate a priority-one response (life-threatening emergency, lights and siren). In some systems, the appropriate response may include a fire-department basic-life-support first responding unit, a paramedic engine company, and a transporting ambulance. Other systems may require only a paramedic ambulance. This form of call-screening, when done appropriately, saves time and money because only the necessary resources are sent. It also limits the liability associated with lights and siren response to possible life-threatening incidents. Many private and public EMS systems throughout the United States use the priority dispatching system.

* **EMD** emergency medical dispatcher.

* **priority dispatching** system using medically-approved questions and predetermined guidelines to determine the appropriate level of response.

FIGURE 5-5 Priority dispatching and pre-arrival medical instruction have enhanced the efficiency of the EMS system.

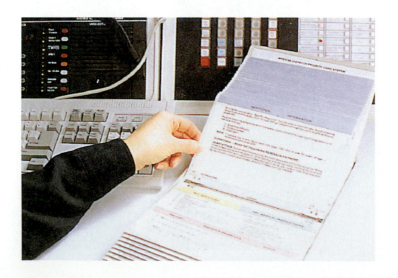

Prearrival Instructions Many EMS systems provide **prearrival instructions**, a service that is considered the standard of care. Prearrival instructions complement the call screening process in a priority dispatch system. As the dispatcher sends the appropriate response, the caller remains on the line and receives prearrival instructions for suitable emergency measures such as cardiopulmonary resuscitation or hemorrhage control. During prearrivals, the dispatcher also can obtain further information for the responding units. In the case of cardiac arrest, the dispatcher can relay information concerning the presence of a living will, a "Do Not Resuscitate" (DNR) form, or other advanced directives. In another case, a unit en route to a baby who had stopped breathing could reduce their response speed if they learned that the child had started breathing and was conscious. Prearrival instructions have saved many lives since 1974. They also are useful for comforting a distressed caller or providing emotional support to bystanders, family members, or the patient himself.

Call Coordination and Incident Recording After sending the appropriate response and providing prearrival instructions, the emergency medical dispatcher's main duties are support and coordination. He will provide the responding units with any additional resources needed and record information about the call such as times, locations, and units involved. Your dispatcher can be your best friend. He can assign the resources you need to manage an incident—additional medical personnel to help with a cardiac arrest, for instance, or the fire department to provide specialized rescue. He also may facilitate communication with other agencies, hospitals, communication centers, and support services.

Discussion with Medical Direction Physician After conducting your assessment and initiating care as outlined by your local protocols, you will contact the medical direction physician to discuss the case. Following consultation, he may give you further orders for interventions such as medications or other medical procedures. The many ways to conduct this communication include the radio, telephone, and cellular phone. Taping these communications for use later is advisable. For example, if a discrepancy arose as to your orders, you could always refer to the tape, which never lies. At this point, you continue treatment and prepare your patient for transport. You will contact your dispatcher, who will record when you leave the scene and when you arrive at your destination.

Your professional relationship with your medical direction physicians must be based on trust. Transmitting clear, concise, controlled reports will encourage your medical direction physicians to accept your assessments and on-scene treatment plans. Your ability to communicate effectively on the radio will cast a large part of your professional reputation. The general radio procedures and standard

Transmitting clear, concise, controlled reports will encourage your medical direction physicians to trust your assessments and on-scene treatment plans.

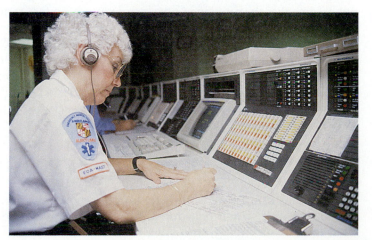

FIGURE 5-6 The dispatcher determines the appropriate level of response according to established guidelines.

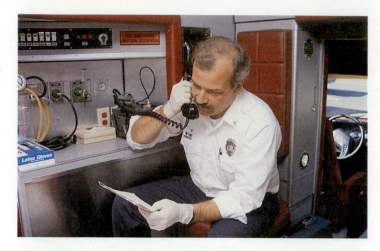

FIGURE 5-7 You will discuss each case with the medical direction physician and follow his instructions for patient care.

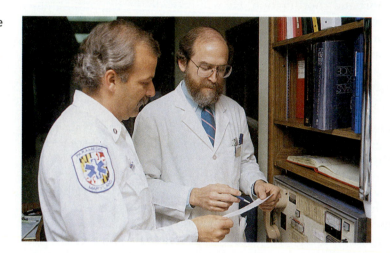

FIGURE 5-8 On arrival at the emergency department, you will give receiving personnel a formal, verbal briefing.

Never leave your patient until you formally transfer responsibility for his care.

format sections later in this chapter offer guidelines for communicating with your medical direction physician and transmitting patient information (Figure 5-7).

Transfer Communications As you transfer care of your patient to the receiving facility staff, you must give the receiving nurse or physician a formal verbal briefing (Figure 5-8). This report should include your patient's vital information, chief complaint and history, physical exam findings, and any treatments rendered. Do not assume that the receiving nurse heard your radio report and knows of your patient. Some systems require the receiving nurse to sign the prehospital care report (PCR) to verify and document the transfer of care. In any case, never leave your patient until you have completed some type of formal transfer of care, because you may be charged with abandonment. Many systems likewise require the medical direction physician to sign the PCR for any medications administered by paramedics, especially if they included controlled substances such as morphine or diazepam. In all cases, end your documentation with transfer of care information on your PCR.

COMMUNICATION TECHNOLOGY

EMS systems can use all of today's various communication technologies. These include the more traditional forms of radio communication as well as innovations in radio technology and other media.

RADIO COMMUNICATION

Many types of radio transmission are possible, with new technologies being developed every day. Usage may vary from system to system. This section discusses some of the more common technologies in use today.

Simplex The most basic communications systems use **simplex** transmissions. These systems transmit and receive on the same frequency and thus cannot do both simultaneously (Figure 5-9). After you transmit a message, you must release the transmit button and wait for a response. This slows communication because you have to wait for all traffic to stop before you can speak. It also makes the system more formal and prevents open discussion. Simplex communication systems are most effective on the scene, when the incident commander or EMS dispatcher must transmit orders or directions without interruption. Most dispatch systems and on-scene communications use simplex transmissions.

Duplex **Duplex** transmissions allow simultaneous two-way communications by using two frequencies for each channel (Figure 5-10). Each radio must be able to transmit and receive on each channel. For example, on channel one, a hospital base station might transmit on 468.000 megahertz (MHz) and receive on

✳ **simplex** communication system that transmits and receives on the same frequency.

✳ **duplex** communication system that allows simultaneous two-way communications by using two frequencies for each channel.

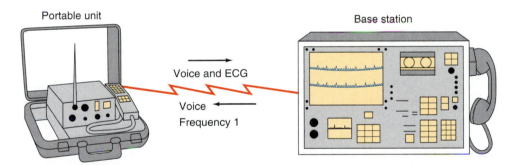

FIGURE 5-9   Simplex communications systems transmit and receive on the same frequency.

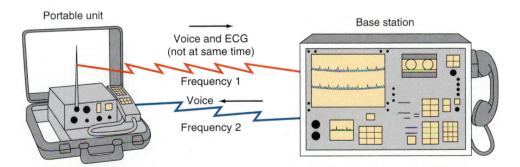

FIGURE 5-10   Duplex communications systems use two frequencies for each channel.

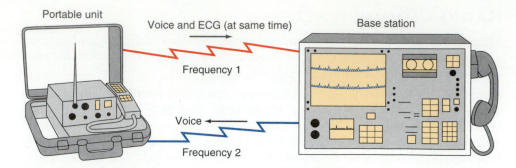

Portable unit

Voice and ECG (at same time) →

Base station

Frequency 1

Voice ←

Frequency 2

FIGURE 5-11 Multiplex systems can transmit voice and data at the same time.

478.000 MHz. Field radios would then transmit on 478.000 MHz and receive on 468.000 MHz—just the opposite. Either party could then transmit and receive on the same channel simultaneously.

Duplex systems work like telephone communications. Many areas use them for communications between the field paramedic and the medical direction physician. The duplex system's major advantage is that one party does not have to wait to speak until the other party finishes his transmission. This allows a much freer discussion and consultation between physician and paramedic. For example, the medical direction physician can interrupt your report with an important question or concern. On the other hand, this ability to interrupt can be a disadvantage when abused.

Duplex systems all allow you to transmit either voice messages or data such as ECG strips.

Multiplex Multiplex systems are duplex systems with the additional capability of transmitting voice and data simultaneously (Figure 5-11). This enables you to carry on a conversation with the medical direction physician while you are transmitting an ECG strip. Speaking while you are transmitting the ECG strip, however, causes much interference on the ECG strip.

✱ multiplex duplex system that can transmit voice and data simultaneously.

Trunking Many communications systems operating in the 800 MHz range use **trunking** to hasten communications. Trunked systems pool all frequencies. When a radio transmission comes in, a computer routes it to the first available frequency. The computer routes the next transmission to the next available frequency, and so on. When a transmission terminates, that frequency becomes available and reenters the pool of unused frequencies. Trunking thus frees the dispatcher or field unit from having to search for an available frequency.

✱ trunking communication system that pools all frequencies and routes transmissions to the next available frequency.

Digital Communications Voice transmission can be time-consuming and difficult to understand. The trend toward combining radio technology with computer technology has encouraged a shift from voice (analog) to **digital communications**. Digital radio equipment is becoming increasingly popular in emergency services communication systems. This technology translates, or encodes, sounds into digital code for broadcast. Digital transmission is much faster and much more accurate than analog transmission. Since the messages are transmitted in condensed form, they help to ease the overcrowding of radio frequencies. Also, because you need a decoder to translate digital transmissions back into voice, scanners cannot monitor them. Your communications, therefore, are considerably more secure than over the radio. Many cellular phone companies now

✱ digital communications data or sounds are translated into a digital code for transmission.

use digital transmissions. Future technology will link patient-monitoring devices to a small computer equipped with a radio for transmission.

The **mobile data terminals** in many emergency vehicles are a basic form of digital communications. They are mounted in the vehicle cab and wired to the radio. When a data transmission such as the address of the incident comes in, the terminal displays the message on a screen or prints it in hard copy. Responders can reply by punching a button to send a message such as "en route," "arrived," or "transporting to the hospital." Though somewhat restrictive and primitive, these terminals have reduced on-air time to a minimum even in the busiest systems. It is important to remember, however, that voice communications will always have a place in emergency services. Crews will always need to speak to one another, to physicians and nurses, or to dispatchers.

* **mobile data terminal** vehicle-mounted computer keyboard and display.

ALTERNATIVE TECHNOLOGIES

Among the more common alternatives to radio communications are the cellular telephone, the facsimile machine, and the computer.

Cellular Telephone Many EMS systems have found that **cellular telephones** are a cost-effective way to transmit essential patient information to the hospital (Figure 5-12). Cellular technology is available in even the most remote areas of the country. A cellular telephone service is divided into regions called cells. These cells are radio base stations, with which the mobile telephone communicates. When the transmission leaves one cell's range, another cell picks it up immediately, without interruption.

* **cellular telephone system** telephone system divided into regions, or cells, that are served by radio base stations.

Like duplex radio transmissions, cellular phones make communication less formal, promote discussion, and reduce on-line times. They further allow the medical direction physician to speak directly with the patient and offer the further advantages of being widely available and highly reliable. Because the ECG signal is digitized, the hospital receives a better signal than if it were transmitted over radio waves. The telephones themselves are inexpensive, but cellular telephone systems charge a monthly fee for their use. Their major disadvantage is that each cell can handle only a limited number of calls. Geography can interfere with the cellular telephone's signals, and in large metropolitan areas the cells often fill up and become unavailable, especially during peak hours. Other disadvantages are that anyone with a scanner can monitor conversations on analog cellular phones; cellular phones require an external antenna; and the cellular phone system will deny access to a cell if you do not know or forget the personal identification number (PIN). Despite their limitations, cellular telephones have become a popular medium for dispatching, on-scene, and medical direction communications.

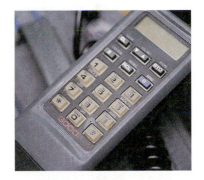

FIGURE 5-12 Cellular telephones have made it possible to transmit high quality facsimiles, computer data, and 12-lead ECGs.

Facsimile A **facsimile machine** (fax) provides a quick way to send printed information. This machine "reads" the printed information, digitizes it line-by-line, and transmits it to another machine, which then decodes it and prints a facsimile of the original. A fax machine enables health care agencies to exchange medical information immediately. Future systems will allow EMS responders to access a patient's medical record from a general data base; responders or database operators will be able to send the same information to the receiving facility. With some electronic run sheet systems, you will be able to transmit your patient information to the receiving hospital long before you arrive. This technology's one obvious limitation is that both the sending and the receiving agency must have access to a fax machine and a telephone line.

* **facsimile machine** device for electronically transmitting and receiving printed information.

Computer Computers have entered every aspect of our daily lives. In emergency services communications, they have revolutionized system management and incident data collection. Most dispatchers no longer enter data via pen and pencil, time stamping machines, or typewriters. They can make a permanent record of any incident's events in real time. Computers also make research faster and easier. For example, if you wanted to determine the day of the week when most cardiac calls happen, or what time of day is busiest, or which area of a city needs more coverage, you could retrieve the pertinent data from your computerized records immediately. You can program your system to provide whatever type of data you want, in whatever format you desire. It also eliminates the need to enter retrospective data when conducting research. For example, the times, locations, and particulars of a call already will be in the computer files for immediate retrieval during a research project. A computer's limitations include its own power, speed, and capacity, as well as its operator's ability. Also, rigidly programmed machines that function only in certain restrictive ways can limit your flexibility.

New Technology

New technology is being developed every day. The National Aeronautics and Space Administration (NASA) has pioneered communications that allow television viewers to hear and see astronauts in space. Ground crews can monitor each astronaut's biological function and maintain a permanent record throughout the trip. And they have been doing this for decades.

In comparison to other industries, public safety communication systems are nearly archaic. Most EMS agencies still document patient assessment and care with hand-written run sheets, and some use radio equipment so old that replacement tubes are no longer available. But times are changing rapidly. Time constraints, storage space, and congested radio traffic necessitate developing new systems that will allow paramedics to transmit, receive, and store vital patient information quickly and reliably. Someday computer-based technology, digital satellite transmission, and electronic storage and retrieval of patient information will replace radio communications, written documentation, and file cabinets filled with EMS run sheets. These technologies are costly, but they already exist.

* **touch pad** computer on which you enter data by touching areas of the display screen.

Current documentation systems already allow you to record all aspects of your EMS response electronically, by use of a **touch pad.** With pen-based reporting systems you can record patient information on a handheld computer. These systems do away with written documentation and capture information in real time, eliminating your need to estimate times after the call. Some systems integrate diagnostic technology and enable you to transmit ECG and pulse oximetry readings to the hospital before arrival. Such advanced knowledge of diagnostic test results from the field may radically change a medical direction physician's decisions and reduce the time needed to make an in-hospital diagnosis and begin therapy. Transmitting a 12-lead ECG, for example, will reduce the time before paramedics in transit or receiving emergency department personnel can begin cardiac muscle-saving thrombolytic therapy for the patient with a suspected myocardial infarction. In some cases paramedics will be able to start therapy en route. Other systems allow you to receive important medical information from your patient's permanent record while on the scene or in transit. For instance, at the home of a patient with an altered mental status and no family to relate his history, you might access his medical records and attain his history via a computerized data base. In this type of system, the transferring facility, the receiving hospital, and you can all access this information simultaneously.

* **slander** to orally defame another person.

* **libel** to defame another person in writing.

A disadvantage of electronic recording systems is the absence of a "paper record" of the incident, should the information be accidentally erased or destroyed. The legal guidelines that apply to written and spoken communication also apply to electronic reporting. You must maintain patient confidentiality, you must be objective, and you must not **slander** or **libel** another person.

REPORTING PROCEDURES

As a paramedic, you must effectively relay all relevant medical information to the receiving hospital staff. Initially, you might do this over the radio or by cellular telephone. Later, when you deliver your patient to the emergency department, you can give additional information in-person to the appropriate receiving hospital personnel.

One of your most important skills will be gathering essential patient information, organizing it, and relaying it to the medical direction physician. The medical direction physician will then issue appropriate orders for patient care. The amount and type of information you relay to the medical direction physician will depend on the type of technology you use, your patient's priority, and your local communication **protocols**. For example, if communications in your region are not secured (private) you must limit the type of information you can communicate without breaching patient confidentiality. The acuteness of your patient's clinical status and the amount of local radio traffic also may determine the length of your report. For a critical patient you may give a brief report while you tend to your patient's medical needs. For a complicated medical emergency, you may wish to communicate a greater share of the results of your history and physical exam to the medical direction physician.

> *One of your most important skills will be gathering essential patient information, organizing it, and relaying it to the medical direction physician.*
>

* **protocol** predetermined, written guidelines for patient care.

STANDARD FORMAT

Communicating patient information to the hospital or to the medical direction physician is a crucial function within the EMS system. Verbal communications, which may occur via radio or land-line, give the hospital enough information on your patient's condition to prepare for his care. These communications also should initiate the medical orders you need to treat your patient in the field. A standard format for transmitting patient assessment information helps to achieve those goals in several ways. First, it adds to the medical communications system's efficiency. Second, it helps the physician to assimilate information about the patient's condition quickly. Third, it assures that medical information is complete. In general, your verbal reports to medical direction should include the following information:

- Identification of unit and provider
- Description of scene
- Patient's age, sex, and approximate weight (for drug orders)
- Patient's chief complaint and severity
- Brief, pertinent history of the present illness or injury (OPQRST)
- Pertinent past medical history, medications, and allergies (SAMPLE)
- Pertinent physical exam findings
- Treatment given so far/request for orders
- Estimated time of arrival at the hospital
- Other pertinent information

The formats and contents of reports for medical and trauma patients differ to include only the information relevant to either type of emergency. Reports for medical patients emphasize the history in the beginning of the report; reports for trauma patients emphasize the injuries and the physical exam.

After transmitting your report, you will await further questions and orders from the medical direction physician. Upon arrival, your spoken report will give essential patient information to the provider assuming care. It should include a brief history, pertinent physical findings, treatment, and responses to that treatment.

GENERAL RADIO PROCEDURES

Using the radio properly will make your communications skillful and efficient. All of your transmissions must be clear and crisp, with concise, professional content (Figure 5-13). Always follow these guidelines for effective radio use:

1. Listen to the channel before transmitting to assure that it is not in use.
2. Press the transmit button for one second before speaking.
3. Speak at close range, approximately two–three inches, directly into, or across the face of, the microphone.
4. Speak slowly and clearly. Pronounce each word distinctly, avoiding words that are difficult to understand.
5. Speak in a normal pitch, keeping your voice free of emotion.
6. Be brief. Know what you are going to say before you press the transmit button.
7. Avoid codes unless they are part of your EMS system.
8. Do not waste air time with unnecessary information.
9. Protect your patient's privacy. When appropriate:
   - Use telephone rather than radio.
   - Turn off external speaker.
   - Do not use your patient's name; doing so violates FCC regulations.
10. Use proper unit or hospital numbers, and correct names or titles.
11. Do not use slang or profanity.
12. Use standard formats for transmission.
13. Be concise in order to hold the attention of the person receiving your radio report.
14. Use the **echo procedure** when receiving directions from the dispatcher or orders from the physician. Immediately repeating each statement will confirm accurate reception and understanding.
15. Always write down addresses, important dispatch communications, and physician orders.
16. When completing a transmission, obtain confirmation that your message was received and understood.

✱ **echo procedure** immediately repeating each transmission received during radio communications.

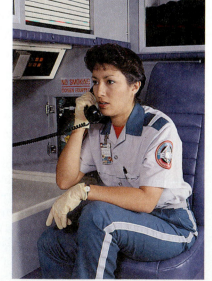

FIGURE 5-13   The professionalism of your communications reflects on the professionalism of your patient care.

Occasionally, communications equipment will not function properly. Even a weak battery can disrupt clear communication. If you are far from the base station, particularly if you have a portable radio, try to broadcast from higher terrain. Structures that contain steel and concrete can interfere with radio transmission. Simply moving outside the building or near a window may improve communications. If that does not work, try to telephone.

MODEL VERBAL REPORTS

The following examples demonstrate professional verbal reports for a medical patient and for a trauma patient. Neither report takes more than forty-five seconds, and each gives the medical direction physician enough information to make an initial diagnosis and prepare for arrival. As you read them, consider how they follow the principles of effective communication discussed throughout this chapter, and note their differences in format and information.

Medical Patient

Paramedic Identification:	This is NAVAC ambulance 4, Paramedic Smith.
Patient Identification:	We have a 63-year-old, 70-kg alert male, patient of Dr. Welby.
Subjective Data:	He complains of sudden onset of substernal chest pain radiating to the neck for the past half hour. He also complains of shortness of breath and nausea. He has a past history of cardiac problems and takes nitroglycerin, Isordil, and Procardia XL.
Objective Data:	He appears in moderate distress at this time, clutching his chest, but able to speak in full sentences. Vitals: BP—138/80; pulse—88 and regular; respirations 24 and slightly labored; skin warm and dry. He has clear lung sounds bilaterally, no JVD, peripheral edema or ascites. ECG shows sinus rhythm with an occasional unifocal PVC. Pulse oximetry is 92% on room air.
Plan:	We have him on oxygen at 15 liters-per-minute via nonrebreather mask, we have a saline lock in place, and have given him 2 baby aspirin and 3 nitros with no relief. Request permission to administer 1–3 milligrams of morphine IV until relief of pain. Our ETA is 20 minutes.

Content Review

ELEMENTS OF MEDICAL PATIENT REPORT
- Paramedic identification
- Patient identification
- Subjective data
- Objective data
- Plan

Trauma Patient

Paramedic Identification:	This is DeWitt Rescue 7, Paramedic Jones.
Patient Identification:	We have a 23-year-old unresponsive female.
Mechanism of Injury:	She was the unbelted driver in a high-speed, head-on one-car versus telephone pole accident with severe damage to the car and intrusion into the passenger compartment.

Content Review

ELEMENTS OF TRAUMA PATIENT REPORT
- Paramedic identification
- Patient identification
- Mechanism of injury
- Injuries
- Plan

Injuries: She has a major head and chest trauma and shows signs of decompensated shock. Vitals are BP—76 by palpation; pulse—120 weak and regular, carotid only; respirations 40 and shallow; skin cool, pale, and clammy. She has a depressed skull fracture in the left parietal region, and a right-sided flail chest. Her pupils are unequal and slow to react, no drainage from the ears or nose, no Battle's sign or raccoon's eyes. Trachea is midline, no JVD. She shows paradoxical chest wall movement and is cyanotic with diminished lung sounds on the right side. Pulse oximetry is 88% on room air.

Plan: We have the patient fully immobilized, have stabilized the flail segment and are assisting ventilation with a bag-valve mask and supplemental oxygen. We have an IV of normal saline running wide open and are starting a second line. Our ETA is 20 minutes.

REGULATION

* **Federal Communications Commission** agency that controls all nongovernmental communications in the United States.

* **very high frequency** radio frequency band from 30 to 300 megahertz

The **Federal Communications Commission** (FCC) controls and regulates all nongovernmental communications in the United States. This includes AM and FM radio, television, aircraft, marine, and mobile land frequency ranges. The FCC has designated frequencies within each radio band for special use. They include public safety frequencies in both the **very high frequency** band (VHF) and the ultrahigh frequency band (UHF). The FCC's primary functions include:

* Licensing and allocating radio frequencies.
* Establishing technical standards for radio equipment.
* Licensing and regulating the technical personnel who repair and operate radio equipment.
* Monitoring frequencies to assure appropriate usage.
* Spot-checking base stations and dispatch centers for appropriate licenses and records.

The FCC requires all EMS communications systems to follow appropriate governmental regulations and laws. You must stay abreast of and obey any FCC regulations that apply to your communications.

SUMMARY

As one of the fundamental aspects of prehospital care, accurate communications help ensure an EMS system's efficiency. Communications begin when the citizen accesses the EMS system and end when you complete your patient report. Your spoken messages must be understandable, and your written messages must be legible. All of your communications must be concise and complete and conform to national and local protocols. The more sophisticated and advanced your EMS system grows, the more sophisticated and advanced its communications—and, accordingly, your communications skills—must become.

YOU MAKE THE CALL

A call comes into your unit for a "possible heart attack" on State Route 11. You and your partner climb into Palermo Rescue, a nontransport first-response vehicle. Your response time is about ten minutes. Upon arrival, a family member meets you. He leads you into the den of a small farm house. Here you see your patient sitting in an overstuffed chair. You note that your patient is a 69-year-old male in obvious distress.

You begin questioning your patient to develop a history. As he speaks, you immediately notice that he has difficulty breathing. He complains of severe chest pain, which began about 30 minutes ago. With his hand, he indicates that the pain is pressure-like and substernal. He also indicates that it radiates to his left arm and jaw. He describes a history of heart disease, including two prior heart attacks. Three years ago, he had cardiac bypass surgery. He currently takes Lanoxin, Lasix, Capoten, and an aspirin a day. He is allergic to Mellaril.

You and your partner complete your assessment. Your patient says he weighs about 250 pounds. He is alert, but anxious. He exhibits jugular venous distention and bibasilar crackles. His abdomen is nontender. His distal pulses are good. Vital signs include: blood pressure 210/110 mmHg, pulse of 70 per minute and regular, and respirations of 20 breaths per minute and mildly labored. Pulse oximetry is 93% on supplemental oxygen. During your assessment, your patient becomes progressively more dyspneic. The transporting ambulance arrives and the paramedic asks you to give a radio report to the receiving hospital based on your assessment while she prepares her patient for transport.

- Based on the information above, organize and prepare your radio report to inform the receiving hospital of your patient's condition.

See Suggested Responses at the back of this book.

FURTHER READING

Clawson, Jeff J. "Emergency Medical Dispatch." In *Principles of EMS Systems,* 2nd ed., edited by W.R. Roush, 263–289. Dallas: American College of Emergency Physicians, 1994.

Clawson, Jeff J., and Kate Dernocoeur. *Principles of Emergency Medical Dispatch.* Englewood Cliffs, N.J.: Brady, 1988.

Delbridge, Theodore R., and Paul Paris. "EMS Communications." In *Principles of EMS Systems,* 2nd ed., edited by W.R. Roush, 245–261. Dallas: American College of Emergency Physicians, 1994.

Mackay, Michele. "Bandwidths, Frequencies, and Megahertz." *JEMS* 22 (May 1997): 42–49.

Marshall, Loren. "Electronic Visions: The Future of EMS Communications Is Now." *JEMS* 19 (March 1994): 54–63.

Stanford, Todd M. *EMS Report Writing: A Pocket Reference.* Englewood Cliffs, N.J.: Brady, 1992.

Steele, Susi B. *Emergency Dispatching: A Medical Communicator's Guide.* Englewood Cliffs, N.J.: Brady, 1993.

Stratton, Samuel J. "Triage by Emergency Medical Dispatchers." *Prehospital and Disaster Medicine* 7 (July-September 1992): 263–268.

ON THE WEB

Visit Brady's Paramedic Website at www.bradybooks.com/paramedic.

CHAPTER 6

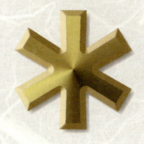

Documentation

Objectives

After reading this chapter, you should be able to:

1. Identify the general principles regarding the importance of EMS documentation and ways in which documents are used. (pp. 272–274)
2. Identify and properly use medical terminology, medical abbreviations, and acronyms. (pp. 275,277–285)
3. Explain the role of documentation in agency reimbursement. (p. 274)
4. Identify and eliminate extraneous or nonprofessional information. (p. 290)
5. Describe the differences between subjective and objective elements of documentation. (pp. 290–292)
6. Evaluate a finished document for errors and omissions and proper use and spelling of abbreviations and acronyms. (pp. 287,289-290)
7. Evaluate the confidential nature of an EMS report. (p. 300)
8. Describe the potential consequences of illegible, incomplete, or inaccurate documentation. (pp. 287,289-300)

Continued

9. Describe the special documentation considerations concerning patient refusal of care and/or transport. (pp. 296–297)

10. Demonstrate how to properly record direct patient or bystander comments. (p. 286)

11. Describe the special considerations concerning mass casualty incident documentation. (pp. 298-299)

12. Demonstrate proper document revision and correction. (pp. 289-290)

13. Given a prehospital care report form and a narrative patient care scenario, record all pertinent administrative information using a consistent format, identify and record the pertinent, reportable clinical data for each patient, correct errors and omissions, using proper procedures, and note and record "pertinent negative" clinical findings. (pp. 272–300)

CASE STUDY

Tom Brewster is nervous. He has never been to a deposition before, and though everyone has assured him that he is not the target of any legal action, he has to wonder what the lawyers want from him.

As he sits outside the conference room, he goes over the call in his head. It was about 2:30 in the morning. He and Eric Billings, his partner, had just finished cleaning up from a GI bleeder when they were dispatched to the single vehicle crash. The driver had gone off the left side of the road, crossed a ditch, and smashed into a tree. He had been lucky. He was out of the car, standing on the side of the road, and did not seem to have any serious injuries. He told Tom and Eric, "I think I'm fine, I just fell asleep and ran off the road." Still, they had performed an initial assessment followed by a rapid trauma assessment, immobilized the man, administered oxygen, and transported him to the emergency department. Tom rode in the back with the patient. On the way to the hospital he checked the glucose level, started an IV as a precaution, and applied a cardiac monitor.

"Everything was normal," Tom now thinks. "What did I miss?" He has reread his prehospital care report a hundred times. Though it has been three years, he now remembers almost every detail of the call. Until two weeks ago, he had almost completely forgotten about it. All too soon, the lawyers call

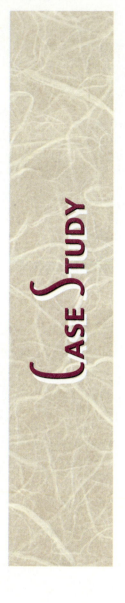

Tom into the conference room, introduce themselves, and swear him to honesty. One of the lawyers begins. "Do you recall the crash that occurred on the evening in question?"

"Yes, I do," Tom replies. He recounts that upon their arrival at the scene, the driver was out of the vehicle. Tom states that they managed him like any other trauma patient and he had no obvious injuries or indications of illness.

"Did the gentleman tell you he is diabetic?"

"No," Tom answers, "but we checked his blood sugar, and it was normal."

"Did he tell you he has heart problems?"

"No," Tom says again, "but we did put him on the heart monitor, and his rhythm was normal."

"Did he tell you he ran off the road because he passed out?"

"No, he told me he fell asleep." Tom feels better. He has the answer to every question, and he has the PCR to back him up.

After a few more questions, the lawyers dismiss Tom and allow him to leave. He has no idea what they were getting at, but he does know that he answered every question honestly. He wonders if he would have had all the answers if the case had been from six or eight years ago. He has really worked on his documentation in the last few years, and he knows he would have never remembered all those details without the help of his PCR.

Six weeks later Tom gets a letter from the lawyer thanking him for his testimony. It turns out the patient was suing his private doctor for not "recognizing his obvious diabetes and heart problems. He claimed these illnesses caused him to be involved in the motor vehicle accident, and it resulted in serious injury." Tom's testimony—and his PCR—have been pivotal in getting the case dismissed.

INTRODUCTION

Document exactly what you did, when you did it, and the effects of your interventions.

Your PCR reflects your professionalism.

In this age of litigation, treating your patient and documenting his care are separate but equally important duties. Your written **prehospital care report (PCR)** is the only truly factual record of events. When written correctly it accurately describes your assessment and care throughout the emergency call. It documents exactly what you did, when you did it, and the effects of your interventions. It can be your best friend or your worst enemy in a court proceeding.

Your PCR is your sole permanent, complete written record of events during the ambulance call. The dispatch center may have a record of the call times and audio tapes of radio transmissions, and your patient will have his memory of the call. You and other responders also may have some recollections about the call. Your PCR, however, will always be considered the most comprehensive and reliable record of the event. In addition, it reflects your professionalism. A well-written, thorough PCR suggests a thorough, efficient assessment and quality care. A sloppy, incomplete PCR suggests sloppy, inefficient care.

USES FOR DOCUMENTATION

Your PCR will be a valuable resource for a variety of people. They include medical professionals, EMS administrators, researchers, and occasionally, lawyers.

MEDICAL

Hospital staff (nurses and physicians) may need more information from you than they can get before you have to take another call. For example, they may want a chronological account of your patient's mental status from the time you arrived on the scene. Your PCR can tell the emergency department staff of your patient's condition before he arrived at the hospital. It serves as a baseline for comparing assessment findings and detecting trends that indicate improvement or deterioration. The surgical staff will want to know the mechanism of injury and other pertinent findings during your initial assessment of your patient and the scene.

If your patient is admitted to the hospital, the floor or intensive care unit staff may need more information about his original condition than he can remember. In addition, your PCR provides them with information from people at the scene to whom they might not have access—family, bystanders, first responders, or other witnesses. Knowing about the circumstances that led to the event or the mechanism of injury may also help rehabilitation specialists to provide better therapy. Your PCR becomes an important document that helps ensure your patient's continuous effective care (Figure 6-1).

* **Prehospital Care Report PCR** the written record of an EMS response.

Your PCR is an important document that helps ensure your patient's continuity of care.

Prehospital Care Report

Agency Name	ARLINGTON RESCUE		MILEAGE			
Dispatch Information	CARDIAC	END	2 4 4 9 6		CALL REC'D	0 7 0 5
		BEGIN	2 4 4 7 6		ENROUTE	0 7 0 7
Call Location	124 CYPRUS ST 2nd FLOOR	TOTAL	0 0 0 2 0		ARRIVED AT SCENE	0 7 1 9

USE MILITARY TIMES

CHECK ONE: ☑ Residence ☐ Health Facility ☐ Farm ☐ Indus. Facility ☐ Other Work Loc. ☐ Roadway ☐ Recreational ☐ Other

LOCATION CODE: 0 1 2 4

CALL TYPE AS REC'D	MECHANISM OF INJURY
☑ Emergency	☐ MVA (✓ seat belt used) N/A ☐ Knife
☐ Non-Emergency	☐ Fall of _____ feet ☐ Machinery
☐ Stand-by	☐ Unarmed assault ☐ _____
	☐ GSW

FROM SCENE: 0 7 3 8
AT DESTIN: 0 7 5 4
IN SERVICE: 0 8 1 0
IN QUARTERS: 0 8 3 2

FIGURE 6-1 The run data in a prehospital care report is vital to your agency's efforts to improve patient care.

ADMINISTRATIVE

EMS administrators must gather information for quality improvement and system management. Information regarding **response times,** call location, the use of lights and siren, and date and time is vital to evaluating your system's readiness to respond to life threatening emergencies. It also is essential to providing information of community needs. The quality improvement or quality assurance committee will use PCRs to identify problems with individual paramedics or with the EMS system. In some agencies, the billing department will need to determine which services are billable. Insurance carriers may need to know more about the illness or injury to process the claim. Some states will use your PCR data to allocate funding for regional systems.

RESEARCH

Your PCR provides the basis for continuously improving patient care in your EMS system.

Your PCR may give researchers useful data about many aspects of the EMS call. For example, they may analyze your recorded data to determine the efficacy of certain medical devices or interventions such as drugs and invasive procedures. They also may use the data to cut costs, alter staffing, and shorten response times. Some systems use computerized or electronic PCRs and a computerized database to analyze the data (Figure 6-2). Regardless of the method you use, your written documentation provides the basis for continuously improving patient care in your EMS system.

LEGAL

A complete, accurate, and objective account of the emergency call may be your best and only defense in court.

Your PCR becomes a permanent part of your patient's medical record. Lawyers may refer to it when preparing court actions, and in a legal proceeding it might be your sole source of information about the case. You may be called upon to testify in a case where your PCR becomes the central piece of evidence in your testimony. Or your PCR may serve as evidence in a criminal case and help determine the accused's innocence or guilt. Each state has its own laws regarding the length of time the hospital must keep its records.

Always write your PCR as if you knew you would have to refer to it someday in a court proceeding. Describe your patient's condition when you arrived and during your care, and note his status upon arrival at the hospital. Always document his condition before and after any interventions, and avoid writing any subjective opinions such as "the patient is intoxicated, obnoxious, and looks like a crack-addict." After your PCR is written, ask your partner to review it for completeness and accuracy. A complete, accurate, and objective account of the emergency call may be your best and only defense against a plaintiff's attorney who will try to find inconsistencies and ambiguities in your account.

GENERAL CONSIDERATIONS

Every EMS system has its own specific requirements for documentation. The type of call record used also varies from system to system. Some systems use reports with check boxes, some **bubble-sheets,** computer scannable reports

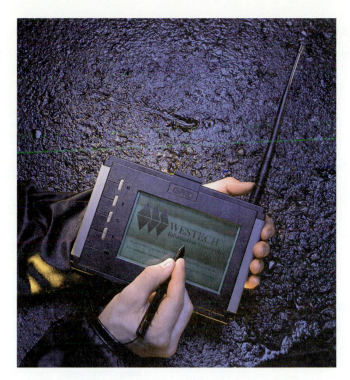

FIGURE 6-2 The handheld electronic clipboard enables you to enter your prehospital care report directly into a computer.

on which you record patient information by filling in boxes or "bubbles" (Figure 6-3 on next page). Still others may use computerized documentation. The particular type of operational data collected, such as time intervals, will also differ among systems. For example, proprietary EMS agencies may require more billing information than community-based volunteer agencies. The general characteristics of a well-written PCR, though, remain constant among all agencies and systems.

MEDICAL TERMINOLOGY

An essential component of good documentation is the appropriate use of medical terminology. Medical terms, though sometimes difficult to spell, transform your report into a universally accepted medical document. Learning the meanings and correct spellings of the medical terms that you will use in your PCRs is essential. Misused or misspelled words reflect poorly on your professionalism and may confuse the report's readers.

If you do not know how to spell a word, look it up or use another word. Many paramedics carry pocket-size medical dictionaries in their ambulances for this purpose. Using "plain English" is acceptable when you do not know the appropriate medical term or its correct spelling. "Chest" is just as accurate as "thorax" and better than "thoracks." "Belly" is not as professional as "abdomen," but it is still better than "abodemin."

ABBREVIATIONS AND ACRONYMS

Medical abbreviations and acronyms allow you to increase the amount of information you can write quickly on your report (Table 6-1 on pages that follow). They also pose problems, however, (*discussion continues following Table 6-1*)

Content Review

CHARACTERISTICS OF A WELL-WRITTEN PCR
- Appropriate medical terminology
- Correct abbreviations and acronyms
- Accurate, consistent times
- Thoroughly documented communications
- Pertinent negatives
- Relevant oral statements of witnesses, bystanders, and patient
- Complete identification of all additional resources and personnel

If you do not know how to spell a word, look it up or use another word.

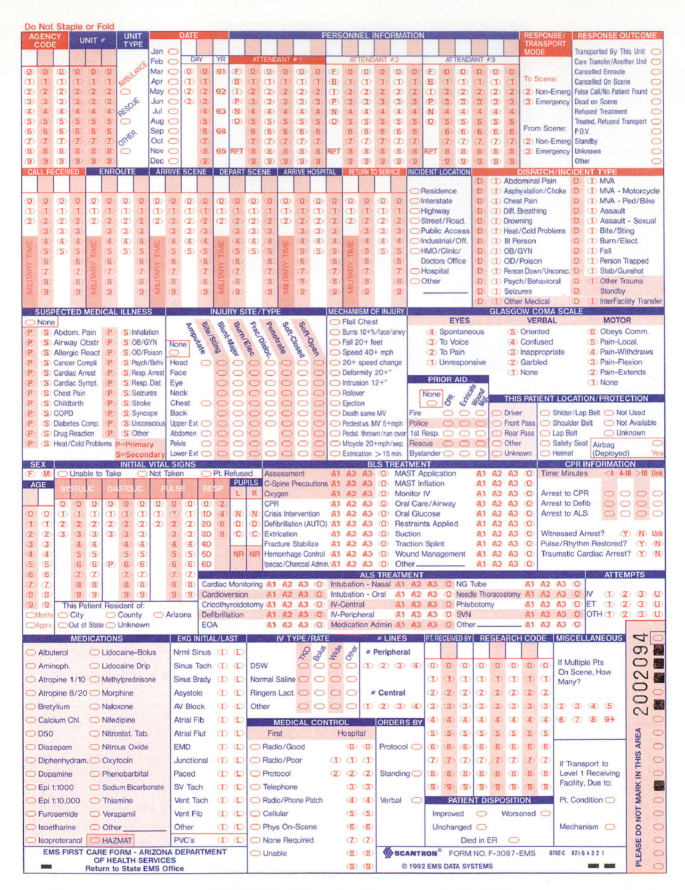

FIGURE 6-3 This prehospital care report's format allows a computer to scan its information.

Table 6-1	**STANDARD CHARTING ABBREVIATIONS**

Patient Information/Categories

Asian	A
Black	B
Chief complaint	CC
Complains of	c/o
Current health status	CHS
Date of birth	DOB
Differential diagnosis	DD
Estimated date of confinement	EDC
Family history	FH
Female	♀
Hispanic	H
History	Hx
History and physical	H&P
History of present illness	HPI
Impression	IMP
Male	♂
Medications	Med
Newborn	NB
Occupational history	OH
Past history	PH
Patient	Pt
Physical exam	PE
Private medical doctor	PMD
Review of systems	ROS
Signs and symptoms	S/S
Social history	SH
Visual acuity	VA
Vital signs	VS
Weight	Wt
White	W
Year-old	y/o

Body Systems

Abdomen	Abd
Cardiovascular	CV
Central nervous system	CNS
Ear, nose, and throat	ENT
Gastrointestinal	GI
Genitourinary	GU
Gynecological	GYN
Head, eyes, ears, nose, and throat	HEENT
Musculoskeletal	M/S
Obstetrical	OB

Table 6-1	STANDARD CHARTING ABBREVIATIONS (continued)

Body Systems *(continued)*

Peripheral nervous system	PNS
Respiratory	Resp

Common Complaints

Abdominal pain	abd pn
Chest pain	CP
Dyspnea on exertion	DOE
Fever of unknown origin	FUO
Gunshot wound	GSW
Headache	H/A
Lower back pain	LBP
Nausea/vomiting	n/v
No apparent distress	NAD
Pain	pn
Shortness of breath	SOB
Substernal chest pain	sscp

Diagnoses

Abdominal aortic aneurysm	AAA
Abortion	Ab
Acute myocardial infarction	AMI
Adult respiratory distress syndrome	ARDS
Alcohol	ETOH
Atherosclerotic heart disease	ASHD
Chronic obstructive pulmonary disease	COPD
Chronic renal failure	CRF
Congestive heart failure	CHF
Coronary artery bypass graft	CABG
Coronary artery disease	CAD
Cystic fibrosis	CF
Dead on arrival	DOA
Delirium tremens	DTs
Deep vein thrombosis	DVT
Diabetes mellitus	DM
Dilation and Curettage	D&C
Duodenal ulcer	DU
End-stage renal failure	ESRF
Epstein-Barr virus	EBV
Foreign body obstruction	FBO
Hepatitis B virus	HBV
Hiatal hernia	HH
Hypertension	HTN
Infectious disease	ID
Inferior wall myocardial infarction	IWMI
Insulin-dependent diabetes mellitus	IDDM
Intracranial pressure	ICP

Diagnoses (continued)

Mass casualty incident	MCI
Mitral valve prolapse	MVP
Motor vehicle crash	MVC
Multiple sclerosis	MS
Non-insulin-dependent diabetes mellitus	NIDDM
Organic brain syndrome	OBS
Otitis media	OM
Overdose	OD
Paroxysmal nocturnal dyspnea	PND
Pelvic inflammatory disease	PID
Peptic ulcer disease	PUD
Pregnancies/Births (gravida/para)	G/P
Pregnancy-induced hypertension	PIH
Pulmonary embolism	PE
Rheumatic heart disease	RHD
Sexually transmitted disease	STD
Transient ischemic attack	TIA
Tuberculosis	TB
Upper respiratory infection	URI
Urinary tract infection	UTI
Venereal disease	VD
Wolff-Parkinson-White syndrome (disease)	WPW

Medications

Angiotensin-converting enzyme	ACE
Aspirin	ASA
Bicarbonate	HCO_3^-
Birth control pills	BCP
Calcium	Ca^{++}
Calcium channel blocker	CCB
Calcium chloride	$CaCl_2$
Chloride	Cl^-
Digoxin	Dig
Dilantin (phenytoin sodium)	DPH
Diphendydramine	DPHM
Diphtheria-Pertussis-Tetanus	DPT
Hydrochlorothiazide	HCTZ
Lactated Ringer's, Ringer's Lactate	LR, RL
Magnesium sulfate	Mg^{++}
Morphine sulfate	MS
Nitroglycerin	NTG
Nonsteroidal antiflammatory agent	NSAID
Normal saline	NS
Penicillin	PCN
Phenobarbital	PB
Potassium	K^+
Sodium bicarbonate	$NaHCO_3$

Table 6-1	**STANDARD CHARTING ABBREVIATIONS** (continued)

Medications *(continued)*

Sodium chloride	NaCl
Tylenol	APAP

Anatomy/Landmarks

Abdomen	Abd
Antecubital	AC
Anterior axillary line	AAL
Anterior cruciate ligament	ACL
Anterior-posterior	A/P
Distal interphalangeal (joint)	DIP
Dorsalis pedis (pulse)	DP
Gallbladder	GB
Intercostal space	ICS
Lateral collateral ligament	LCL
Left lower lobe	LLL
Left lower quadrant	LLQ
Left upper lobe	LUL
Left upper quadrant	LUQ
Left ventricle	LV
Liver, spleen, and kidneys	LSK
Lymph node	LN
Medial collateral ligament	MCL
Metacarpalphalangeal (joint)	MCP
Metatarsalphalangeal (joint)	MTP
Midaxillary line	MAL
Posterior axillary line	PAL
Posterior cruciate ligament	PCL
Proximal interphalangeal (joint)	PIP
Right lower lobe	RLL
Right lower quadrant	RLQ
Right middle lobe	RML
Right upper lobe	RUL
Right upper quadrant	RUQ
Temporomandibular joint	TMJ
Tympanic membrane	TM

Physical Exam/Findings

Arterial blood gas	ABG
Bilateral breath sounds	BBS
Blood sugar	BS
Breath sounds	BS
Cardiac injury profile	CIP
Central venous pressure	CVP
Cerebrospinal fluid	CSF
Chest X-ray	CXR
Complete blood count	CBC

Physical Exam/Findings *(continued)*

Computerized tomography	CT
Conscious, alert, and oriented	CAO
Costovertebral angle	CVA
Deep tendon reflexes	DTR
Dorsalis pedis (pulse)	DP
Electrocardiogram	EKG, ECG
Electroencephalogram	EEG
Expiratory	Exp
Extraocular movements (intact)	EOMI
Fetal heart tones	FHT
Full range of motion	FROM
Full term normal delivery	FTND
Heart rate	HR
Heart sounds	HS
Heel-to-shin (cerebellar test)	H→S
Hemoglobin	Hgb
Inspiratory	Insp
Jugular venous distention	JVD
Laceration	lac
Level of consciousness	LOC
Moves all extremities (well)	MAEW
Nontender	NT
Normal range of motion	NROM
Palpation	Palp
Passive range of motion	PROM
Point of maximal impulse	PMI
Posterior tibial (pulse)	PT
Pulse	P
Pupils equal and reactive to light	PEARL
Pupils equal, round, reactive to light and accomodation	PERRLA
Range of motion	ROM
Respirations	R
Tactile vocal fremitus	TVF
Temperature	T
Unconscious	unc
Urinary incontinence	UI

Miscellaneous Descriptors

After (post-)	$\bar{p}$
After eating	pc
Alert and oriented	A/O
Anterior	ant.
Approximate	≈
As needed	prn
Before (ante-)	$\bar{a}$
Before eating (*ante cibum*, before meal)	a.c.
Body surface area (%)	BSA

Table 6-1   STANDARD CHARTING ABBREVIATIONS (continued)

Miscellaneous Descriptors *(continued)*

Celsius	C°
Change	Δ
Decreased	↓
Equal	=
Fahrenheit	F°
Immediately	stat
Increased	↑
Inferior	inf.
Left	Ⓛ
Less than	<
Moderate	mod.
More than	>
Negative	−
No, not, none	∅
Not applicable	n/a
Number	No or #
Occasional	occ
Pack years	pk/yrs, p/y
Per	/
Positive	+
Posterior	post.
Postoperative	PO
Prior to arrival	PTA
Radiates to	→
Right	Ⓡ
Rule out	R/O
Secondary to	2°
Superior	sup.
Times (for 3 hours)	× (×3h)
Unequal	≠
Warm and dry	W/D
While awake	WA
With (*cum*)	c̄
Within normal limits (*or* we never looked)	WNL
Without (*sine*)	s̄
Zero	0

Treatments/Dispositions

Advanced cardiac life support	ACLS
Advanced life support	ALS
Against medical advice	AMA
Automated external defibrillator	AED
Bag-valve mask	BVM
Basic life support	BLS
Cardiopulmonary resuscitation	CPR
Carotid sinus massage	CSM

Treatments/Dispositions (continued)

Continuous positive airway pressure	CPAP
Do not resuscitate	DNR
Endotracheal tube	ETT
Estimated time of arrival	ETA
External cardiac pacing	ECP
Intermittent positive-pressure ventilation	IPPV
Long spine board	LSB
Nasal cannula	NC
Nasogastric	NG
Nasopharyngeal airway	NPA
No transport—refusal	NTR
Nonrebreather mask	NRM
Nothing by mouth	NPO
Occupational therapy	OT
Oropharyngeal airway	OPA
Oxygen	O_2
Per square inch	psi
Physical therapy	PT
Positive end-expiratory pressure	PEEP
Short spine board	SSB
Therapy	Rx
Treatment	Tx
Turned over to	TOT
Verbal order	VO

Medication Administration/Metrics

Centimeter	cm
Cubic centimeter	cc
Deciliter	dL
Drop(s)	gtt(s)
Drops per minute	gtts/min
Every	q
Grain	gr
Gram	g, gm
Hour	h, hr, or °
Hydrogen-ion concentration	pH
Intracardiac	IC
Intramuscular	IM
Intraosseous	IO
Intravenous	IV
Intravenous push	IVP
Joules	j
Keep vein open	KVO
Kilogram	kg
Liter	L
Liters per minute	LPM, L/min
Microgram	mcg
Milliequivalent	mEq

Table 6-1 STANDARD CHARTING ABBREVIATIONS (continued)

Medication Administration/Metrics *(continued)*

Milligram	mg
Milliliter	ml
Millimeter	mm
Millimeters of mercury	mmHg
Minute	min
Orally	po
Subcutaneous	SC, SQ
Sublingual	SL
To keep open	TKO

Cardiology

Atrial fibrillation	AF
Atrial tachycardia	AT
Atrioventricular	AV
Bundle branch block	BBB
Complete heart block	CHB
Electromechanical dissociation	EMD
Idioventricular rhythm	IVR
Junctional rhythm	JR
Modified chest lead	MCL
Normal sinus rhythm	NSR
Paroxysmal atrial tachycardia	PAT
Paroxysmal supraventricular tachycardia	PSVT
Premature atrial contraction	PAC
Premature junctional contraction	PJC
Premature ventricular contraction	PVC
Pulseless electrical activity	PEA
Supraventricular tachycardia	SVT
Ventricular fibrillation	VF
Ventricular tachycardia	VT
Wandering atrial pacemaker	WAP

You must be familiar with your local EMS system's acronyms and abbreviations.

because they can have multiple meanings. For instance, their meanings can vary in different areas of medicine. Is "CP" chest pain, cardiovascular perfusion, or cerebral palsy? Is "CO" cardiac output or carbon monoxide? Is "BLS" basic life support or burns, lacerations, and swelling? These are all common abbreviations with more than one accepted meaning. Furthermore, many abbreviations are specific to one community. You must be familiar with those used in your local EMS system.

Abbreviations and acronyms can cause considerable confusion when someone unfamiliar with the call reads your report. Health care professionals who are not familiar with local customs or with emergency medicine might not understand them. One way to clarify the meaning of a new abbreviation or acronym is to write it out the first time you use it, followed by the abbreviation or acronym in parenthesis. After that, you can use the abbreviation alone throughout the report. The following examples illustrate how abbreviations and acronyms can shorten your narratives. In standard English the report might be written:

> The patient is a 54-year-old conscious and alert male who complains of sudden onset of chest pain and shortness of breath which started 20 minutes ago. He has taken 2 nitroglycerin with no relief. He denies any nausea, vomiting, or dizziness. He has a past history of coronary artery disease, a heart attack 3 years ago, and high blood pressure. He takes nitroglycerin as needed, Procardia XL, hydrochlorothiazide, and potassium. He has no known drug allergies.

Using abbreviations and acronyms, the same report might be written:

> Pt. is 54 y/o CAO male c/o sudden onset CP/SOB × 20 min. Pt took NTG × 2 s̄ relief. ∅ n/v, dizziness. PH: CAD, AMI × 3y, HTN. Meds: NTG prn, Procardia XL, HCTZ and K^+; NKDA.

TIMES

Incident times are another important but perilous part of the PCR. The times you record on your PCR are considered the official times of the incident. For medical and legal purposes, you must ensure their accuracy.

The PCR typically has spaces for the time the call was received, the dispatch time, the time of arrival at the scene, time of departure from the scene, time of arrival at the hospital, and time back in service. Other time intervals are important, as well. The time you and your crew arrived at the patient's side is often very different from the time the ambulance arrived at the scene—when your patient is on the fourth floor of a building without an elevator, for example, or in a field several hundred yards from the road. Whatever the reason, document in your report any significant discrepancies between your arrival at the scene and your arrival at the patient. The times of vital signs assessment, medication administration, certain medical procedures as local protocols require, and changes in patient condition are also important and require accurate documentation.

One common problem with documenting times is inconsistencies among the dispatch center clock, the ambulance clock, and your watch. Imagine a report that documents that the ambulance arrived on scene at 20:32 according to the dispatch time, that CPR was started at 20:29 according to your watch, and the first defibrillation was administered at 20:43 according to the defibrillator's internal clock. While we may recognize this phenomenon and tend to discount the accuracy of the recorded times, they are nonetheless the official, legal times. Whenever possible, therefore, record all times from the same clock. When that is not possible, be sure that all the clocks and watches you use are synchronized. If they cannot be synchronized and the documented times seem to conflict with each other, explain this in your narrative. A simple statement such as "All time intervals on the scene were documented using my watch, all other times are those reported by the dispatch center" will suffice.

Whenever possible, record all times from the same clock.

COMMUNICATIONS

Your communications with the hospital are another important item to document. Though your system may make voice recordings of those communications, the recordings are usually not kept indefinitely. Again, the PCR will likely be the only permanent record of your discussion with the medical direction physician. Specifically, you should document any medical advice or orders you receive and the results of implementing that advice and those orders. In some situations you

Document any medical advice or orders you receive and the results of implementing that advice and those orders.

might need to document what you reported to the physician and/or discussed with him, so the reader will be able to understand the decision-making process. Finally, always document the physician's name on your PCR and, if possible, have him sign it to verify your treatments.

PERTINENT NEGATIVES

The patient assessment and medical interventions are the essence of the EMS event and become the core of your PCR. We will discuss specific approaches to documenting assessment and interventions later in this chapter, but some general rules apply regardless of the method.

Document all findings of your assessment, even those that are normal. Although the positive findings are usually of most interest, some negative findings—known as pertinent negatives—are also important. For example, if your respiratory distress patient does not have swollen ankles or crackles, that helps rule out a field diagnosis of congestive heart failure. Or if your patient with a broken leg does not have loss of sensory or motor function, it suggests he has no serious neurologic injury. You should include such information in your report.

The pertinent negatives vary for each chief complaint. In general, if a positive assessment finding for any given chief complaint would be important, a negative finding probably is pertinent. Even though these findings do not warrant medical care or intervention, your seeking them demonstrates the thoroughness of your examination and history of the event.

Document all findings of your assessment, even those that are normal.

ORAL STATEMENTS

Also essential to every PCR, regardless of approach, are the statements of witnesses, bystanders, and your patient. They help to document the mechanism of injury, your patient's behavior, the events leading up to the emergency, and any first aid or medical care others rendered before you arrived. They also may include information regarding the disposition of personal items such as wallets or purses. At crime scenes, document safety-related information such as weapons disposition. Your PCR may be the only written report of what happened to a murder weapon. Other details such as where you first saw a victim, what position he was in, and the time you arrived on the scene may be crucial evidence someday in a criminal proceeding.

Whenever possible, quote the patient—or other source of information—directly. Clearly identify the quotation with quotation marks, and identify its source. For example:

> Bystanders state the patient was "acting bizarre and threatening to jump in front of the next passing car."

ADDITIONAL RESOURCES

Document all of the resources involved in the event. If an air-medical service transported your patient, your documentation should include your assessment and all interventions up to the point when you transferred care. Identify the air-medical service and your patient's ultimate destination, if you know it. If other EMS, fire, rescue/extrication, or law enforcement agencies were involved in the call, document their roles. This can be particularly important in mutual aid calls, when many different agencies cooperate in your patient's care. Also include personnel from the coroner's or medical examiner's office for dead-on-arrival (DOA) scenes.

If a physician stops to help, identify him by name and document his qualifying credentials. If one of your medical direction physicians is on the scene and directs care, document his activities. Likewise document the names, credentials, and activities of any other medically qualified personnel present who offer to help. Your clinical experience and local protocols will determine how you integrate qualified health care workers into your emergency scene. Document that integration carefully.

ELEMENTS OF GOOD DOCUMENTATION

A well-written PCR is accurate, legible, timely, unaltered, and professional. Each of these traits is essential.

COMPLETENESS AND ACCURACY

The accurate PCR should be precise but comprehensive. Include all of the relevant information that anyone might be expected to want later, and exclude superfluous information. For example, if your patient's foot was run over by a lawn mower, reporting that his great toe on that foot had been amputated six years ago would be important; documenting that he had his tonsils removed when he was three years old probably would not. That you applied direct pressure to the bleeding foot is pertinent; that the lawn mower was a John Deere model 6354 is not.

Many PCRs provide check boxes and a space for written narratives (Figure 6-4 on next page). You should complete both the narrative and check-box sections of every PCR. All check-box sections of a document must show that you attended to them, even if you did not use a given section on a call. The check boxes can help to ensure that routine, common information is recorded for every call, but no PCR has a check box for every possible chief complaint, assessment finding, or intervention.

The narrative is the core of the documentation. Even if you document something in a check-box, repeating that information in the narrative might be worthwhile. By doing so, you can expand on the yes-or-no limitations of the check box to explain the timing, the assessment findings, the circumstances, or the changes in patient condition associated with the indicated action.

Remember that proper spelling, approved abbreviations, and proper acronyms also affect your PCR's accuracy. Misspelled words lose their meaning; many abbreviations are not universally recognized; and several acronyms have more than one meaning. Make sure that the meaning of any abbreviation or acronym is clear.

LEGIBILITY

Poor penmanship and illegible reports lead to poor documentation. Some EMS providers say, "I wrote it, and I can read it. That's all that matters." This is simply not true. The PCR does not exist solely for its author's reference. It is a permanent record that many different people use. Your handwriting must be neat enough that other people can read and understand the report—especially the narrative. It must also be neat enough that you can read and understand it yourself many years from now, long after the event has faded from your memory. Your writing must be heavy enough to transfer to any carbon copies. Using a ballpoint pen whenever possible makes carbon copies more legible and makes it difficult for someone to tamper with the document. Clearly mark the check boxes to eliminate any doubt that a check mark is not just a meaningless scratch. Always remember that other members of the health care team may use the report for medical information, research, or quality improvement.

Your handwriting must be neat enough that other people can read and understand the report.

Prehospital Care Report
FOR BLS FR USE ONLY

Recycled Paper

M	D	Y		RUN NO.		AGENCY CODE		VEH. ID.
DATE OF CALL								

Name		Agency Name		MILEAGE		USE MILITARY TIMES

MILEAGE: END, BEGIN, TOTAL — LOCATION CODE

CALL REC'D, ENROUTE, ARRIVED AT SCENE, FROM SCENE, AT DESTIN, IN SERVICE, IN QUARTERS

Address

Dispatch Information

Call Location

CHECK ONE: ☐ Residence ☐ Health Facility ☐ Farm ☐ Indus. Facility ☐ Other Work Loc. ☐ Roadway ☐ Recreational ☐ Other

Ph #

AGE | DOB M D Y | SEX ☐ M ☐ F

Physician

CALL TYPE AS REC'D.
☐ Emergency
☐ Non-Emergency
☐ Stand-by

COMPLETE FOR TRANSFERS ONLY
Transferred from [ ]
☐ No Previous PCR
☐ Unknown if Previous PCR
Previous PCR Number [ ]-[ ]

CARE IN PROGRESS ON ARRIVAL:
☐ None ☐ Citizen ☐ PD/FD/Other First Responder ☐ Other EMS

MECHANISM OF INJURY
☐ MVA (✓ seat belt used →) ☐ Fall of ___ feet ☐ GSW ☐ Machinery
☐ Struck by vehicle ☐ Unarmed assault ☐ Knife ☐

☐ Extrication required ___ minutes

Seat belt used? ☐ Yes ☐ No ☐ Unknown

Seat Belt Use Reported By ☐ Crew ☐ Patient ☐ Police ☐ Other

CHIEF COMPLAINT

SUBJECTIVE ASSESSMENT

PRESENTING PROBLEM
If more than one checked, circle primary

☐ Airway Obstruction
☐ Respiratory Arrest
☐ Respiratory Distress
☐ Cardiac Related (Potential)
☐ Cardiac Arrest

☐ Allergic Reaction
☐ Syncope
☐ Stroke/CVA
☐ General Illness/Malaise
☐ Gastro-Intestinal Distress
☐ Diabetic Related (Potential)
☐ Pain

☐ Unconscious/Unresp.
☐ Seizure
☐ Behavioral Disorder
☐ Substance Abuse (Potential)
☐ Poisoning (Accidental)

☐ Shock
☐ Head Injury
☐ Spinal Injury
☐ Fracture/Dislocation
☐ Amputation

☐ Major Trauma
☐ Trauma-Blunt
☐ Trauma-Penetrating
☐ Soft Tissue Injury
☐ Bleeding/Hemorrhage

☐ OB/GYN
☐ Burns
Environmental
☐ Heat
☐ Cold
☐ Hazardous Materials
☐ Obvious Death

☐ Other

PAST MEDICAL HISTORY	V I T A L S I G N S	TIME	RESP	PULSE	B.P.	LEVEL OF CONSCIOUSNESS	GCS	R PUPILS L	SKIN	STATUS
☐ None ☐ Allergy to ___ ☐ Hypertension ☐ Stroke ☐ Seizures ☐ Diabetes ☐ COPD ☐ Cardiac ☐ Other (List) ☐ Asthma			Rate: ☐ Regular ☐ Shallow ☐ Labored	Rate: ☐ Regular ☐ Irregular		☐ Alert ☐ Voice ☐ Pain ☐ Unresp.		☐ Normal ☐ Dilated ☐ Constricted ☐ Sluggish ☐ No-Reaction	☐ Unremarkable ☐ Cool ☐ Pale ☐ Warm ☐ Cyanotic ☐ Moist ☐ Flushed ☐ Dry ☐ Jaundiced	C U P S
Current Medications (List)			Rate: ☐ Regular ☐ Shallow ☐ Labored	Rate: ☐ Regular ☐ Irregular		☐ Alert ☐ Voice ☐ Pain ☐ Unresp.		☐ Normal ☐ Dilated ☐ Constricted ☐ Sluggish ☐ No-Reaction	☐ Unremarkable ☐ Cool ☐ Pale ☐ Warm ☐ Cyanotic ☐ Moist ☐ Flushed ☐ Dry ☐ Jaundiced	C U P S
			Rate: ☐ Regular ☐ Shallow ☐ Labored	Rate: ☐ Regular ☐ Irregular		☐ Alert ☐ Voice ☐ Pain ☐ Unresp.		☐ Normal ☐ Dilated ☐ Constricted ☐ Sluggish ☐ No-Reaction	☐ Unremarkable ☐ Cool ☐ Pale ☐ Warm ☐ Cyanotic ☐ Moist ☐ Flushed ☐ Dry ☐ Jaundiced	C U P S

OBJECTIVE PHYSICAL ASSESSMENT

COMMENTS

TREATMENT GIVEN

☐ Moved to ambulance on stretcher/backboard
☐ Moved to ambulance on stair chair
☐ Walked to ambulance
☐ Airway Cleared
☐ Oral/Nasal Airway
☐ Esophageal Obturator Airway/Esophageal Gastric Tube Airway (EOA/EGTA)
☐ EndoTracheal Tube (E/T)
☐ Oxygen Administered @ ___ L.P.M., Method ___
☐ Suction Used
☐ Artificial Ventilation Method ___
☐ C.P.R. in progress on arrival by: ☐ Citizen ☐ PD/FD/Other First Responder ☐ Other
☐ C.P.R. Started @ Time ▶ [ ] Time from Arrest Until C.P.R. ▶ [ ] Minutes
☐ EKG Monitored (Attach Tracing) [Rhythm(s) ___]
☐ Defibrillation/Cardioversion No. Times [ ] ☐ Manual ☐ Semi-automatic

☐ Medication Administered (Use Continuation Form)
☐ IV Established Fluid ___ Cath. Gauge [ ]
☐ Mast Inflated @ Time ___)
☐ Bleeding/Hemorrhage Controlled (Method Used: ___)
☐ Spinal Immobilization Neck and Back
☐ Limb Immobilized by ☐ Fixation ☐ Traction
☐ (Heat) or (Cold) Applied
☐ Vomiting Induced @ Time ___ Method ___
☐ Restraints Applied, Type ___
☐ Baby Delivered @ Time ___ In County ___
   ☐ Alive ☐ Stillborn ☐ Male ☐ Female
☐ Transported in Trendelenburg position
☐ Transported in left lateral recumbent position
☐ Transported with head elevated
☐ Other ___

DISPOSITION (See list)

DISP. CODE [ ]

CONTINUATION FORM USED YES ◀

CREW	IN CHARGE	DRIVER'S NAME	NAME	NAME
	☐ EMT ☐ AEMT #	☐ CFR ☐ EMT ☐ AEMT #	☐ CFR ☐ EMT ☐ AEMT #	☐ CFR ☐ EMT ☐ AEMT #

© COPYRIGHT 1986 NEW YORK STATE DEPARTMENT OF HEALTH

AGENCY COPY/WHITE

EMS 100 (11/86) provided by NYS-EMS PROGRAM
DOH 3822 (6/94)

FIGURE 6-4   Complete both the narrative and check-box sections of every PCR.

> The ~~left~~ right pupil was fixed and dilated

FIGURE 6-5   The proper way to correct a prehospital care report is to draw a single line through the error, write the correct information beside it, and initial the change.

TIMELINESS

As a rule, you should avoid writing your report in the ambulance during transport of your patient for two reasons. First, the bumpy ride makes it difficult to write neatly. More importantly, your time is better spent communicating with your patient and conducting ongoing assessments. Most hospitals have an area where you can sit and complete your paperwork.

Ideally, you should complete your report immediately after you complete the emergency call, when the information is fresh in your mind and you can check with your partner or patient if you have any questions about the events. At times you may be too busy to complete the entire documentation immediately following a call. If so, make notes on scratch paper and write enough of the report that you will be able to finish it completely and accurately later. The sooner you finish it, the more details you are likely to recall and the better the report will be.

Ideally, you should complete your report immediately after you complete the emergency call.

ABSENCE OF ALTERATIONS

Mistakes happen. During a busy shift or in the middle of the night you will check the wrong box, misspell a word, or omit important information. You will be thinking of one medication and write another's name on your report. If you make a mistake writing your report, simply cross through the error with one line and initial it (Figure 6-5). Some systems may expect you to date the correction, as well. Do not scribble over or blacken out any area of the call report. Never try to hide an error. Such foolish tactics only raise the reader's curiosity about what you wrote originally. After crossing out the error, continue with the correct information. If you find the error after you've already written several more sentences, submit an **addendum.**

Whenever possible, have everyone involved in the call read or reread the PCR before you submit it. Make all corrections before you submit the report to the hospital or to the EMS administrative offices. Do not make changes on the original report after you have submitted it. If for any reason you need to make corrections after you have submitted the report, or some portion of it, place an addendum. Simply note on the original report, "See addendum," and attach the addendum to the original report. Write the addendum on a separate sheet of paper or on an official form if one exists. Likewise, if more information comes to your attention after you have submitted the report, write a supplemental narrative on a separate report form.

Write any addendum to your report as soon as you realize that you made an error or that additional information is needed. Note the purpose of the revision and why the information did not appear on your original report. The addendum should document the date and time that it was written, the reason it was written,

Never try to hide an error.

* **addendum** addition or supplement to the original report.

and the pertinent information. Only the original author of a report should attach an addendum, as it is part of the official call record. Agencies should have separate forms for other EMS personnel, supervisors, or citizens who, for some reason, want to contribute to the documentation.

PROFESSIONALISM

Write your report in a professional manner. Remember that someday it may be scrutinized by hospital staff, quality improvement committees, supervisors, lawyers, and the news media. Your patient's family may request, and is entitled to, a copy of your report from your agency. Write cautiously and avoid any remarks that might be construed as derogatory. **Jargon** can be confusing and does little to enhance your image. Do not describe a patient well known to EMS providers as a "frequent flyer." Never include slang, biased statements, or irrelevant opinions. Include only objective information. "The patient smelled of beer and had slurred speech and difficulty walking" are factual statements. "The patient was very drunk" is an inference; even if accurate, it is still just your opinion. **Libel** and **slander** are, respectively, writing or speaking false and malicious words intended to damage a person's character. Always write and speak carefully. A seemingly innocent phrase or comment can come back to haunt you.

NARRATIVE WRITING

The narrative is the part of the written report in which you depict the call at length. Less structured than the check-box or fill-in sections of your report, the narrative allows you the freedom to describe your assessment findings in detail. When other people read your report, they usually will rely on your written narrative for the most relevant information. For example, as you transfer care to the emergency department nurse, she will usually scan your PCR for information concerning your patient's history, vital signs, and physical exam.

NARRATIVE SECTIONS

Any patient documentation includes three sections of importance—the subjective narrative, the objective narrative, and the assessment/management plan.

Subjective Narrative

The subjective part of your narrative typically comprises any information that you elicit during your patient's history. This includes the chief complaint (CC), the history of present illness (HPI), the past history (PH), the current health status (CHS), and the review of systems (ROS). In trauma, this also includes the mechanism of injury, as told to you by your patient or bystanders. The following is a typical subjective narrative on a patient complaining of shortness of breath:

CC: The patient is a 74-year-old conscious black female who complains, "I can't catch my breath."

HPI: Gradual onset of severe shortness of breath for the past 3 hours; began while sitting in living room watching television; nothing provokes or relieves the dyspnea; her son states this is worse than usual for her. She has had a 3-day history of some vague chest discomfort. She denies any chest pressure, nausea, or dizziness.

PH: She has a 5-year history of heart problems and congestive heart failure; hospitalized for this problem 3 times in the past 5 years; no surgeries.

CHS: Meds: Isosorbide, nitroglycerin, furosemide, digoxin, potassium; No known drug allergies; 50 pack/year smoker; non-drinker; non-drug abuser.

ROS: Resp: Unproductive cough for 1 day; audible wheezing; no hx of COPD or asthma; last chest X-ray 1 year ago. Card: no palpitations, pressure, or pain; + orthopnea; + paroxysmal nocturnal dyspnea; + edema for past few days; past ECG 1 year ago. GU: No changes in urinary patterns. Per. Vasc: + pitting edema for few days; cold feet.

Objective Narrative

The objective part of your narrative usually includes your general impression and any data that you derive through inspection, palpation, auscultation, percussion, and diagnostic testing. This includes vital signs, physical exam, and tests such as cardiac monitoring, pulse oximetry, and blood glucose determination.

To document your physical exam you can use either of two approaches—head-to-toe or body systems. While the medical community accepts both extensively, emergency medical services more often uses the head-to-toe approach.

Head-to-Toe The head-to-toe approach is well suited for any call when you perform an entire physical exam, because you document your findings in the same order that you conducted the exam—from head-to-toe. Remember that even though you may have conducted your pediatric assessment from toe-to-head, you should document it in head-to-toe order. This style encourages you to be systematic and thorough. It is appropriate for major trauma and serious medical emergencies, when you examine every body area and system. Include all circulatory and neurological findings within the body area you are documenting. For example, when recording findings in the extremities, include distal neurovascular function. When documenting the head, include the results of cranial nerve testing. The following illustrates the head-to-toe approach for a patient from an automobile accident:

> **Content Review**
>
> **APPROACHES TO THE PHYSICAL EXAM**
> • Head-to-toe
> • Body systems

General: The patient presents in the front seat of the car, in moderate distress with bruises to his forehead and some facial lacerations. Pt. is alert and oriented to self, time, and place.

Vital signs: Pulse—100 strong, regular radial, BP—110/88; Resp—24 non-labored; skin pale and cool.

HEENT: Depression to right frontal bone, minor bleeding controlled prior to arrival; no drainage from ears, nose. No periorbital ecchymosis or Battle's sign; pupils equal and reactive to light; extraocular movements intact, cranial nerves II—XII intact.

Neck: Trachea midline; no jugular vein distention; + cervical spine tenderness.

Chest: Equal expansion; bruises across the chest wall; no deformities; equal bilateral breath sounds.

Abdomen: Soft, non-tender.

Pelvis: Unstable pelvic ring; pain upon palpation.

Extremities: + Circulation, sensory, and motor function in all four extremities; no deformities noted.

Posterior:	No injuries noted.
Labs:	Sinus tachycardia no ectopy, pulse oximetry 97% on supplemental oxygen.

Body Systems The body systems approach focuses on body systems instead of body areas. It is best suited to screening and preadmission exams in which you conduct a comprehensive exam involving all body systems. Each body system has different key components that you should assess and document.

When you use the body systems approach in emergency medicine, you usually will focus only on the system, or systems, involved in the current illness or injury. For example, a patient having an asthma attack would require an in-depth evaluation of the respiratory system. Another patient with lower abdominal pain would need a close examination of the gastrointestinal system. Neither patient would require a full head-to-toe physical exam but, instead, intensive documentation of the affected body system or systems. The body systems approach can be one of the most comprehensive approaches to documentation.

The following illustrates a body systems approach for a patient with chest pain and shortness of breath:

General:	Patient is a healthy-looking female who presents sitting upright in her chair, able to speak in phrases only.
Vital Signs:	Pulse—90; BP—170/80; Resp—28 labored; skin—warm and diaphoretic
HEENT:	+ Lip cyanosis and pursing; some nasal flaring; pink, frothy sputum; jugular veins distended.
Respiratory:	Good respiratory effort; accessory neck muscle use; trachea midline; + intercostal, supraclavicular, suprasternal retractions; = chest expansion; diffuse crackles and wheezing in all lung fields, decreased breath sounds.
Per. Vasc.:	+ Ascites fluid wave; + 2 pitting edema in lower extremities; strong peripheral pulses.
Labs:	Sinus tachycardia with occasional unifocal premature ventricular contractions. Pulse oximetry—92% room air; 97% on supplemental oxygen.

Assessment/Management

* **field diagnosis** what you believe to be your patient's problem, based on your history and physical exam.

In the assessment/management section, you document what you believe to be your patient's problem. This is also known as your **field diagnosis,** or impression. For example, your field diagnosis for a patient with chest pain may be "possible angina or rule/out myocardial infarction." You do not have to make an exact diagnosis. When you are not sure, simply document what you suspect is the general problem. Sometimes, for instance, your field impression might be "rule out acute abdomen, or seizures." *Rule out* identifies possible diagnoses that you believe the emergency physician should evaluate.

Record your complete management plan from start to finish.

Record your complete management plan from start to finish. This includes how you packaged and moved your patient to the ambulance. Did you carry him on a stair-chair or on a backboard fully immobilized or did he walk? List any interventions you completed before contacting your medical control physician. For example, did you control bleeding with direct pressure? Did you start an IV? Then describe any orders from the medical control physician, and always include his name. Describe how you transported your patient and the effects of any interventions such as drug administration or other invasive procedures. Include the results of ongoing assessments and any changes in your patient's condition. Finally, describe your patient's condition when you transferred care to the emergency department staff. The following example is a management plan for a trauma patient with a pelvic fracture whose condition deteriorates en route to the hospital.

On-Scene

Extrication:	Rapid extrication from vehicle, placed supine on backboard
Airway:	Airway cleared with suctioning, nasopharyngeal airway inserted
Breathing:	Oxygen @ 15 liters/min via non rebreather mask
Circulation:	Foot of stretcher raised 30°; bleeding from arm laceration controlled with dry sterile dressing and direct pressure; PASG applied; IV—16 ga. left antecubital area—normal saline run KVO per Dr. Johnson.

Transport

Transported by ground ambulance to University Hospital with full body immobilization supine on long spine board; ETA 10 minutes.

Ongoing:	Patient becomes restless and anxious; VS: pulse—120 weak carotid only, BP—50 palpated, Resp—28, skin: cool, pale, clammy with some mottling; PASG inflated; initial IV run wide open; second IV 16 ga. right antecubital normal saline—run wide open.

Arrival

Patient transferred to ED staff restless; VS: pulse 120, BP—80 palpated, Resp—26, skin—mottled and cool.

GENERAL FORMATS

The mnemonics SOAP and CHART identify two common patterns for organizing a narrative report. These acronyms provide templates for most medical and trauma reports. They help you to arrange your history, physical exam, and management plan into a logical, readable structure. They are widely used because they group information in categories that differentiate between subjective and objective information. For example, someone wanting only to determine your patient's medications can find that list easily in either the SOAP or CHART format. Either pattern is acceptable and effective when used consistently.

SOAP

SOAP stands for *S*ubjective, *O*bjective, *A*ssessment, and *P*lan. The detailed SOAP format includes:

Subjective:	• Chief complaint
	• History of present illness
	• Past History
	• Current health status
	• Family History
	• Psychosocial History
	• Review of systems

Objective:	• Vital Signs
	• General impression
	• Physical exam
	• Diagnostic tests
Assessment:	• Field diagnosis
Plan:	• Standing orders
	• Physician orders
	• Effects of interventions
	• Mode of transportation
	• Ongoing assessment

CHART

Content Review

CHART

- Chief complaint
- History
- Assessment
- Rx (treatment)
- Transport

CHART stands for **C**hief complaint, **H**istory, **A**ssessment, **R**x (treatment), and **T**ransport. The detailed CHART format includes:

Chief Complaint

History:	• History of present illness
	• Past History
	• Current health status
	• Review of systems
Assessment:	• Vital signs
	• General impression
	• Physical exam
	• Diagnostic tests
	• Field diagnosis
Rx:	• Standing orders
	• Physician orders
Transport:	• Effects of interventions
	• Mode of transportation
	• Ongoing assessment

Other Formats

No single narrative format is ideal for all situations.

Use the patient management format for critical patients when you focus on immediately managing a variety of patient problems.

Like patient assessment itself, documentation is not "one-size-fits-all." No one narrative format is ideal for all situations. Two additional formats—patient management and call incident—are appropriate in certain circumstances.

Patient Management The patient management format is preferred for some critical patients, such as those in cardiac arrest, when you focus on immediately managing a variety of patient problems and not on conducting a thorough history and physical exam. This format is a chronological account from the time you arrived on the scene until you transferred care to someone else. It emphasizes your assessment and management of the conditions you found. Simply begin your chart with a description of the event and any other pertinent information and then document your management, starting with your airway, breathing, and circulation (ABCs) assessment. Record everything in real time and in absolute chronological order, and always include the results of your interventions. A patient management chart would look like this:

Patient is an 89-year-old Hispanic male who was found by his wife unconscious on the floor immediately after collapsing. He presents pulseless and apneic.

Time	Intervention
1320	Airway cleared with suctioning; quick look—ventricular fibrillation.
1321	Defibrillation @ 200, 300, 360 joules—no change.
1322	CPR begun; oropharyngeal airway inserted, ventilation with BVM @ 12/min with supplemental oxygen.
1324	IV 18-gauge left antecubital area—normal saline KVO; epinephrine 1:10,000 1 mg IVP.
1325	Defibrillation @ 360 joules—no change; lidocaine 100 mg IVP.
1327	Defibrillation @ 360 joules—patient converts to normal sinus rhythm rate of 72 with strong peripheral pulses, BP—110/76, no spontaneous respirations. ET tube inserted. + lung sounds bilaterally with BVM.
1328	Ventilation continued @ 12/min via BVM; lidocaine infusion 2 mg/min.
1332	Patient transferred to ambulance on stretcher—transported to University Hospital.
1335	Patient has spontaneous respirations @ 20/min, + bilateral breath sounds; becoming more awake; HR—72, BP—120/76.
1340	Arrived at UH—Patient is conscious, alert and oriented with retrograde amnesia.

Call Incident The call incident approach simply emphasizes the mechanism of injury, the surrounding circumstances, and how the incident occurred. Use this approach to begin documenting a trauma call with a significant mechanism of injury. It is most suitable when the events surrounding the call might be significant. It would be inappropriate for a man sitting in his living room with chest pain or for someone who simply cut his finger with a carving knife. You may use this style in both the subjective and objective sections of your PCR. The following example shows call incident documentation for a motor vehicle crash:

Use the call incident approach to begin documenting a trauma call with a significant mechanism of injury.

Subjective: The patient is a 46-year-old conscious and alert white male who was an unrestrained driver in a low-speed, head-on, two-car motor vehicle crash, moderate front-end damage, no passenger compartment intrusion, deformity to windshield, dashboard, and steering wheel. Patient states he "reached for cigarette on floor and when he looked up, there was another vehicle in front of him." He denies any loss of consciousness and can recall all details prior to and immediately following the crash. Patient complains of pain to the head, neck, chest, and hip from being thrown against the dashboard and windshield.

Objective: The patient presents in the front seat of the car, appears in moderate distress with bruises to his forehead, facial lacerations, and a deformed left leg. His left leg is pinned underneath the dashboard with his left foot hooked around the brake pedal. Upon arrival, fire department rescue personnel were holding manual stabilization of his head and neck and stabilizing the vehicle.

These are not the only systems of documentation. Indeed, you may use some combination of these systems or develop a unique format for your regional system. The important thing is for your documentation to be complete, accurate, and consistent. By using the same system to document every call, you will be less likely to accidentally overlook or omit something.

SPECIAL CONSIDERATIONS

Some circumstances create special problems for EMS documentation. Patient refusals, calls where transport is unnecessary, multiple patients, and mass casualties are among the more common examples. In these and other unusual circumstances, take extra care to document everything that happened during the call.

PATIENT REFUSALS

Two types of patients might refuse care. The first type is the person who is not seriously ill or injured and simply does not want to go to the hospital. For example, the belted driver of a minor automobile crash has an abrasion on his knee from striking the dashboard. He is alert and oriented, has no other injuries, and claims he will seek medical attention if it bothers him later. This type of patient usually signs your PCR in a special place marked "Refusal of Care," and you return to service.

The second type of patient is more worrisome. This patient refuses care even though you feel he needs it. This is known as **against medical advice,** or **AMA.** Some legal experts regard AMA as your failure to convince your patient to accept necessary treatment and transport. Such patient refusals are particularly troublesome because they have the most potential to end badly. Still, patients retain the right to refuse treatment or transportation if they are competent to make that decision and are not actively suicidal. While you cannot make a legal determination of competence (sometimes it takes a court decision), document that you believe your patient was competent to refuse care. Though specific laws vary from state to state, your patient will demonstrate competence by his understanding of the circumstances and the risks associated with refusing care and by accepting those risks and the responsibility for refusing care. Assess your patient as thoroughly as possible, with special emphasis on his mental status and behavior. Pay extra attention to any patient suspected of being under the influence of drugs or alcohol. Clearly document that your patient has an adequate mental status and understands your field diagnosis, alternative treatments, and the consequences of refusing care. Also record his reason for refusing care (Table 6-2).

Even after you document your patient's competence, most patient refusals require more thorough documentation than the typical EMS run because the opportunity for and consequences of abandonment charges are tremendous. Simply having your patient sign your PCR is not sufficient. Again, document that you described your patient's injuries to him and that he understood the risks of refusing treatment and transport. Inform him of potential complications from injuries that might not be obvious. Discuss those associated risks also, and document this discussion. Also document any involvement of your patient's family or friends. Since ruling out serious injury is all

✱ against medical advice (AMA) your patient refuses care even though you feel he needs it.

Patients retain the right to refuse treatment or transportation if they are competent to make that decision.

Table 6-2	REFUSAL OF CARE DOCUMENTATION CHECKLIST

❑ Thorough patient assessment

❑ Competency of patient

❑ Your recommendation for care and transport

❑ Explanation to the patient about possible consequences of refusing care, including possibility of death, if appropriate

❑ Other suggestions for accessing care

❑ Willingness to return if patient changes mind

❑ Patient's understanding of statements and suggestions and apparent competence to refuse care based on that understanding

but impossible in the field, you may need to make clear the possibility of your patient's dying. Although this might seem extreme, it plainly conveys that the risks are serious. A patient who was informed that he was at risk of dying, refused care, and subsequently had his leg amputated because of an infection would have a hard time convincing a jury that he did not think the risks were serious.

In many systems, you must contact the medical direction physician before allowing a patient to refuse transport. If you confer with a physician, document any information, advice, or orders that the physician gives you. If your patient speaks directly to the physician, document that as well. Once more, document that your patient understands the circumstances and the risks and still chooses to refuse transport. Note that you instructed him to call an ambulance or go to the emergency department if his condition worsens, or if he just changes his mind. You can ask a bystander or law enforcement officer to witness the patient refusal, although this is not always required.

Your documentation also should include a complete narrative with quotations and statements from others on the scene. For example, if your patient's wife and son plead with him to go to the hospital, include their comments in your report. If your system uses a specific form for patient refusals, complete that paperwork as well (Figure 6-6 on next page). The additional form, however, is not a substitute for a complete documentation of the circumstances.

SERVICES NOT NEEDED

Some systems allow you to determine that your patient does not need ambulance transport. Although such policies help to reduce ambulance utilization rates, the risks of denying transport are even greater than those of patient refusals. In these cases, the documentation must clearly demonstrate that transport was unnecessary. As with patient refusals, document any discussion you have with the emergency department physician and any advice you give to your patient.

Transportation may not be needed for other reasons, as well. Ambulances are often called to minor accidents where no injuries have occurred. When this happens, first responders such as the fire department rescue unit or a police agency might cancel the ambulance. If the ambulance is canceled en route, document the canceling authority and the time of notification. If you arrive on the scene and find no patients, document that. If, when you arrive, you are canceled by on-scene personnel, document that you made no patient contact and record the person and agency who canceled you. The difference is considerable between "no patients found" and "only minor injuries, patients refusing transport." Although they might refuse transport, evaluate people with even the most minor injuries. Consider them patients and document them accurately.

The risks of denying transport are even greater than those of patient refusals.

RELEASE FROM RESPONSIBILITY

DATE _____ 19 _____ TIME _____ a.m.
p.m.

This is to certify that _____

is refusing   ☐ TREATMENT   ☐ TRANSPORTATION

against the advice of the attending Emergency Medical Technician and of the Phoenix Fire Department, and when applicable, the base hospital and the base hospital physician.

I acknowledge that I have been informed of the following:

1. The nature and potential of the illness or injuries.
2. The potential risks of delaying treatment and transportation, up to and including death.
3. The availability of ambulance transportation to a hospital for treatment.

Nevertheless, I assume all risks and consequences of my decision, including further physical deterioration, loss of limb, paralysis, and even death, and hereby release the attending Emergency Medical Technician and the Phoenix Fire Department, and when applicable, the base hospital and the base hospital physician from any ill effects which may result from my refusal.

Witness _____   Signed: **X** _____

Witness _____   Relationship to Patient _____

Refusal must be signed by the patient; or by the nearest relative or legal guardian in the case of a minor, or when patient is physically or mentally incompetent.

☐ Patient refuses to sign release despite efforts of attending Emergency Medical Technician to obtain such signature after informing patient of concerns listed in numbers 1, 2, and 3 above.

GUIDELINES — Patient Refusal Documentation

In addition to those items normally documented (chief complaint, history of present illness, mechanism of injury, physical assessment, etc.) the following items should be recorded, regardless of patient's cooperation:

- Mental Status (orientation, speech, etc.)
- Suspected presence of alcohol or drugs
- Patient's exact words (as much as possible) in the refusal of care OR the signing of the release form
- Circumstances or reasons (including exact words of patient, if possible) for INCOMPLETE ADVISEMENT (risk of injury, abusiveness, unruliness, risk of injury other than from patient, etc.)
- Advice given to patients' guardian(s)

FIGURE 6-6   One example of a refusal of care form.

MASS CASUALTY INCIDENTS

Multiple patients, mass casualties, and disasters all present special documentation problems. The number of patients needing care and transport during such situations may overwhelm you. Often, more than one ambulance crew cares for the many patients. Some EMS personnel may fill only support roles and never actually provide patient care. Obtaining complete patient information might be impossible, and completing documentation for one patient before going on to care for others might be impractical.

In these situations, you must weigh your patients' needs against the demand for complete documentation. Document as much as possible—as quickly as possible—on your PCR. You can complete the documentation later as an addendum. If you cannot remember the particulars of a specific patient or transport, do not guess. Document only what you know to be factual and accurate. A simple note at the end of the documentation explaining the circumstances will account for any missing information.

Some EMS agencies use special forms for multiple patient events, and most provide a general incident report form or record that anyone connected with the call may complete. You should become familiar with local policies and procedures for documenting these situations. Many systems use **triage tags** to record vital information on each patient quickly (Figure 6-7). A triage tag has just enough room for your patient's vital information—name, major injuries, vital signs, treatment, and priority (urgent, non-urgent). You affix it to your patient,

* **triage tags** tags containing vital information, affixed to your patient during a multi-patient incident.

Whatever your local policies regarding multiple patients and mass casualties, document as completely and accurately as possible without detracting from patient care.

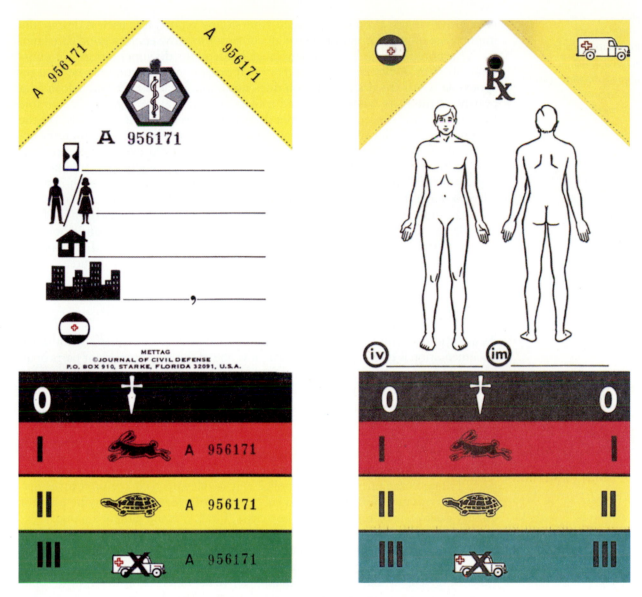

FIGURE 6-7   A triage tag offers a quick way to record vital information.

and it remains there throughout the event; you can transfer its information to your PCR later. Whatever your local policies, document as completely and accurately as possible without detracting from patient care.

CONSEQUENCES OF INAPPROPRIATE DOCUMENTATION

Inappropriate documentation can have both medical and legal consequences. The medical consequences of inadequate documentation are potentially the most serious. Health care providers across several disciplines may refer to your PCR in planning their care for a patient. Do not guess about your patient's medical problems if you are not certain. An inaccurate or incomplete report can affect patient care for many hours, even days, after the ambulance call ends. Failing to document a medication allergy or documenting an incorrect medical history could

Good documentation now enables good care later.

have grave effects. If no one can read your sloppy report, it is useless despite the importance of its information. Good documentation now enables good care later.

The potential legal consequences of inadequate documentation are enormous. If poor documentation results in inappropriate care, you may be held responsible. Or if the documentation does not make it clear that you informed a patient of the risks when he refused transport, you may be legally accountable for any harmful consequences. If the documentation does not explicitly say the patient in ventricular fibrillation was defibrillated immediately, you might be accused of providing inadequate care. Even though you did everything appropriately, poor, incomplete, or inaccurate documentation will encourage anyone who is pursuing a frivolous lawsuit. Good documentation discourages such actions. Always remember that if it is not documented, you did not do it.

Inaccurate, incomplete, illegible documentation also reflects poorly on the EMS provider writing the report. Missing information, misspelled words, and poor penmanship give the impression of a sloppy, incompetent provider. Good documentation, on the other hand, enhances the EMS provider's professional stature.

CLOSING

As a paramedic you will assume responsibility for your documentation. Although documentation is often a begrudged task, it is one of the most important parts of an EMS call. Ensuring that your documentation is complete, accurate, legible, and appropriate is one of your professional responsibilities. As a professional, you should recognize this responsibility and set a positive example for others as you fulfill it.

Your report's confidentiality cannot be overemphasized. Confidentiality is your patient's legal right. Do not discuss your report with anyone not medically connected directly with the case. Generally, you are allowed to share patient information with another health care provider who will continue care, with third-party billing companies, with the police if it is relevant to a criminal investigation, and with the court if it issues a subpoena. Your report also may be used for quality assurance or research. In these cases, block out the patient's name.

Computer charting will certainly become common in the future. Several systems now on the market allow you to enter data electronically, transmit that information to the receiving facility, and immediately receive a printed report. When you use such systems, remember that the principles of effective documentation still apply.

ſUMMARY

Regardless of the system you use for documentation, all EMS records should possess the same basic attributes. Appropriate terminology, proper spelling, accepted abbreviations and acronyms, and accurate times are essential. A description of the patient assessment and interventions, including pertinent negatives and communications with on-line physicians, is equally important. Finally, all of the personnel and resources involved in a call must be documented. The record must be accurate and precise, free of jargon, and neatly written. Corrections should be made properly, including the use of an addendum when appropriate.

Prehospital care providers may use many systems of documentation, including the CHART and SOAP formats. Whatever system you use, it is best if you use the same one consistently. This results in more reliable, complete documentation and reduces the chances of omitting important information. Any of the existing documentation systems can incorporate a head-to-toe assessment of the patient. Special situations such as multiple patients and refusals of transportation require extra attention. They are often the most difficult calls to document, yet they are also the calls for which good documentation can be most valuable. A complete narrative—in addition to any check boxes or filled-in "bubbles"—is the best way to ensure that all the necessary information is documented.

Although EMS providers frequently dislike documentation, it is one of the most important parts of the EMS call. Ensuring that the documentation is complete, accurate, legible, and appropriate is one of an EMS provider's professional responsibilities. Your PCR is the only permanent record of the ambulance call and the only permanent reflection of your professionalism.

YOU MAKE THE CALL

While helping the quality assurance officer in your agency, you come across the following narrative:

"We were dispatched to a 10-48, coroner Main/Spice. Vehicle is upside down. PMD on scene reports no serious injuries. Patient is nasty and abusive. Looks like a drug abuser. Is walking around acting abnoctious. Minor injuries identified and treated per protocol. Police arrested patient. EMS transport not needed."

1. What is wrong with this narrative? (You should be able to identify at least 10 faults).

2. What will you do to make sure your documentation is better than this?

See Suggested Responses at the back of this book.

FURTHER READING

Bevelacqua, Armando S. *Prehospital Documentation: A Systematic Approach.* Upper Saddle River, N.J.: Brady, 1992.

Brown-Nixon, Candace. "Field Documentation Myths." *Emergency Medical Services* 19 (August 1990): 18–21, 68.

Strange, Julie. "Does Your Documentation Reflect Your Care?" *Emergency Medical Services* 19 (August 1990): 23–29.

ON THE WEB

Visit Brady's Paramedic Website at www.bradybooks.com/paramedic.

Suggested Responses to "You Make the Call"

The following are suggested responses to the "You Make The Call" scenarios presented in each chapter of Paramedic Care, Volume 2 Patient Assessment. Each represents an accepted response to the scenario and should not be interpreted as the only correct response.

Chapter 1

1. *List some nonverbal communication techniques that will facilitate open discussion of your patient's problems.*

     Eye contact; body language; a calm, controlled voice; touch; active listening.

2. *Outline the components of the interview that you would use for this patient in the following categories:*

   a) *History of Present Illness*—Use the mnemonic OPQRST—ASPN to gather information concerning Mr. Harmon's current problem. What were you doing when the chest pain started? Did it begin suddenly or gradually? Does anything make the pain better or worse? Can you describe the pain in your own words? How bad is it? Can you rate it on a scale of one to ten? How long have you had the pain? Do you have any shortness of breath, nausea, or dizziness?

   b) *Past History*—Do you have a history of heart problems? Are you being treated for any other medical problems? Have you ever been hospitalized? Have you had any surgeries?

   c) *Current Health Status*—Are you taking any medications (including over-the-counter)? Do you have any allergies to medications? Do you smoke? If so, how many packs per day and for how many years? How much alcohol do you drink in a week? Do you take any recreational drugs such as marijuana, cocaine, or amphetamines? Have you had your cholesterol or triglyceride levels checked? Any other screening tests?

   d) *Review of Systems*

   Cardiac—Have you ever had heart trouble, high blood pressure, rheumatic fever, heart murmurs, chest pain or discomfort, palpitations, shortness of breath, shortness of breath while lying flat, or peripheral edema? Have you ever been awakened from sleep with shortness of breath? Have you ever had an ECG or other heart tests?

   Respiratory—Have you ever had any of the following: wheezing, coughing up blood, asthma, bronchitis, emphysema, pneumonia, TB, or pleurisy? When was your last chest X-ray? Are you coughing now? If so, can you describe the sputum?

   Gastrointestinal—Have you ever had any of the following: trouble swallowing, heartburn, loss of appetite, nausea/vomiting, regurgitation, vomiting blood, indigestion? Have you had abdominal pain, food intolerance, excessive belching or passing of gas? Have you had any black, tarry stools or chronic diarrhea?

Chapter 2

1. How would you begin the exam?

As with any other patient in any other situation, begin with a primary assessment. Make sure your patient has a patent airway, is breathing effectively, has circulatory integrity, and is alert and oriented. Identify and correct any abnormalities in his airway, breathing, and circulation (ABCs). Only then should you continue with a history and physical exam.

2. What is your differential field diagnosis?

A differential field diagnosis is a list of possible reasons for your patient's complaint. In this case, you would suspect a distal bone fracture, a ligament sprain, a joint dislocation, or a muscle or tendon strain.

3. What elements of the history are appropriate to ask this patient?

Has your patient ever experienced muscle or joint pain, stiffness, arthritis? If so, ask her to describe the location or symptoms. Has she ever sprained her ankle before? Previous sprains weaken ligaments surrounding the ankle joint and are prone to further sprains.

4. Outline your physical exam.

First remove both shoes and inspect the foot and ankle for obvious deformities, redness, and swelling. Compare your findings to the uninjured ankle. Then feel around the entire joint and pinpoint any areas of tenderness and swelling. Now test for range of motion. If your patient is in significant pain, or these movements cause further pain, do not perform them in the field. Ask your patient to bring her foot upward (dorsiflexion). Normal dorsiflexion is 20°. Then have her point it downward (plantar flexion). Normal plantar flexion is 45°. Now provide some resistance and ask her to repeat both movements. Note any difficulties or pain. While stabilizing the ankle with one hand, grasp the heel with the other hand and invert the foot, then evert it. Normal inversion is 30°, normal eversion 20°. Now ask her to perform the same movements against resistance. These four procedures test the stability of the ankle joint. A sprained ankle will cause your patient pain when the injured ligament is stretched or torn. Since the lateral ligaments are smaller and weaker than the medial ligaments, lateral sprains are more common, causing severe pain upon inversion and plantar flexion.

Chapter 3

1. Outline each phase of your patient assessment for this patient.

Scene survey: Survey the scene for hazards and ensure it is safe to enter. Form a general impression from the first look at your patient. Note his posture, facial expressions, skin color, and degree of distress.

Initial assessment: Assess his airway, breathing, and circulation; provide immediate oxygen therapy as you ascertain the history.

Focused history and physical exam: Ascertain chief complaint, history of present illness, past history, and current health status. Assess for lip cyanosis and pursing, accessory muscle use, and retractions. Note the respiratory rate and quality. Observe the inspiratory and expiratory phases. Inspect, palpate, auscultate, and percuss the chest. Obtain baseline vital signs.

Ongoing exam: Reevaluate airway, breathing, and circulation. Reassess the chief complaint and the effects of interventions. Reassess vital signs every five minutes. Alter priority determinations and management plans as necessary.

Chapter 4

1. *Would you give him the aspirin?*

No, never. This patient obviously has a neurological problem, not a simple headache. His clinical condition requires a full history and physical exam with emphasis on the neurological exam.

2. *Describe the knowledge base necessary to manage this situation.*

You would need to know the anatomy and physiology of the brain, the pathophysiology and classic signs and symptoms of neurological diseases. You would also need to recall the principles of emergency management of acute neurological disease.

3. *How would you proceed from this point?*

At this point, convince the man to be evaluated and transported to the hospital. Conduct a full history and physical exam and treat him accordingly.

Chapter 5

"This is Palermo Rescue, paramedic Randy Griffin. We have a 69-year-old, 115-kg male with chest pain and difficulty breathing that began approximately 1:00 PM. He describes the pain as pressure-like, and it radiates to the left arm and jaw. He suffered immediate dyspnea and orthopnea. He has a history of heart disease, including two prior MIs and a bypass three years ago. He currently takes Lanoxin, Lasix, Capoten, and aspirin. He is allergic to Mellaril.

On physical exam, we find him to be morbidly obese and in moderate distress. He is diaphoretic and pale. He has bilateral basilar crackles and prominent JVD. His distal pulses are strong and he has +2 pitting edema. Vital signs are as follows: BP-210/110, Pulse 70, respirations 20, pulse ox 93% on supplemental O_2. ECG shows sinus rhythm with no ectopy. We are administering oxygen via nonrebreather mask, we have started an IV of normal saline running KVO, we have administered 2 baby aspirin, 3 nitro, and 4 mg of morphine without relief of the pain."

Chapter 6

1. *What is wrong with this narrative?*

What is a "10-48"? Is this the same in every EMS system?
Was the ambulance dispatched to the corner of Main and Spice?
Was the ambulance dispatched to the coroner, at Main and Spice?
Was the ambulance dispatched to the main coroner, whose name is Spice?
What is "PMD"?
"Patient is nasty and abusive" is judgmental.
"Looks like a drug abuser" is judgmental.
"Abnoctious" should be spelled "obnoxious."
"Obnoxious" is judgmental.
What exactly are the injuries?
Exactly what treatment, if any, was rendered?
Was EMS transport not needed because the patient was not hurt, or because the police transported him?
Did the patient go to the hospital or to jail?

2. *What will you do to make sure your documentation is better than this?*

Avoid using codes.
Practice spelling and use only words you can spell correctly.
Do not use abbreviations that are unclear; spell out terms the first time you use them, followed by the abbreviation in parenthesis.
Do not be judgmental.
Describe the head-to-toe assessment completely.
Be particularly careful and complete in no-transport situations.

Glossary

ABCs airway, breathing, and circulation.

ACLS advanced cardiac life support.

active listening the process of responding to your patient's statements with words or gestures that demonstrate your understanding.

acuity the severity or acuteness of your patient's condition.

algorithm schematic flow chart that outlines appropriate care for specific signs and symptoms.

ALS advanced life support.

anticipatory thinking ahead.

ascites bulges in the flanks and across the abdomen, indicating edema caused by congestive heart failure.

auscultation listening with a stethoscope for sounds produced by the body.

autonomic nervous system part of the nervous system that controls involuntary actions.

Babinski response big toe dorsiflexes and the other toes fan out when sole is stimulated.

Battle's sign black and blue discoloration over the mastoid process

blood pressure force of blood against arteries' walls as the heart contracts and relaxes.

borborygmi loud, prolonged, gurgling bowel sounds indicating hyperperistalsis.

bradycardia pulse rate lower than 60.

bradypnea slow breathing.

bronchophony abnormal clarity of patient's transmitted voice sounds.

Broselow Tape a measuring tape for infants that provides important information regarding airway equipment and medication doses based on your patient's length.

bruit sound of turbulent blood flow around a partial obstruction.

CAGE questionnaire a questionnaire designed to determine the presence of alcoholism.

cardiac monitor machine that displays and records the electrical activity of the heart.

cardiac output the amount of blood the heart ejects each minute, measured in ml.

cellular telephone system telephone system divided into regions, or cells, that are served by radio base stations.

chief complaint the pain, discomfort, or dysfunction that caused your patient to request help.

chief complaint the reason the ambulance was called.

circulation assessment evaluating the pulse and skin and controlling hemorrhage.

clinical judgment the use of knowledge and experience to diagnose patients and plan their treatment.

closed-ended questions questions that elicit a one- or two-word answer.

communication the process of exchanging information between individuals.

convergent focusing on only the most important aspect of a critical situation.

crackles light crackling, popping, nonmusical sounds heard usually during inspiration.

crepitation (or crepitus) crunching sounds of unlubricated parts in joints rubbing against each other.

critical thinking thought process used to analyze and evaluate.

Cullen's sign discoloration around the umbilicus (occasionally the flanks) suggestive of intra-abdominal hemorrhage.

decerebrate posturing arms and legs extended.

decorticate posturing arms flexed, legs extended.

delirium an acute alteration in mental functioning that is often reversible.

dementia a deterioration of mental status that is usually associated with structural neurological disease.

depression a mood disorder characterized by hopelessness and malaise.

detailed physical exam careful, thorough process of eliciting the history and conducting a physical exam.

diastole phase of cardiac cycle when ventricles relax.

diastolic blood pressure force of blood against arteries when ventricles relax.

differential field diagnosis the list of possible causes for your patient's symptoms.

digital communications data or sounds are translated into a digital code for transmission.

diuretic a medication that stimulates the kidneys to excrete excess water.

divergent taking into account all aspects of a complex situation.

duplex communication system that allows simultaneous two-way communications by using two frequencies for each channel.

dysmenorrhea menstrual difficulties.

dyspnea the sensation of having difficulty in breathing.

echo procedure immediately repeating each transmission received during radio communications.

egophony abnormal change in tone of patient's transmitted voice sounds.

EMD emergency medical dispatcher.

facsimile machine device for electronically transmitting and receiving printed information.

Federal Communications Commission agency that controls all nongovernmental communications in the United States.

field diagnosis prehospital evaluation of the patient's condition and its causes.

focused history and physical exam problem-oriented assessment process based on initial assessment and chief complaint.

general impression your initial, intuitive evaluation of your patient.

glucometer tool used to measure blood glucose level.

Grey-Turner's sign discoloration over the flanks suggesting intra-abdominal bleeding.

HEENT head, eyes, ears, nose, and throat.

hematemesis vomiting blood.

hematuria blood in the urine.

hemoptysis coughing up blood.

HEPA high-efficiency particulate air.

hypertension blood pressure higher than normal.

hyperthermia increase in body's core temperature

hypotension blood pressure lower than normal.

hypothermia decrease in body's core temperature.

impulsive acting instinctively without stopping to think.

index of suspicion your anticipation of possible injuries based upon your analysis of the event.

initial assessment prehospital process designed to identify and correct life-threatening airway, breathing, and circulation problems.

inspection the process of informed observation.

intermittent claudication intermittent calf pain while walking that subsides with rest.

Korotkoff sounds sounds of blood hitting arterial walls.

lesion any disruption in normal tissue.

libel to defame another person in writing.

major trauma patient person who has suffered significant mechanism of injury.

manometer pressure gauge with a scale calibrated in millimeters of mercury (mmHg).

mechanism of injury combined strength, direction, and nature of forces that injured your patient.

mobile data terminal vehicle-mounted computer keyboard and display.

multiplex duplex system that can transmit voice and data simultaneously.

nocturia excessive urination at night.

open-ended questions questions that allow your patient to answer in detail.

ophthalmoscope handheld device used to examine interior of eye.

orthopnea difficulty in breathing while lying supine.

otoscope handheld device used to examine interior of ears and nose.

pack/year history a way to quantify your patient's smoking history by multiplying number of packs smoked per day by the number of years smoking.

palpation using your sense of touch to gather information.

paroxysmal nocturnal dyspnea sudden onset of shortness of breath at night.

patient assessment problem-oriented evaluation of patient and establishment of priorities based on existing and potential threats to human life.

percussion the production of sound waves by striking one object against another.

perfusion passage of blood through an organ or tissue.

periorbital ecchymosis black and blue discoloration surrounding the eye sockets.

pitting depression that results from pressure against skin when pitting edema is present.

pleural friction rub the squeaking or grating sound of the pleural linings rubbing together.

polyuria excessive urination.

prearrival instructions dispatcher's instructions to caller for appropriate emergency measures.

prehospital care report (PCR) the written record of an EMS response.

primary problem the underlying cause for your patient's symptoms.

priority dispatching system using medically-approved questions and predetermined guidelines to determine the appropriate level of response.

proactive acting to prevent or deal with potential problems before they occur.

protocol standard that includes general and specific principles for managing certain patient conditions.

PSAP public safety access point.

pseudo-instinctive learned actions that are practiced until they can be done without thinking.

pulse oximeter noninvasive device that measures the oxygen saturation of blood.

pulse pressure difference between systolic and diastolic pressures.

pulse quality strength, which can be weak, thready, strong, or bounding.

pulse rate number of pulses felt in one minute.

pulse rhythm pattern and equality of intervals between beats.

quality of respiration depth and pattern of breathing.

radio band a range of radio frequencies.

radio frequency the number of times per minute a radio wave oscillates.

rapid trauma assessment quick check for signs of serious injury.

reactive acting on problems after they occur.

referred pain pain that is felt at a location away from its source.

reflective acting thoughtfully, deliberately, and analytically.

respiration exchange of oxygen and carbon dioxide during inhalation and exhalation in the lungs and at the cellular level.

respiratory effort how hard patient works to breathe.

respiratory rate number of times patient breathes in one minute.

review of systems a list of questions categorized by body system.

rhonchi continuous sounds with a lower pitch and a snoring quality.

scene safety doing everything possible to ensure a safe environment.

semantic related to the meaning of words.

semi-Fowler's position sitting up at 45°.

simplex communication system that transmits and receives on the same frequency.

slander to orally defame another person.

sphygmomanometer blood pressure measuring device comprising a bulb, a cuff, and a manometer.

standing orders treatments you can perform before contacting the medical control physician for permission.

stethoscope tool used to auscultate most sounds.

stridor predominantly inspiratory wheeze associated with laryngeal obstruction.

stroke volume the amount of blood the heart ejects in one beat.

subcutaneous emphysema crackling sound caused by air just underneath the skin.

systole phase of cardiac cycle when the ventricles contract.

systolic blood pressure force of blood against arteries when ventricles contract.

tachycardia pulse rate higher than 100.

tachypnea rapid breathing.

ten-code radio communications system using codes that begin with the word ten.

tenderness pain that is elicited through palpation.

thrill vibration or humming felt when palpating the pulse.

tidal volume amount of air one breath moves in and out of lungs.

tinnitus the sensation of ringing in the ears.

touch pad computer on which you enter data by touching areas of the display screen.

trunking communication system that pools all frequencies and routes transmissions to the next available frequency.

turgor normal tension in the skin.

ultrahigh frequency radio frequency band from 300 to 3,000 megahertz.

very high frequency radio frequency band from 30 to 300 megahertz

visual acuity wall chart/card wall chart or handheld card with lines of letters used to test vision.

vital statistics height and weight.

wheezes continuous, high-pitched musical sounds similar to a whistle.

whispered pectoriloquy abnormal clarity of patient's transmitted whispers.

Index

Abbreviations and acronyms, 275–85
Abdomen
    of children and infants, 163
    in detailed physical exam, 228
    examination of, 89
    field assessment of, 217–19
    quadrants of, 89
    rapid trauma assessment of, 211–12
Abdominal aorta, 92, 93
Abdominal arteries, 93
Abdominal organs, examination of, 90–95
Abdominal pain, field assessment of, 219
Abdominal palpation, 93–97
Abdominal reflexes, 155, 158
Abducens nerve (CN-VI), 139, 144
Accessory nerve (CN-XI), 145, 147
Accommodation, 63, 64
Achilles tendon, 155
Acoustic nerve (CN-VIII), 66, 142, 145
Acromioclavicular (AC) joint, 110
Acronyms and abbreviations, 275–85
Active listening, 9
Acuity, patient, 237–38
Addendum, 289
Adolescents, general appearance and behavior, 160
Against medical advice (AMA), 296
Airbags, 203
Airway assessment, 191–98. See also Breathing
    ongoing, 231–32
Alcohol, history taking on use of, 15
Alertness of patient, 190
Algorithms, patient care, 238, 239
Allergies, history taking on, 15
Altered mental status, field assessment of, 218–19
Anger, history taking and, 20
Anisocoria, 64
Ankles, examination of, 115–17
Anticipatory approach to decision making, 243
Anus
    in detailed physical exam, 229
    examination of, 99–100
Anxiety, history taking and, 20

Aorta, 84
    abdominal, 92
Appearance
    of children and infants, 158–59
    in general survey, 41
    neurological exam and, 134–36
Arterial blood pressure, 86, 88
Arteries. See also specific arteries
    abdominal, 93
Ascites, 94, 97
Assessment/management section of narratives, 292
Assessment of patient, 174–75. See also Focused history and physical exam; Initial assessment; Ongoing assessment; Scene size-up
    basic components of, 174
    critical thinking skills and, 240
Atrial gallop, 89
Attention, neurological exam and, 137
Auricle, 65
Auscultation, 32–33
Autonomic nervous system, 243
AVPU mnemonic, 190

Babinski response, 155
Bag-valve masks, 192, 195, 208, 211
Balance, 149, 151
Barrel chest, 78
Battle's sign, 66, 226
Beau's lines, 56
Behavior, neurological exam and, 134–36
Bell's palsy, 145
Biceps, 153
Biot's respirations, 198
Blindness, history taking and, 23
Blood glucose, 220
Blood pressure
    arterial, 86, 88
    cardiovascular examination and, 86, 88
    measurement of, 35–37, 43–46
Body odors, examination of, 42
Body substance isolation, 175, 177–79
Body systems approach to physical examination, 292
Body temperature, 37
    skin temperature, 51
    taking of, 46
Borborigmy, 94
Bowel sounds, 94

Brachial artery, 128
Brachial pulse, 196
Brachioradialis, 154
Bradycardia, 33
    in children and infants, 163
Bradypnea, 35
Brain stem, 134
Breathing. See also Airway assessment
    examination of, 77–79
    ongoing assessment of, 232
Breathing assessment, 198–99
Breath odors, examination of, 42
Breath sounds, 81–82
Bronchiolitis, 195
Bronchophony, 82
Broselow Tape, 42
Bruits, 86, 87, 94, 96
Bubble sheets, 274–75

CAGE questionnaire, 15
Call incident approach to narratives, 295–96
Capillary refill reliably, 196
Cardiac cycle, 85
Cardiac monitoring, 220
Cardiac monitors, 47–48
Cardiac output, 85–86
Cardiovascular system
    of children and infants, 163
    in detailed physical exam, 228
    examination of, 83–89
    field assessment of, 217
    history taking on, 18
Carotid arteries, 74, 75, 86
Carotid pulse, 34, 43, 86, 87, 199
Carpal tunnel syndrome, 106, 108
Cartilage, 101
Cataracts, 65
Cellular telephones, 263
Cerebellar system, 148
Cerebellum, 134
Cerebral cortex, 134
Cerebrum, 134
CHART format for organizing narratives, 294
Chest
    in detailed physical exam, 228
    examination of, 77–83
        anterior chest, 82–83
        posterior chest, 79–82
    field assessment of, 217–19
    funnel, 78
    rapid trauma assessment of, 205–11
Chest pain, 216–18

Cheyne-Stokes respirations, 198
Chief complaint, 5, 11–12, 215
Childhood diseases, in history taking, 14
Children, physical examination of, 158–64
    abdomen, 163–64
    anatomy, 160
    building patient and family rapport, 158
    cardiovascular system, 163
    chest and lungs, 162–63
    general appearance and behavior, 158–60
    head and neck, 160–62
    nervous system, 164
    recording examination findings, 164–65
Circulation assessment, 128–30, 195, 199–200
Clarification, in patient interview, 9
Clinical decision making, 236–47. See also Critical thinking process
Clinical judgment, 236–37
Closed-ended questions, 8
Clubbing, 56
CN-III (oculomotor nerve), 139, 141, 144
CN-II (optic nerve), 139, 141
CN-I (olfactory nerve), 138, 140, 146
CN-IV (trochlear nerve), 139, 141, 144
CN-IX (glossopharyngeal nerve), 145
CN-VI (abducens nerve), 139, 144
CN-VII (facial nerve), 145
CN-VIII (acoustic nerve), 142, 145
CN-V (trigeminal nerve), 144
CN-XI (accessory nerve), 145, 147
CN-XII (hypoglossal nerve), 147
CN-X (vagus nerve), 143, 145
Cocaine abuse, 70
Cochlea, 66
10-code systems, 254
Cog-wheel rigidity, 148
Colon, 90
Communications, 250–68
    basic model for, 253–54
    defined, 253
    digital, 262–63
    EMS response, 257–60
    with the hospital, documentation of, 285–86
    overview of, 252
    regulation of, 268
    transfer, 260
    verbal, 254–56

Communication technology, 260–64
Computers, 263–64
Concept of your patient and the scene, forming a, 245
Confrontation of patient, 10
Conjunctiva, 59, 64
Conjunctivitis, 64
Contractile force, 86
Control, maintaining, 244
Convergent approach to decision making, 243
Coordination, 151
Cornea, 60, 64, 65
Corneal reflex, 63, 65
Crackles, 81
Cranial nerves, 59, 137–47. See also specific nerves
    in detailed physical exam, 229
Cranium, 59
Crash scenes, 183
Crepitation (crepitus), 103–4
Crime scenes, 183
Critical decisions, 236
Critical thinking process (critical decision making), 244–47
Critical thinking skills, 240–43
Crying, history taking and, 21
Cullen's sign, 94, 211, 228
Current health status, 215
Cyanosis, lip, 226

Daily life, history taking on, 17
Decerebration, 191
Decision making, clinical. See Clinical decision making; Critical decisions
Decortication, 191
Deep tendon reflexes, 153
Deep vein thrombosis (DVT), 133
Delirium, history taking and, 21–22
Dementia, history taking and, 21–22
Depression, history taking and, 21
Detailed physical exam, 223–31
    abdomen, 228
    anus and rectum, 229
    cardiovascular system, 228
    chest and lungs, 228
    eyes, 226
    head, 223–26
    mouth and pharynx, 226–28
    musculoskeletal system, 229
    neck, 228
    nose and sinuses, 226
    pelvis, 228
    peripheral vascular system, 229
    recording exam findings, 231
    vital signs, 231
Diagnosis, field. See Field diagnosis
Diaphragm, 77, 79
Diaphragmatic excursion, 79, 81
Diastole, 85

Diastolic blood pressure, 35
Diet, history taking on, 16
Differential field diagnosis, 5, 241
Digestive organs, 90
Digestive system, 90
Digital communications, 262–63
Disorientation, neurological exam and, 137
Distal interphalangeal (DIP) joints, 104, 105, 108
Distress, signs of, 41
Divergent approach to decision making, 243
Documentation, 272–300. See also Narratives; Prehospital care report (PCR)
    abbreviations and acronyms in, 275–85
    of communications with the hospital, 285–86
    consequences of inappropriate, 299–300
    elements of good, 287–90
    general considerations, 274–75
    mass casualty incidents and, 298–99
    medical terminology in, 275
    refusal of care by patients and, 296
    special considerations, 296–99
    unnecesary services and, 297
    uses for, 273–74
Dress, examination of, 42
Drugs, history taking on use of, 15
Duodenum, 90
Duplex transmissions, 261–62
Dysmenorrhea, 18
Dyspnea, 18

Earaches, 66
Ear canal, 65
    discharge (otorrhea) from, 66
    examination of, 66
Eardrum (tympanic membrane), examination of, 65, 66–67
Ears
    of children and infants, 161
    in detailed physical exam, 226
    examination of, 65–67
Echo procedure, 266
Edema, in legs, 131
Egophony, 82
Elbows, examination of, 106–7, 109, 110
Emergency medical care, for responsive medical patients, 221
Emergency medical dispatcher (EMD), 252, 258
Empathy with patient, 10
Emphysema, subcutaneous, 204, 205
EMS response communications, 257–60

Endocrine system, history taking on, 19
Endotracheal intubation, 193, 195, 231
Environmental hazards, history taking on, 16
Epididymis, 91
Esophageal Tracheal CombiTube, 194, 195
Esophagus, 90
Eustachian tubes, 66
Examination. See Physical examination
Exercise, history taking on, 16
External ears, 66
Extrapyramidal tract, 148
Extremities, field assessment of, 218
Eye goggles, 179, 182–84
Eyelashes, 59, 64
Eyelids, 59, 64
Eyes
    in detailed physical exam, 226
    examination of, 59
    external, 59, 64
    internal, 60

Face, examination of, 59
Facial expressions
    examination of, 42
    neurological exam and, 136
Facial nerve (CN-VII), 145
Facilitation, in patient interview, 9
Facsimile machine (fax), 263
Fallopian tubes, 91
Family history, 16
Family of patient, history taking and, 23
Federal Communications Commission (FCC), 268
Feelings, asking about, in patient interview, 10
Feet, examination of, 115–17, 131
Female genitalia
    in detailed physical exam, 228
    examination of, 95, 98
    history taking on, 18
Female reproductive organs, 91, 92
Femoral artery, 128
Field assessment. See Patient assessment
Field diagnosis, 237, 292
    differential, 241
Fingernails, 55–57
Focused history and physical exam, 174, 201–23
    of isolated-injury trauma patients, 213–14
    of major trauma patients, 202–13
        history, 213
        mechanism of injury, 202–3
        rapid trauma assessment, 203–12
        vital signs, 212

of responsive medical patients, 214–21
of unresponsive medical patients, 221–23
Friends of patient, history taking and, 23
Frontal lobe, 134
Funnel chest, 78

Gag reflex, 195
Gait, 149
    examination of, 42
Gallbladder, 90
Gastrointestinal system, 18
    history taking on, 18
General impression, 186
    initial assessment and, 188
General state of health, 14
Genitalia. See Female genitalia; Male genitalia
Gingiva, 70
Glasses, safety, 179, 183
Glenohumeral joint, 110–12
Glossopharyngeal nerve (CN-IX), 145
Gloves, latex or vinyl, 177, 179
Glucometers, 48
Glucose (blood glucose level), determination of, 48, 220
Gonorrhea, 98, 99
Grey-Turner's sign, 94, 211, 228
Grooming
    examination of, 42
    neurological exam and, 135
Gurgling, 194

Hair, examination of, 53–55
Hair loss, 53–54
Hands, examination of, 104–6
Hazardous materials, 181, 182
Head
    of children and infants, 160
    in detailed physical exam, 223–26
    examination of, 57–59
    rapid trauma assessment of, 204
Head-tilt/chin lift maneuver, 190, 193
Head-to-toe approach to physical examination, 291–92
Health, apparent state of, 42
Hearing acuity, checking, 66
Hearing loss, 145
Hearing problems, history taking and, 22
Heart. See also Cardiovascular system
Heart sounds, 85–88
HEENT (head, eyes, ears, nose, and throat), 17–18, 216, 218, 219
Height, measurement of, 42
Heimlich maneuver, 195
Helmets, 179, 183
Hematemesis, 18
Hematologic system, history taking on, 19
Hematuria, 18
Hemoptysis, 18

HEPA masks, 179
Hips, examination of, 119–24
History taking, 5–23. *See also* Interview, patient
    anger and hostility and, 20
    anxious patients and, 20
    blind patients and, 23
    comprehensive, 11–19
        chief complaint, 11–12
        current health status, 14–15
        past history, 13–17
        preliminary data, 11
        present illness, 12–13
        primary problem, 12
    confusing behaviors or histories and, 21–22
    crying by patient and, 21
    depression and, 21
    hearing problems and, 22
    intoxication of patient and, 21
    language barriers and, 22
    limited intelligence and, 22
    major trauma patients, 213
    multiple symptoms and, 20
    overly talkative patients and, 19–20
    reassurance and, 20
    responsive medical patients, 214–21
    review of systems, 17–19
    on sensitive topics, 10–11
    sexual, 11
    sexually attractive or seductive patients and, 21
    silence and, 19
    talking with families or friends and, 23
Home situation, history taking on, 16–17
Hostility, history taking and, 20
Hygiene, personal
    examination of, 42
    neurological exam and, 135
Hypertension, 36
Hyperthermia, 37
Hypoglossal nerve (CN-XII), 147
Hypotension, 36
Hypothermia, 37

Immunizations, history taking on, 16
Impulsive decisions, 242
Index of suspicion, 186
Infants, physical examination of, 158–64
    abdomen, 163–64
    anatomy, 160
    building patient and family rapport, 158
    cardiovascular system, 163
    chest and lungs, 162–63
    general appearance and behavior, 158–60
    head and neck, 160–62

    nervous system, 164
    recording examination findings, 164–65
Inguinal canal, 91
Initial assessment, 174, 186–201
    airway assessment, 191–98
    breathing assessment, 198–99
    circulation assessment, 199–200
    general impression, 188
    mental status, 188–91
    priority determination, 200–201
    steps in, 187
Inner ear, 66
Inner ear infection (otitis), 65, 66
Insight, neurological exam and, 137
Inspection, 29–30
Intermittent claudication, 18
Interpretation, in patient interview, 10
Interpreting data, critical thinking process and, 245–46
Interview, patient, 5
    asking questions in, 8
    introductions in, 7–8
    language and communication in, 9
    patient's first impression of paramedic and, 6
    setting the stage for, 5–6
Intoxication, history taking and, 21
Iris, 60
Isolated-injury trauma patients, focused history and physical exam of, 213–14

Jargon, 290
Joints, 100–103
Judgment, neurological exam and, 137
Jugular veins, 74, 75, 88

Kidneys, 90–91
Knees, examination of, 118–19
Korotkoff sounds, 35
Kussmaul's respirations, 198

Labia majora, 95
Labia minora, 95, 98
Lacrimal glands, 59
Language. *See also* Speech
    neurological exam and, 136
    in patient interview, 9
Language barriers, history taking and, 22
Large intestine. *See* Colon
Lawyers, prehospital care report (PCR) and, 274
Legal uses of prehospital care report (PCR), 274
Legs, examination of, 131
Leisure activities, history taking on, 16
Lens, 60

Lesions, skin, 51–52
Level of consciousness, 41
Libel, 264, 290
Lip cyanosis, 226
Listening, active, 9
Liver, 90
Location of all patients, 185
Lungs
    in detailed physical exam, 228
    examination of, 77–79, 81–83
Lymph nodes, 128, 130, 131
    examination of, 74–76
Lymph system, 93, 128

Major trauma patients, focused history and physical exam of, 202–13
    history, 213
    mechanism of injury, 202–3
    rapid trauma assessment, 203–12
    vital signs, 212
Male genitalia, 98
    in detailed physical exam, 228
    history taking on, 18
Male reproductive system, 91, 92
Malleus, 66
Management plan, 236–39, 243, 244, 246, 292
Manometer, 39
Masks
    bag-valve, 192, 195, 208, 211
    HEPA, 179
Mass casualty incidents, documentation of, 298–99
Mass casualty plan, 185
Mastoiditis, 66
Mastoid process, 65
MCP (metacarpophalangeal) joints, 104–6, 108
Mechanism of injury, 184, 185–86
    in major trauma patients, 202–3
Medical direction physician, 259–60
Medic alert tags, 208, 212
Medical history. *See* History taking
Medical terminology, 275
Medications, history taking on, 15
Memory, neurological exam and, 137
Mental checklist, 244
Mental status, 134–37, 188
    in detailed physical exam, 229
    field assessment of, 218–19
    ongoing assessment of, 231
Mesentery arteries, 92
Mesentery veins, 90
Metacarpophalangeal (MCP) joints, 104–6, 108
Middle ear, 65–66

Mobile data terminals, 263
Model verbal reports, 267–68
Mons pubis, 95
Mood, neurological exam and, 136
Motor activity, examination of, 42
Motor system
    in detailed physical exam, 229
    examination of, 147–51
Mouth
    of children and infants, 161
    detailed physical exam of, 226–28
    examination of, 70–74
Mucous membrane, 67
Multiplex systems, 262
Muscle atrophy, 148
Muscle bulk, 148
Muscle strength, 149, 151
Muscle tone, 148, 149
Musculoskeletal system
    of children and infants, 164
    in detailed physical exam, 229
    examination of, 100–127
        ankles and feet, 115–17
        elbows, 106–7, 109, 110
        hips, 119–24
        knees, 118–19
        shoulders, 110–14
        spine, 124–27
        wrists and hands, 104–6, 108, 109
    history taking on, 18

Nails, 55–57
Narratives, 287, 290–96
    assessment/management section of, 292
    call incident approach to, 295
    CHART format for organizing, 294
    objective, 291
    patient management format for organizing, 294–95
    SOAP format for organizing, 293–94
    subjective, 290–91
Nasopharyngeal airway, 192, 195
Neck
    of children and infants, 160–62
    in detailed physical exam, 228
    examination of, 74–77
    field assessment of, 216–17
    rapid trauma assessment of, 204–5
Needle cricothyrotomy, 194, 195
Nervous system
    autonomic, 243
    examination of. *See* Neurological exam

Neurological exam, 133–58
    areas covered by, 133
    of children and infants, 164
    cranial nerves, 59,
        137–47, 229. *See also
        specific nerves*
    in detailed physical
        exam, 229
    facial expressions, 136
    in the field, 218–19
    grooming and personal
        hygiene, 135–36
    insight and judgment, 137
    memory and attention, 137
    mental status and speech,
        134–37
    mood, 136
    motor system, 147–51
    reflexes, 153–58
    sensory system, 151–53
    speech and language, 136
    thought and perceptions,
        136–37
Neurologic system, history taking
on, 19
Nocturia, 18
Nonverbal communication, 7
Nose
    in detailed physical
        exam, 226
    examination of, 67, 69–70
Nystagmus, 64–65

Objective narrative, 291–92
Occipital lobe, 134
Ocular muscles, 59
Oculomotor nerve (CN-III), 60,
64, 139, 141, 144
Olfactory nerve (CN-I), 138,
140, 146
Ongoing assessment, 231–33
Onset of illness, in history
taking, 12
Onycholysis, 56
Open-ended questions, 8
Ophthalmic artery, 60
Ophthalmoscope, 39, 63, 65
Optic nerve, 60
Optic nerve (CN-II), 139, 141
Oropharyngeal airway, 192, 195
Orthopnea, 18
Ossicles, 66
Osteoporosis, 101, 103
Otitis (inner ear infection), 65, 66
Otoscope, 39, 66
Outer ear, 65
Ovaries, 91

Painful stimuli, responsiveness
to, 191
Palliation of symptoms, in history
taking, 12–13
Palpation, 30–31
Pancreas, 90
Parietal lobe, 134
Parkinson's disease, 148
Paronychia, 56
Paroxysmal nocturnal dyspnea, 18
Past medical history, 215

Patient acuity, 237–38
Patient assessment, 174–75. *See
also* Focused history and physical
exam; Initial assessment
        Ongoing assessment; Scene
        size-up
            basic components
                of, 174
            critical thinking
                skills and, 240
Patient history. *See* History
PCR. *See* Prehospital care report
Pelvis
    in detailed physical exam,
        228–29
    field assessment of, 218
    rapid trauma assessment
        of, 212
Penis, 98
Perceptions, neurological exam
and, 136–37
Percussion, 31–32
Perfusion, 36
Periorbital ecchymosis, 226
Periorbital ecchymosis (raccoon
eyes), 59
Peripheral pulse, 130–31
Peripheral vascular system
    in detailed physical
        exam, 229
    examination of, 128–33
    history taking on, 18
Peripheral vision, 61, 62
Personal hygiene
    examination of, 42
    neurological exam
        and, 135
Pharyngeotracheal lumen airway,
193, 195
Pharynx, 72
    detailed physical exam of,
        226–28
Physical abuse, history taking
on, 10
Physical examination, 28–165.
See also Focused history and
physical exam
    abdomen (abdominal
        organs), 89–95
    anus, 99–100
    approach and overview,
        28–41
    body systems approach
        to, 292
    cardiovascular system,
        83–89
    chest and lungs, 77
        anterior chest,
            82–83
        posterior chest,
            79–82
    detailed, in the field,
        223–31
    ears, 65–67
    equipment for, 37–40
    eyes, 59–65
    general approach to,
        40–41
    general survey, 41–48

    hair, 53–55
    head, 57–59
    head-to-toe approach
        to, 291
    of infants and children,
        158–64
            abdomen, 163–64
            anatomy, 160
            building patient
                and family
                rapport, 158
            cardiovascular
                system, 163
            chest and lungs,
                162–63
            general appearance
                and behavior,
                158–60
            head and neck,
                160–62
            nervous system, 164
            recording
                examination
                findings, 164–65
    mouth, 70–74
    musculoskeletal system,
        100–127
            ankles and feet,
                115–17
            elbows, 106–7,
                109, 110
            hips, 119–24
            knees, 118–19
            shoulders, 110–14
            spine, 124–27
            wrists and hands,
                104–6, 108, 109
    nails, 55–57
    neck, 74–77
    nervous system, 133
    nose, 67, 69–70
    peripheral vascular
        system, 128–33
    skin, 49–52
    techniques of, 29–37
            auscultation, 32–33
            inspection, 29–30
            measurement of
                vital signs, 33–37
            palpation, 30–31
            percussion, 31–32
Pigeon chest, 78
PIP (proximal interphalangeal)
joints, 104, 105
Pitting, 131
Plantar reflex, 155
Pleural friction rubs, 82
PMI (point of maximum
impulse), 84, 87, 88
Pneumatic antishock garment,
197
Point of maximum impulse
(PMI), 84, 87, 88
Point-to-point testing, 151
Polyuria, 18
Popliteal artery, 128
Position sense, 149
Posterior body, field assessment
of, 212, 218, 219

Posture
    examination of, 42
    neurological exam and, 135
Prearrival instructions, 259
Prehospital care report (PCR),
255, 260, 272–73. *See also*
Documentation
    absence of alterations in,
        289–90
    administrative uses of, 274
    completeness and accuracy
        of, 287
    incident times in, 285
    legal uses of, 274
    legibility of, 287
    medical uses of, 273
    narratives in, 287, 290–96
    oral statements in, 286–87
    pertinent negatives in, 286
    professionalism of, 290
    research uses of, 274
    timeliness of, 289
Preload, 86
Preschoolers, general appearance
and behavior, 159–60
Pressure, thinking under,
243–44
Primary problem, 12
Priority determination, 200–201
Priority dispatching, 258
Prostate gland, 92
Protocols, 238, 239–40
Provocation of symptoms, in
history taking, 12–13
Proximal interphalangeal (PIP)
joints, 104, 105
Pseudo-instinctive level, raising
your technical skills to, 243
Psoriasis, 56
Psychiatric illnesses, history
taking on, 14
Psychiatric system, history taking
on, 19
Puberty, 98
Public safety access point (PSAP),
257–58
Pulmonary artery, 84
Pulse, 199
    carotid, 34, 43, 86, 87
    peripheral, 130–31
    taking of, 33–34, 43
Pulse oximeter, 46–47
Pulse oximetry, 220
Pulse pressure, 36
Pupils, 60, 64
Pyramidal tract, 148

Quadriceps, 154
Questions, in patient interview, 8

Raccoon eyes (periorbital
ecchymosis), 59
Radial artery, 128
Radial pulse, 196, 199
Radio, guidelines for using,
266
Radio bands, 255
Radio frequencies, 255
Radio technologies, 261–63

Rapid trauma assessment, 203–12
of abdomen, 211–12
of chest, 205–11
of extremities, 212
of head, 204
of neck, 204–5
of pelvis, 212
of posterior body, 212
Rapport, with children and infants, 158
Rapport with patients, 5–11
Reactive approach to decision making, 243
Reassurance, patients needing, 20
Rectum, 99
in detailed physical exam, 229
Referred pain, 13
Reflection, in patient interview, 9
Reflective decisions, 242
Reflexes
assessment of, 153–58
in detailed physical exam, 229
Refusal of care by patients, 296–97
Religious beliefs, history taking on, 17
Reporting procedures, 265–68
Reports. See Documentation; Prehospital care report (PCR)
Research uses of prehospital care reports (PCRs), 274
Respiration, 34–35
measurement of, 43
quality of, 35
Respiratory arrest, 195
Respiratory effort, 35
Respiratory rate, 35
Respiratory system, history taking on, 18
Response times, information regarding, 274
Retina, 60
Review of systems, 17–19
Rhonchi, 81
Romberg test, 151
Rotator cuff, 110, 111

Safety, of emergency scene, 179–85
Safety glasses, 179, 183
Safety measures, history taking on use of, 16
Scale, 39–40
Scalp, 57
Scanning the situation, 244
SCBA (self-contained breathing apparatus), 181, 183
Scene safety, 176, 179–85
Scene size-up, 175–86
body substance isolation, 177–79

components of, 176–77
location of all patients, 185
nature of the illness, 186
scene safety and, 179–85
Sclera, 60, 64
Screening tests, history taking on, 16
Scrotum, 98
Self-contained breathing apparatus (SCBA), 181, 183
Semi-Fowler's position, 204–5
Sensory system
assessment of, 151–53
in detailed physical exam, 229
Sexual development, 42
Sexual history, 11
Sexually attractive or seductive patients, history taking and, 21
Shoulders, examination of, 110–14
Sigmoid colon, 90
Significant others, history taking on, 16–17
Simplex transmissions, 261
Sinuses
in detailed physical exam, 226
paranasal, 67
Sizing up the scene. See Scene size-up
Skin
color of, 42, 50
examination of, 42, 49–52
history taking on, 17
mobility and turgor of, 51
moisture of, 50–51
temperature of, 51
texture of, 51
Skin lesions, 42, 51–52
Skull, examination of, 57, 59
Slander, 264, 290
Sleep patterns, history taking on, 16
Small intestine, 90
Smoking, history taking on, 15
SOAP format for organizing narrative reports, 293–94
Speech
in detailed physical exam, 229
neurological exam and, 136, 147
Sphygmomanometer, 38–39
Spinal cord, 124–25
Spine, examination of, 124–27
Spleen, 93
Splitting, 88
Standing orders, 238, 239
Sternocleidomastoid muscles, 147
Stethoscope, 37–38
Stomach, 90
Stridor, 82, 195

Stroke volume, 86
Subcutaneous emphysema, 204, 205
Subjective narrative, 290–91
Substance abuse, history taking on, 15–16
Synovial capsule, 101, 102
Systole, 85
Systolic blood pressure, 35

Tachycardia, 33
in children and infants, 163
Tachypnea, 35
Tactile fremitus, 79
Tandem walking, 149
Technology, communication, 260–64
Teeth, 70, 72
Temperature, body, 37
skin temperature, 51
taking of, 46
Temporal lobe, 134
Temporomandibular joint (TMJ), 57, 59
Tenderness, 13
Tendon reflexes, deep, 153
Tendons, 100
Terminal hair, 53
Terminology
communication, 256
medical, 275
Terry's nails, 56
Testes, 91, 98
Thinking
critical. See Critical thinking process
under pressure, 243–44
Thinking skills, critical, 240–43
Thoracic aorta, 93
Thorax, examination of, 77–79, 83
Thought, neurological exam and, 136–37
Thrills, 86
Thyroid gland, 74, 75
Tidal volume, 35
Tinnitus, 17
Tobacco, history taking on use of, 15
Toddlers. See also Children
general appearance and behavior, 159
Tongue, 70, 72
Tongue blade, 72
Touch pad computer, 264
Trachea, 74–76, 82
Transfer communications, 260
Trapezius muscles, 145, 147
Trauma patients, 174, 175. See also Major trauma patients
isolated-injury, 213–14
verbal reports for, 267–68
Tremor, 148

Triage, 184, 185
Triage tags, 298–99
Triceps, 154
Trigeminal nerve (CN-V), 144
Tripodding, 82
Trochlear nerve (CN-IV), 139, 141, 144
Trunking, 262
Turgor of skin, 51
Tympanic membrane (eardrum), examination of, 65, 66–67

Ulnar artery, 128
Ultrahigh frequency (UHF) radio, 255
Unresponsive medical patients, focused history and physical exam of, 221–23
Unresponsive patients, 191
Ureters, 91
Urethra, 91
Urinary system, 90–91
history taking on, 18
Urine, 91

Vagina, 98
Vaginal discharge, 98
Vagus nerve (CN-X), 143, 145
Vas deferens, 91, 92
Vellus hair, 53
Venous pressure, 86, 88
Ventilation, 195
Ventricular gallop, 88
Verbal communication, 254–56
Verbal reports, model, 267–68
Verbal stimuli, responsiveness to, 190–91
Very high frequency band (VHF), 268
Visual acuity, 60, 62
Visual acuity card, 60
Visual acuity wall chart, 60, 62
Visual fields, 60–61
Vital signs
baseline, 220
in detailed physical exam, 231
measurement of, 33, 43–46
Vital statistics, 42

Washing hands, 175, 177
Weight, measurement of, 42
Wheezing, 81, 195
Whispered pectoriloquy, 82
Wrists, examination of, 104–6, 108, 109
Written communication, 255–56